Contemporary obstetric and gynecologic nursing

Contemporary obstetric and gynecologic nursing

Edited by

LEOTA KESTER McNALL, R.N., M.N.

Associate Professor, Department of Nursing,
California State University,
Los Angeles, California

with 51 illustrations

The C. V. Mosby Company

ST. LOUIS • TORONTO • LONDON   1980

Copyright © 1980 by The C. V. Mosby Company

All rights reserved. No part of this book may be reproduced in any manner without written permission of the publisher.

Printed in the United States of America

The C. V. Mosby Company
11830 Westline Industrial Drive, St. Louis, Missouri 63141

Library of Congress Cataloging in Publication Data

Main entry under title:

Contemporary obstetric and gynecologic nursing.

    Bibliography: p.
    Includes index.
    1. Gynecologic nursing. 2. Obstetrical nursing. I. McNall, Leota Kester, 1939-
[DNLM: 1. Genital diseases, Female—Nursing. 2. Obstetrical nursing. WY156.7 C761]
RG105.C56   610.73'678   79-27333
ISBN 0-8016-3325-7

C/M/M 9 8 7 6 5 4 3 2 1   03/B/345

Contributors

Guy E. Abraham, M.D.
Professor of Obstetrics and Gynecology, University of California School of Medicine, Los Angeles, California

Kathryn C. Bemmann, M.D.
Assistant Clinical Professor of Psychiatry, Medical College of Wisconsin, Milwaukee, Wisconsin

Salee Berman, R.N., O.G.N.P.
Co-Founder and Co-Director of "NACHIS" Natural Childbirth Institute, Culver City, California

Victor M. Berman, M.D., J.F.A.C.O.B.G.
Co-Founder and Co-Director of "NACHIS" Natural Childbirth Institute, Culver City, California

Ede Marie Buerger, R.N., M.S.
Clinical Nurse Specialist, Neonatal Intensive Care Unit, Loma Linda University Medical Center, Loma Linda, California

Susan C. Bundy, B.S.
Counselor, The Women's Center, Inc., Waukesha, Wisconsin

Colleen Conway, R.N., C.N.M., Ph.D.
Associate Professor, Graduate Programs, Department of Nursing, California State University, Long Beach, Long Beach, California

Maureen O. Doran, R.N., M.S.N., C.S.
Psychiatric Nursing Clinical Specialist, Veteran's Administration Hospital; Clinical Assistant Professor, University of Colorado School of Nursing, Denver, Colorado

Elizabeth Elmer, M.S.W.
Associate Professor of Child Psychiatry, Department of Psychiatry, School of Medicine, University of Pittsburgh, Pittsburgh, Pennsylvania

Steven G. Gabbe, M.D.
Associate Professor of Obstetrics and Gynecology, Director of Jerrold R. Golding Division of Fetal Medicine, Hospital of the University of Pennsylvania, Philadelphia, Pennsylvania

Velvia M. Garner, R.N., M.S.N., A.N.P.
Assistant Professor, University of Colorado School of Nursing, Denver, Colorado

Loretta Ivory, C.N.M., M.S.
Director, Midwifery Services, Denver Birth Center, Denver, Colorado

Frank A. Manning, M.D., F.R.C.S. (C)
Assistant Professor, Department of Obstetrics and Gynecology, University of Southern California School of Medicine, Los Angeles, California

André J. Nahmias, M.D., M.A., M.P.H.

Professor of Pediatrics and Chief, Infectious Diseases and Immunology; Professor of Pathology, Associate Professor of Preventive Medicine and Community Health, Emory University School of Medicine, Atlanta, Georgia

Lawrence D. Platt, M.D.

Assistant Professor, Department of Obstetrics and Gynecology, University of Southern California School of Medicine, Los Angeles, California

Thomas F. Rocereto, M.D.

Interim Chairman, Department of Obstetrics and Gynecology, Cooper Medical Center, Camden, New Jersey

Judith P. Rooks, C.N.M., M.S., M.P.H.

Assistant Professor, Department of Obstetrics and Gynecology; Associate Director, Oregon Program for Reproductive Health, Health Sciences Center, Portland, Oregon

Louise Sipos, R.N., B.A.

Research Associate, Division of Maternal-Fetal Medicine, Department of Obstetrics and Gynecology, University of Southern California School of Medicine, Los Angeles, California

Barbara Star, Ph.D.

Assistant Professor, School of Social Work, University of Southern California, Los Angeles, California

Aarolyn M. Visintine, M.D.

Senior Research Associate, Department of Pediatrics, Division of Infectious Diseases and Immunology, Emory University School of Medicine, Atlanta, Georgia

Preface

With the expanding scope of nursing practice, professional opportunities and responsibilities of practitioners have taken on greater dimensions and, therefore, require an understanding of a broader range of issues pertinent to the health care of women. Further, women in today's society desire more from health care than the system has been providing, especially care that is sensitive to individual needs and the experiences of being a woman. Thus the purpose of this collection of contributions is to present theoretical knowledge, research findings, and therapeutic strategies that, from a multiprofessional approach, will assist the practitioner in meeting the challenges and demands of both the health care system and the consumers of that system.

Contemporary Obstetric and Gynecologic Nursing is divided into four parts. Part One emphasizes the significance of the women's movement in promoting quality health care for women, the cultural aspects of health and illness behaviors associated with childbearing among selected ethnic groups, and the psychophysical preparations for childbirth. Part Two focuses on the methods and problems of assessing fetal size and growth, the significance of evaluating developmental behaviors of the neonate, and research findings regarding the TORCH syndrome of perinatal infections. Part Three deals with the physiologic, psychosocial, and legal issues of assault and battery in both infants and women, with a special focus on nursing implications. Part Four focuses on the prevention, detection, and management of selected obstetric and gynecologic problems, including sexual dysfunction, premenstrual tension, vulvovaginitis, cervical pathology, significance of the pubococcygeal muscle, and the use of real-time ultrasound in obstetrics and gynecology. The contributors and I hope to appeal to health care professionals in a variety of health care systems and ultimately to the health care consumers who benefit from their endeavors.

Leota Kester McNall

Contents

PART ONE

Women's health care

1 The women's movement and its effect on women's health care, 3
Judith P. Rooks

2 Cultural aspects of health and illness behaviors in childbearing, 27
Velvia M. Garner

3 Psychophysical preparations for childbirth, 40
Colleen Conway

PART TWO

Fetal and neonatal development

4 Assessment of fetal size and growth, 59
Steven G. Gabbe

5 Developmental profile of the neonate, 69
Ede Marie Buerger

6 The TORCH syndrome of perinatal infection, 86
Aarolyn M. Visintine and André J. Nahmias

PART THREE

Problems of assault and battery

7 Infant battery, 103
Elizabeth Elmer

8   Battered women, 121
    Barbara Star

9   Sexual assault: social, legal, medical, and psychologic aspects, 136
    Kathryn C. Bemmann and Susan C. Bundy

PART FOUR
Selected Ob/Gyn problems and issues

10 Sexual dysfunction, 159
    Maureen O. Doran

11 The premenstrual tension syndromes, 170
    Guy E. Abraham

12 Diagnosis of vulvovaginitis in the adult female, 185
    Loretta Ivory

13 Differential diagnosis of cervical pathology, 200
    Thomas F. Rocereto

14 A guide to a healthy pubococcygeus muscle: kegeling, not cutting, 216
    Salee Berman and Victor M. Berman

15 Real-time ultrasound in obstetrics and gynecology, 229
    Louise Sipos, Lawrence D. Platt, and Frank A. Manning

Contemporary obstetric and gynecologic nursing

PART ONE

Women's health care

In her discussion of the women's movement and its effects on women's health care, Rooks emphasizes the significant effect the movement has had on promoting quality health care for women, especially in the areas of contraception and abortion legislation, the physician-client relationship as it pertains to women's rights and responsibilities regarding their own health care, and the current trend to change women's health care by changing health care providers. Consideration is given to the significance of the expanding roles of nurses.

Garner describes some of the traditional beliefs and practices of Hispanics, Blacks, Asians, and Native Americans and their impact on the cultural aspects of health and illness behaviors, pregnancy, and childbirth. Of particular importance is the need to recognize that both nurse and client belong to subcultures representing diverse lifestyles and beliefs and that each acts according to a set of behaviors characteristic of their respective groups.

Conway, in a discussion of the psychophysical preparations for childbirth, describes various methodologies of pain relief during labor, including systematic relaxation, cognitive control, cognitive rehearsal, the Hawthorne effect, and systematic desensitization. The implications for nursing are directed toward maintaining safety for both mother and infant and providing for the woman's emotional need to make the most of her childbearing experience.

CHAPTER 1

The women's movement and its effect on women's health care

Judith P. Rooks

INTRODUCTION

Despite substantial, recent improvements in their status, all women in the United States are affected by the remaining general, diffuse, institutionalized, and sometimes subtle discrimination between males and females that exists in almost every aspect of our culture. Differences in men's and women's roles in sex, marriage, and the family underlie discrimination against women in employment, education, religion, politics, the arts, science, and athletics. The purpose of the women's movement is to break down the system of sexual discrimination and to help women achieve full adult status in our society with the same opportunities and responsibilities as men.

The organized women's rights movement in the United States began with a conference convened by Lucretia Mott and Elizabeth Cady Stanton at Seneca Falls, New York, in 1848. This event and the social movement that followed were influenced by at least three important factors: (1) with time, popular understanding of the democratic principles of the American and French Revolutions evolved so that an increasing proportion of the people believed that the basic equality of mankind included women as well as men, (2) many of the nineteenth century feminist leaders were Quakers because the Quakers educated women and practiced sexual equality, and (3) some women who had been active in the fight for emancipation of slaves were barred because of their sex from the 1840 World Anti-Slavery Conference in London. Having participated in a movement based on the equality of all people, they were outraged that the principle for which they had fought was not applied to them.[45]

By 1870 more than 300,000 women were working in America's factories. Many of these women, as well as many children, worked long hours for very low pay under unsafe and unhealthy conditions. Feminists concluded that women's right to vote was an essential weapon for correction of these abuses. Suffrage for women became "The Cause." Soon groups of women throughout the country formed to fight for women's suffrage and to improve conditions for women in their own communities.[28] During the last half of the nineteenth century and the first two decades of the twentieth century, American women led active and vigorous campaigns for suffrage and for a wide range of social improvement and public health programs aimed primarily at helping the poor and improving conditions for children.

Female citizens of the United States received the right to vote when the nineteenth amendment to the Constitution was ratified in 1920. Much of the vigor of the women's movement dissipated after that victory. It did not re-emerge as a major social force until the late 1960s when the women's movement gathered strength along with the civil rights movement, protest against United State's participation in the Vietnamese war, and the emergence of a youth counterculture. Some of the intelligent, well-educated, young women involved in these causes gradually became aware that even within antiauthoritarian, equality-oriented movements, they were second-class citizens because of their sex. They began to slowly and painfully help each other understand the socialization processes, emotions, and experiences that caused not only their male colleagues, but *they themselves,* to have different and lower expectations of women than they had of men. Although women in the movement rallied around demands for repeal of restrictive abortion laws and other changes in laws and bureaucratic practices, the women's movement was different from the other concurrent social causes and protests because the first changes the movement required were internal changes within the women themselves. Occasional well-publicized marches and demonstrations provided observable evidence of the movement. However the most important activities of this phase of the women's movement were intrapsychic, interpersonal, and group experiences that gradually affected, in varying degrees, the way most women in the country thought and felt about themselves as people.

The early movement for equality for women was closely associated with efforts to improve the conditions and health of poor women and children. Although the modern women's movement is deeply involved with women's health and health care issues, the emphasis on poor women and their problems is less apparent now. The current movement has been criticized for consisting mainly of well-educated, middle or professional-class white women who have not made adequate efforts to include poor and ethnic minority women and who do not adequately understand or address these women's special problems and needs.

It is difficult to describe social movements because they evolve in response to the changes they create. It is particularly hard to describe the women's movement because it is amorphous. Many women (and men) do not know whether they are in it or not. There is no membership list and no way to join. No one has been designated to speak for the movement, and there is no approved set of policies and goals. Many different groups of women use a variety of means to reach similar or disparate goals and yet contribute to the same overall "movement."

This chapter is not a recitation of the criticisms women have made of health care in the United States. It is an attempt to describe the effects that activities of the women's movement have produced on women's health care. This is a difficult task because the effects of the women's movement have been inextricably meshed with those of other significant changes in our society since the early 1960s. Consumerism, concern about pollution and rapid population growth, increasing bureaucracy, rapid increases in the cost of health care, changes in sexual mores, loss of respect for institutionalized authority, and rapid advances in technology (especially in contraception) along with an apparent increased desire for natural products and a simpler lifestyle are all factors that have effected and are effecting the changes ascribed here to the women's movement itself, which has probably been the most important influence on the specific changes that will be described in this chapter. For many, the major effects of the women's movement have been quite personal and profound.

CONTRACEPTION AND ABORTION: HEALTH SERVICES NECESSARY FOR EQUALITY FOR WOMEN

The ability to control when and under what circumstances they will conceive and bear children is a basic prerequisite to equality for women and a primary goal of the women's movement. Although socialization is the major cause of the great differences between the roles played by most men and women in our society, the major reasons for sexist socialization of children probably stem primarily from three undeniable biologic facts: (1) women in general are smaller and have less muscular strength than men, (2) heterosexual intercourse may result in pregnancy for women, but not for men, and (3) women, having carried and given birth to their babies, usually develop strong attachments to their children immediately after birth. Although fathers may develop similarly strong attachments to their children, they can avoid it if they wish. Thus, women are less likely than men to reject responsibility for their children's care.

The last two differences alone are enough to explain why gender-specific self-concepts and behavior patterns developed and were passed on to countless generations of girls and boys. As a result, there are different standards for male than for female sexual behavior, and female children tend to be socialized to be more dependent, passive, home-centered, and other-oriented than male children and are not encouraged as much as males to strive for long-term educational or career goals or to seek important jobs.

Now that machines perform many tasks that previously required strong muscles, muscular strength is a less important biologic factor in today's society. The women's movement is now trying to overcome the other two biologic barriers to sexual equality by making it possible for women as well as men to have sexual intercourse without fear of pregnancy and childbirth and by encouraging fathers and mothers to share equally in all phases of parenting and childcare from the moment of birth.

Contributions of the women's movement to fertility control

Margaret Sanger (1879-1966), a nurse, feminist, and author of "Providing Women with Birth Control," was the most important early leader of the family planning movement in the United States. In 1916, Sanger and her sister, also a nurse, started the first birth control clinic in America, in Brooklyn, New York, using contraband diaphragms they had smuggled into the country from Germany. They were arrested, tried, convicted, and jailed under a state law that prohibited dissemination of contraceptive information and devices except for the prevention or cure of disease. Sanger's case was reviewed by the New York Court of Appeals in 1918. Although the Appeals Court did not overturn her conviction, the Court's opinion on her case led to a broader interpretation of the conditions for which physicians could legally prescribe contraceptive devices. The legal opinion that resulted from Sanger's arrest was a critical factor in making it possible to establish effective birth control clinics in the United States.[30] Sanger was not only a major leader of the family planning movement in this country, but throughout the world. She introduced the now well-known family planning slogan, "every child a wanted child,"[30] wrote and lectured widely on the importance of birth control, distributed pamphlets on family limitation, and was a prime mover in creating organizations and initiating programs to provide contraceptive methods to women. She was also a life-long feminist, initiating publication of a magazine entitled *Woman Rebel* in 1914, and later writing a book entitled *Women and the New Race*.[33]

Despite the efforts of Sanger and her many male colleagues in the family planning movement, until the early 1960s, sexual abstinence, the rhythm method, barrier contraceptives, and illegal abortion were virtually the only available means for avoiding unwanted pregnancies and births. Although not illegal, voluntary surgical sterilization of women was restricted by a recommendation of the American College of Obstetricians and Gynecologists (ACOG) that a woman's request for surgical sterilization should not be honored unless her age multiplied by the number of her living children equalled or exceeded 120.[1] Thus sterilization was available to women 40 years of age or older with three children, women 30 years of age or older with four children, and women 24 years of age or older with five children, but not to younger women with fewer children.

A "contraceptive revolution" began in the early 1960s when the oral contraceptive pill and the intrauterine device (IUD) became available. By 1965 contraception was used by 67% of white American women who had married before 25 years of age, were of childbearing age, and were still married to the same husband. Of those using contraception, 47% were using pills, IUDs, or male or female sterilization—the effective "modern" methods. By 1975, 79% of such couples were using contraception, and 74% of those couples used the modern methods.[60]

The need for abortions: removing the legal barriers

Neither the new contraceptives nor the increased access to sterilization, which resulted after ACOG dropped its recommended restrictions, were enough to completely satisfy the family planning movement's goal of "every child a wanted child" or the feminist goal of making women as able as men to have sexual lives without fear of unwanted pregnancies and children. Legal abortion was necessary to achieve both these goals.

Contraception alone is not enough for many reasons. Most women are fertile for at least 30 years, (from approximately 13 years of age to 45 years of age or older), and few American women now want more than three children. Although the mean age of women at first marriage is increasing in the United States,[60] as of 1976 more than half (55%) of never-married, teenage girls in the United States had experienced sexual intercourse at least once.[18] Thus, most women are at risk for unwanted pregnancy for 20 to 30 years. If all sexually active women used contraceptive methods that were 95% effective (for example, IUDs) during 20 years of exposure to unwanted conception, they would still experience an average of one unwanted pregnancy per woman (5% pregnant per year times 20 years). The most effective temporary contraceptives—the pill and IUD—are both associated with rare but sometimes serious and even fatal complications; therefore, some women are afraid to use them, or try to use them, but make mistakes. It is easy for a woman to forget her pills when she goes away for the weekend, to misplace them, or to run out of pills. Some women do not use contraceptives because they were not planning to have sex, yet become pregnant and request abortions. This happens frequently in new relationships, especially those involving teenagers. Without abortions, women's vulnerability to unpredictable, unwanted pregnancies remains—diluted but not dispelled by contraception.

As of January 1, 1970, abortion was illegal except to save a pregnant woman's life in 41 of the 50 states. A 1969 U.S. District Court Decision had made legal abortion available virtually on request in the District of Columbia,[60] and nine states had abortion statutes based on a model abortion law that had been proposed in 1957 by the American Law Institute (ALI). With minor differences, the laws in those nine states allowed physicians to perform abortions when necessary to protect a woman's life or health, to prevent the birth of a deformed baby, or when the pregnancy resulted from rape. The decision that a woman could have an abortion, however, was made by physicians, rather than by the woman herself. Although the procedures varied somewhat, ALI abortion laws commonly required that three physicians certify the existence of the condition that made a woman eligible for a legal abortion and that a committee of physicians representing the hospital agree that the abortion was necessary. Since most women who wanted and needed abortions had not been raped, had no reason to think they were carrying deformed fetuses, and were in good health, most of the few who obtained legal abortions under these laws did so by professing mental illness. Of the 12,417 legal abortions reported for the entire United States in 1969, 91% were done for "mental health" reasons.[18] The re-emerging women's movement rallied around the need to provide women with access to safe and dignified legal abortions.

During 1970, three more states enacted ALI-type abortion laws, but four states—Hawaii, Alaska, New York, and Washington—enacted an entirely new kind of abortion law that contained no legal restrictions on obtaining an abortion. These laws would not have been enacted except for the political climate created by the women's movement.

On December 13, 1971, the United States Supreme Court heard arguments by two women lawyers in cases involving the abortion statutes of Texas and Georgia. Sarah Weddington argued on behalf of Jane Roe, an unmarried pregnant woman from Texas. Margie Pitts Hames argued on behalf of Mary Doe, a married woman in Atlanta who already had three children and believed that she would be emotionally and economically unable to care for another child. On January 22, 1973, the Court ruled that both the Texas and Georgia abortion laws were unconstitutional on several grounds, thus nullifying these and similar laws in every state. Although state abortion laws still vary slightly, for practical purposes the 1973 Supreme Court decisions now comprise the abortion law of the United States. Those decisions prohibit states from enacting laws that interfere with a woman's right to have an abortion during the first trimester (13 weeks) of pregnancy, except that the state may require that abortions be performed only by physicians. The state may regulate the conditions under which abortions during the second trimester (approximately the fourteenth through twenty-sixth week) of pregnancy are performed to the extent that the regulations are in the interest of protecting the health of women having abortions. However, the state may not enact laws that restrict the reasons for which a second trimester abortion may be performed. The state may regulate or forbid abortions in the third trimester of pregnancy, except when they are necessary to preserve a pregnant woman's life or health.[55]

The Supreme Court abortion decisions have had far-reaching effects on women's lives and health and on many aspects of our whole system of health care. Prior to the abortion law changes that occurred between 1969 and 1973, physicians' and nurses' only professional contact with abortion involved women who were admitted to hospitals with hemorrhage, torn uteri, and/or serious infections resulting from illegal abortions. Health professionals tended to view these women as pitiable victims and/or culprits of a despicable and lowly crime. Every year since 1976, at least one million women have had legal abortions within this country's health care system. One million new patients in the system each year created a marketing environment that promoted innovation and rapid changes of attitude. Although previous clinical recommendations stated that abortions be performed as in-patient procedures (frequently 3-day hospitalizations) with use of general anesthesia, cervical dilatation, and sharp curettage,[56] American physicians quickly adopted simpler abortion procedures developed in China and Eastern Europe and learned that early abortions could be performed safely on an out-patient basis in free-standing (nonhospital) clinics, without use of general anesthesia. Out-patient abortion clinics, established under the control or influence of women, paid as much attention to "abortion counseling" and the patients' psychologic well-being as they did to the actual surgery. Abortion clinics became big business, some of which were dependent on feminist-controlled referral services that could make or break them depending on feminist judgments about the appropriateness of the clinic personnel's behavior toward patients. For most participating health professionals (generally young, social change-oriented physicians and nurses), working in an abortion clinic is a unique learning experience. Although some abortion clinics remain procedure- and money-oriented businesses, legal abortion has been an important training ground for changing the relationships between nurses, physicians, and patients.

Serving as "watchdogs": an interdependent but vigilant cooperation with medical family planners

Because reproduction is a physiologic body process, the profession of medicine is inextricably involved in its control. Thus all women depend on physicians (predominantly men) for the means to meet this basic need. Resentment over this dependence, along with blatant sexism, arrogance, insensitivity, greed, and careless practice on the part of some physicians and overzealous, incautious enthusiasm for some female forms of contraception on the part of the medical family planning movement have collectively resulted in well-publicized attacks on medicine by many feminists. In 1972, Frankfort stated the feminist critique of male-dominated medicine in her best-selling book, *Vaginal Politics,* which "raised the consciousness" of millions of women about sexism in the health care system.[29]

Despite this antagonism, the women's movement and physician involvement in family planning are entwined in an intricate cycle of cause and effect. Both family planning and feminism have derived great benefit from a long history of cooperative interdependence between women's rights activists and physicians involved in the world-wide birth control/family planning effort.

The achievements of Sanger, Weddington, and Hames are only highlights of the contributions the women's movement has made to the control of human fecundity.

Although feminists contributed much to this effort, the equality of women is only one of many motivations for birth control and family planning. A wide variety of people have contributed to the development and mass-marketing of contraceptives, the provision of widespread clinical family planning services, and the removal of legal, bureaucratic, and economic barriers to contraception, abortion, and sterilization. Sanger, Weddington, and Hames could not have achieved their breakthroughs without the cooperation and independent contributions of countless other men and women, some motivated by the feminist goal of giving women control over their lives through fertility control, but others motivated by such diverse concerns as population control, eugenics, profit, personal professional advancement, reduction of welfare rolls, and provisions for the well-being of children.

As a result of the efforts of all these people, contraception is now readily available to women in the United States; as of 1974 only about 19% American women between 18 and 44 years of age were not using contraception. Now that this goal has been largely accomplished, many feminists have stepped back from the family planning/birth control movement, to serve it in a different way—as "watchdogs" drawing attention to its faults and excesses. This is a necessary and important function, especially given the strength of some of the other forces promoting fertility control. It is a difficult function, the issues are complicated, and as illustrated by the following examples, the problems are often without completely satisfactory solutions.

1. Many feminists would like to see more effort toward development and promotion of male methods of contraception. This desire is based on the belief that men should share in the responsibility, inconveniences, expense, and health risks of contraception, which women now primarily assume. In fact, increasing numbers of men are doing just that; male sterilization has become extremely popular, especially among couples with stable marriages.[60] However, the use of condoms, in spite of their theoretical effectiveness and lack of health risks, has declined, while IUD use, which involves some risk to a woman's health, has increased.[34] The low reliance on condoms for contraception is not necessarily a result of male resistance. One large family planning program that actively promoted distribution of condoms to teenage boys found that they were not only willing to use them, but were also willing to assume a major share of responsibility for preventing unwanted births.[6] It may be that failure to use male methods of contraception is largely a result of female preference, especially preference for methods that women can control. Women know that if a man forgets or fails to use a condom, he is not the one at risk of becoming pregnant.

2. There is need for a better female contraceptive—something as effective and easy to use as the pill, but without its frequent unpleasant side effects and infrequent but serious complications. Spokeswomen for the feminist movement have been critical of drug companies and physicians for using women in experiments to develop and test new products and methods for contraception. As they have pointed out, if the experiment is successful, the companies may get richer and the scientists more famous, but if the drug or procedure fails, it is the women on whom it was used who have taken the risks. Nevertheless, if a better female-controlled contraceptive is ever to be developed, women will have to be willing to have it tested on them.

3. In 1973, it was learned that two black teenage girls in Montgomery, Alabama, had been surgically sterilized without their knowledge or consent and without their

mother's informed consent by a local white physician who considered them mentally retarded. It was also learned that Aiken, South Carolina's only two physicians routinely informed pregnant women on Medicaid, who already had two or more children, that they would not deliver their babies unless the women agreed to postpartum surgical sterilization. As a result of these disclosures, leaders of the women's, civil rights, and civil liberties movements demanded that new laws and regulations be created to prevent women from being sterilized without their truly informed and freely given consent. Furthermore, as of March 8, 1979 new legislation prevents federal funding of sterilizing surgery for any woman who is less than 21 years of age, mentally retarded, or does not sign a special consent form at least 30 days before the procedure.[57] These restrictions will prevent some poor women with special problems from being able to exercise control over their fertility, which is a major goal of the women's movement. For instance, a young woman who is mentally retarded enough to be unable to use barrier contraceptive methods reliably and is without means for private medical care may have medical problems that contraindicate her use of either an IUD or oral contraception. Her inability to have her request for sterilization honored may result in her either becoming pregnant against her wishes or may cause her family or other guardians to restrict her life in ways that deprive her of desired social and sexual interaction with males.

CHANGING THE PHYSICIAN-PATIENT RELATIONSHIP BY CHANGING PATIENTS: INFORMATION, RIGHTS, AND RESPONSIBILITIES

The dictionary defines a *patient* as "an individual awaiting or under medical care and treatment," "the recipient . . . of services," or "one that is acted upon."[59] A *client* is defined as "a person who engages the professional services of another."[49] Although many *patients* are also *clients* who actively engaged the health services they receive, the two terms are not interchangeable. An essential connotation of *patient* is passivity—a patient is acted upon, the object of other's efforts. *Client* implies a *voluntary* and willing *participation*. Clients can discharge the person they have engaged and take their business elsewhere; patients passively accept whatever services are offered.

Being a patient is well suited to the sick role, which Parsons and others have described as having an incapacity for which the sick person cannot be held responsible, relinquishing some of their rights, being exempted from some of the responsibilities of normal adulthood, being dependent and needing help, regressing to a less mature stage of psychologic adaption, and losing status.[47] This sick patient role has been an inherent part of acute or serious illness and may be a necessary phase in successful adaption to such illness, leading to recovery.[44]

The "all-knowing, all-powerful physician role" is a perfect and sometimes necessary complement to the role of the seriously or acutely ill patient. The stereotypic physician-patient relationship—a kind but authoritarian physician who relates paternalistically to a grateful and dependent patient—may be almost unavoidable in some situations. However, in most instances it is counterproductive for the preventive and health maintenance care that constitutes the bulk of health services required by normal premenopausal women. Such women require relatively frequent use of health services—for family planning, treatment of gynecologic conditions, screening (pap smears and breast exams), and childbearing. In addition, they are usually the family member who deals with the frequent health care needs of children. Most of these health service situations do not involve acute or serious illness and are better served by a different kind of relationship between the patient and the physician.

The women's movement is attempting to change the sterotypic relationship between physicians and their female patients *primarily by changing the behavior of women as patients*. The change is needed to avoid embarrassment and injury to women's self-respect and dignity; to give women greater control over their health care to improve the quality of the care (and thus indirectly to improve their health); and to enhance women's exercise of informed, free choice regarding those aspects of their sexual, reproductive lives and health that require medical monitoring or intervention. The major means by which women in the movement are effecting this desired change include: (1) creating alternative sources of accurate health and medical information, (2) promulgating the concept that the patient has an absolute right to control what happens to her (or his) body and therefore must give informed, noncoerced consent for (or may refuse) any aspect of medical care and treatment, and (3) emphasizing the limitations of technologic medicine and the necessity for women (and men) to take responsibility for their own health by learning and practicing healthy living habits.

An alternative source of accurate health information

The basic energy of the women's movement during the past decade stems from a greater understanding by an increasing number of women of the ways sexism has affected them personally. This understanding has come about largely through self-disclosure and discussions between women in small and intimate groups. Within such groups many women learned that the feelings of dependency, childlikeness, indignity, and frustrated anger they had experienced individually as patients were not the result of some unique personal inadequacy, but were the common experiences of their friends. One such group was formed in Boston following a women's conference in 1969. They decided to fight their feelings of dependence with knowledge, by learning about their bodies themselves. They researched medical- or health-related subjects they thought women needed to understand and summarized what they learned in a series of clearly written and illustrated papers. Their papers presented not only the facts women needed to know about their sexual and reproductive functions, but also the feelings—good, bad, and indifferent—that women experience at different times about all aspects of their sexual and reproductive lives. The papers were the basis of a course that the group conducted for other women in Boston. Eventually the papers were published—*Our Bodies, Ourselves*[11] is now available throughout the United States and in eight other countries. Two million copies have been sold. In the book, women can find up-to-date, accurate, easy to understand information on almost any aspect of their sexual and reproductive lives and health, including illustrations of a woman's body and sexual organs that are not ugly, repulsive, or obscene; many women feel badly about themselves and their lives sometimes—you are not the only one—you are normal; very few questions about sex, contraception, or reproduction have only one right answer—there are pros and cons to all the alternatives, and different answers are "best" for different women—you are probably the only one who can really decide what is best for you; if the issue is *your health,* only you have *the right* to decide; women are smart enough to understand everything they need to know to make the major decisions about their own health care; medical science does not have all the answers; physicians may overstate their opinions as fact, their preferences as necessity; how you live (eat, exercise, relate to other people) affects how healthy you will be; you are responsible for your own health.[11]

Our Bodies, Ourselves is being translated into Spanish and has been put into braille. The information in it and information made available more recently by other alternative (nonhealth care establishment) sources are a cornerstone of the effect the women's movement is having on women's health care. With this information, healthy women cannot be stereotypic "patients"; and if the patient does not act like a patient, the physician has to change also. Relationships are dynamic; one element cannot change without affecting the other. If the patient is generally informed, is not afraid of the unknown, is not ashamed of her body, is confident in requesting the information and services she wants, and is aware of her right to request further explanation or a second opinion, to refuse part or all of a proposed diagnostic or treatment regimen, or to discharge one physician and engage another, the physician's role has to change also.

These roles *are* changing, not for all women or all physicians and not as much as many women want, but substantially. At the 1978 Annual Meeting of the American College of Obstetricians and Gynecologists, one session was called "The Great Debate: Who's Running the Show?" Its purpose was to discuss what role women should play in their own health care. Although the session was well attended, there was little debate. The panelists spoke in favor of women's right to abortion, commented on the remarkable success of *Our Bodies, Ourselves,* and stated that obstetricians-gynecologists should treat women as partners in their own health care. These attitudes and statements would have been debated 5 years earlier but were received with almost no opposition in 1978. The only real debate was in response to a remark from a woman (not a physician) in the audience that the professional code against physicians advertising makes it difficult for women to "shop" for an appropriate doctor, that women, for instance, need to be able to determine (without paying for an office visit) whether a specific obstetrician allows husbands in the delivery room, uses the Leboyer method, has a high cesarean section rate, or uses electronic monitoring on all patients in labor. In response to this statement, several physicians said that women should receive answers to such questions only from their physicians, who can simultaneously teach them the need for frequent use of procedures (such as electronic fetal monitoring and cesarean sections), which the women may incorrectly oppose. In November, 1978, the Federal Trade Commission ruled that the American Medical Association and its local societies' ethical prohibitions on physicians' advertising violates the Federal Trade Commission Act and is illegal.[2] Thus the issue that raised debate at the 1978 ACOG meeting will probably be accepted with relative equanimity in a few more years.

Informed consent

The women's movement, evolving legal concepts and case law regarding physicians' and others' (that is, pharmaceutical companies) responsibilities for untoward results of medical treatments and procedures, and the complications of oral contraceptives made the 1970s the start of a new era in informed consent for medical care and procedures. The birth control pill was put on the market in 1960. Women were told that it was "safe, virtually 100 percent effective, simple to use and reversible."[21] Ten years later Senator Gaylord Nelson (D-Wis.) held 9 days of well-publicized hearings before the Senate Small Business Committee's Monopoly Subcommittee, during which the pill was purported to cause cancer, suicide, psychosis, divorce, diabetes, overweight, underweight, loss of libido, chronic fatigue, blindness, and hypertension. Expert witnesses testified that almost none of the nearly nine million American women using the pill at that time were well-informed about its risks.[52] Associations between the pill and some of the ill effects cited during the Nelson hearings have never been scientifically proved. However since that time the pill has been found to increase women's risk of still other serious, even fatal conditions, including strokes, heart attacks, and other thromboembolic diseases,[20, 42, 43, 53] noncancerous but sometimes fatal liver tumors,[51] gall stones, and pyelitis.[53] All witnesses and Senators who participated in the hearings agreed that more research was needed to determine the risks associated with all methods of contraception.[52]

Soon after the hearings, the Food and Drug Administration (FDA) announced that it would develop literature to inform users of the pill of the risks associated with oral contraception and would require that the literature be put in all pill packages. Although drug companies had previously been required to make facts on drug risks available to *physicians,* this was only the second time the FDA required that such information be made available to the people who *use* the drugs.* It was an important step in the concept of informed consent for health care. The idea that a patient should be thoroughly informed of the risks, benefits, and *alternatives* to any proposed form of medical therapy and has the right to refuse even "necessary" treatment is now being clarified. Although this concept is far from being a true precept of health care practices in this country, much of the credit for the progress that has been made belongs to the women's movement. The reproductive health care of women has experienced the most significant advances in actualizing the concept of informed consent. In May 1977 the FDA required that literature to inform patients of the contraindications, risks, and effectiveness of IUDs be included with every IUD marketed in the United States.[25] Two months later, it required similar "patient package inserts" for all estrogen products (the "morning after pill" and estrogen replacement therapy for postmenopausal women).[26] In 1978, patient package inserts were required for products containing progestogens (the "mini-pill" and depo-provera.)[27] The FDA is in the process of mandating similar patient-oriented literature for several prescription drugs not associated with women's reproductive health. New federal rules specifying procedures that must be followed in obtaining informed consent from women prior to sterilization procedures to be paid for by government funds are also important precedents.

Assuming responsibility for one's own health

Underlying the change the women's movement is attempting to produce in the role of women as patients or as "health care clients" is the belief that individuals are responsible for their own health care. Publication of *Our Bodies, Ourselves* in 1971 was the beginning of a diffuse but sustained effort by women in the movement to accept and fulfill that responsibility by educating

---
*FDA required that an insert warning against overuse be inserted in packages containing isoproterenol inhalent spray in 1968.

themselves and others toward the goals of (1) adopting healthy life habits and (2) developing women's movement sources of needed health care when the necessary services are either unavailable within the traditional health care system (for instance, counselling and support services for rape victims) or when available care is thought to be inappropriate (that is, providing home births as an alternative to hospital delivery).

Self-help clinics. In 1971 a group of feminists running a women's health center in Los Angeles developed a "self-help clinic" program that was widely publicized through both underground and mass media and through a nationwide tour to demonstrate the self-help clinic concept to women in other parts of the country. A self-help clinic is a group of women who meet to share experiences, knowledge, and feelings about the sexual, reproductive, and other aspects of their bodies and their health. Because a woman's internal sex organs are normally hidden from her view, an important part of a woman's experience at a self-help clinic is learning about this part of female anatomy by physical examination of another woman and learning to examine her own vagina and cervix by using a plastic speculum and a mirror.

Although the women who originated the first self-help clinic designed a rather formal program that included training in self-diagnosis and treatment of common minor ailments (such as vaginitis) by inexpensive home remedies (such as yogurt) and learning to perform menstrual extraction, these activities are no longer necessarily implied by the term *self-help. Menstrual extraction,* taught as part of a Los Angeles feminist women's health care self-help clinic, is performed by inserting a plastic catheter through the cervical os and aspirating the endometrial lining using negative pressure created by withdrawing the plunger of a large syringe. If the procedure is used after menstrual bleeding has started, it removes all the tissue at once so that the woman avoids having her normal menstrual period. If it is used when the menstrual period is due but has not started, it is a means of self-induced abortion. Although this procedure received much publicity in the early 1970s, the safety of regular self- or friend-induced menstrual extraction has not been adequately studied, and it is neither practiced nor advocated widely within the women's movement. Although neither self-diagnosis and treatment of vaginal and cervical disease nor menstrual extraction proved popular to a broad segment of women, the idea of providing opportunities for women to see their own cervices and vaginas has gained fairly wide acceptance. Some physicians, nurse-midwives, and nurses now keep a mirror available and routinely have women undergoing pelvic examinations look at their own cervices.

NORMALIZING WOMEN'S SEXUAL FUNCTIONS

A third health-related goal of the women's movement is to redefine full and active sexuality of women as "normal" and to remove the aura of illness from the female processes of menstruation, pregnancy, childbirth, and menopause.

Women, as sexual people

The double standard for sexual behavior includes not only the expectation that women should be more chaste than men, but also the belief that sexual satisfaction is both less natural and less important to women than to men. The assumption that it is more "normal" for females to have unsatisfactory sex lives is supported by the fact that there is a high prevalence of sexual dissatisfaction among women. The 1953 report of the study of *Sexual Behavior in the Human Female* (the "Kinsey Report") based on 5940 interviews conducted between 1938 and 1953 found that 25% of the married women interviewed experienced no coital orgasms during the first year of marriage. Eleven percent of those married 20 years had never experienced orgasm during marital coitus.[40] The major goals of the women's movement regarding female sexuality are summarized below:

1. *Women and their health advisors should stop accepting lack of sexual satisfaction as normal.* The effect of this attitude of acceptance is that millions of women believe that chronic sexual dissatisfaction is simply their fate and that nothing can be done about it. They try to submerge their sexual needs and to write off that aspect of their personalities.

2. *Treatment should be available to women for whom sex is unsatisfying.* The degree of sexual satisfaction experienced by many if not most women can be enhanced by the simple, inexpensive treatment of providing them with accurate knowledge about the anatomy and physiology of male and female sexual arousal and orgasm; correcting misinformation (such as the myth that it is normal for women to find sex unsatisfying or that a "real woman" can have orgasm without clitoral stimulation); giving them permission and encouragement to initiate sex when they want it and to communicate verbally and nonverbally to their partners what kinds of erotic stimulation they like, how much they want, and when; and giving them permission and even instruction to masturbate.

3. *Women should not judge their own sexual satisfaction by the measurement established by and based on the experience of men, that is, orgasm is the only important thing.* Although women's sexuality is no weaker or less important than men's, it is different. There is extreme variation in what is sexually satisfying for women. For some women at some times, the phase of sexual arousal may be more important than orgasm itself. Women (and men) may sometimes want the comfort and pleasure of holding, cuddling, and caressing without the stimulation and exertion of coitus. Women's orgasms vary greatly (from woman to woman and from time to time) in intensity and in the extent to which they are satisfying and fulfilling; the most intense orgasms are not necessarily the most fulfilling.

The major requests the women's movement makes of health professionals (other than those in mental health) toward achieving the three goals stated above are: (1) to stop telling sexually dissatisfied women that their condition is normal and irrevocable, (2) to inform them that help is available and to refer them for counselling, and (3) to deal with the patient's problems or requests without making value judgments about the woman's personal choices (for example, to stop referring to women who have had many sexual partners as "promiscuous," while not using that term for similarly sexually active men).

By and large the women's movement has not requested that the regular health care system try to provide treatment for women with sexual dysfunctions. Although they do not want these conditions to be considered "normal," they also do not want them to be defined as within the physician's province of "disease." Also, because the high prevalence of women's sexual problems is seen as a result of sexism and the double sexual standard, many women believe that the movement itself offers the best opportunity for cure.

Many nurses, social workers, and other women who originally worked as counselors in family planning or abortion clinics or abortion referral services later expanded their interest to include the entire subject of women's sexuality and intimate relationships (with other women as well as with men). Some of these women then received additional formal education through graduate studies in social work, psychology, psychiatric nursing, or counseling or through special programs to train sex therapists. Others developed considerable noncredentialed expertise simply through experience and sharing of knowledge with other women. A cadre of experienced, feminist-oriented sex counselors and therapists now provide services to women on a group or one-to-one basis through programs offered in a variety of non-health care settings such as local YWCAs and colleges and sometimes in association with health services such as family planning or abortion clinics, that are comfortable with the basic premises of the women's movement. However, less "liberated" women are also being reached, directly or indirectly, with the message that sexual dissatisfaction is not a natural and untreatable condition that women should simply accept. Women's magazines such as *Glamour, Redbook,* and *McCalls* now frequently carry articles supporting the goals of the women's movement. All women (except for the poor) now have a better chance than previously to find help within the confines of the traditional health care system. Many factors in society, including the women's movement, have combined to create demand and pressure for better education of professionals. These demands have resulted in inclusion of information about sexuality in both undergraduate and graduate educational programs for nurses and physicians and in more and better treatment of sexual problems by obstetricians-gynecologists, psychiatrists, family physicians, and other members of the health care team.

Removing the aura of abnormality and illness from the female organs and their functions

The women's movement wants the health professions, which are society's accepted authorities on what is normal and healthy versus what is abnormal and sick, to stop reinforcing common beliefs that women's vaginas are naturally foul smelling and dirty and need to be regularly cleansed (by douching), that menstruation makes women slightly crazy, irrational, and sick, and that menopause is a time of mental and sometimes physical illness. Some feminists believe that the practice of using drapes to block a woman's view of her own pelvic examination (not done when men's testicles are examined) should be discontinued because it reinforces many women's feelings that the area between their legs is ugly and obscene. Many feminists believe that pregnancy and childbirth should be treated as normal processes unless or until proven otherwise, which is to say that there should be much less "treatment" during pregnancy and birth.

Menstruation. Throughout history many cultures and religions have considered the menstrual discharge to render women unclean or impure during and for some time following menstruation.[61] Many women in this country were taught as girls to refer to their menstrual periods as "the curse." Probably because it involves discomfort and bleeding, many young girls think of menstruation as a monthly illness during which they assume variations of the "sick role." Not long ago, menstruation was routinely accepted as a reason to excuse girls from physical education classes, and women believed that, for health reasons, they should abstain from heavy physical activity, baths, swimming, and coitus while they were experiencing menstrual bleeding. The "premenstrual tension," emotional lability, and/or depression that some women experience secondary to water retention and other hormone-induced changes immediately preceding and during menstruation led to a common belief that all women were emotionally unstable to some degree while menstruating. This belief has been used as one reason (among others) for considering women unfit to occupy positions that could not be safely held by a person subject to frequent periods of mild insanity. Some otherwise normal women with uterine or other pathology (for example, endometriosis) experience so much pain that they are physically incapacitated during menses, and it has been found that women are more apt to be admitted to mental hospitals and commit crimes during the premenstrual or menstrual period than during the rest of their menstrual cycles.[61] Nevertheless, acceptance of the idea that menstruation is a time of vague physical and mental illness has declined sharply in the past 15 years with the aid of both feminists and the medical profession.

Another request of the women's movement is that the symptoms women experience during menstruation be legitimized by finding their specific physical causes and making them widely known, perhaps leading to determining safe palliative treatments to alleviate the symptoms, and removing the suspicion of hypochondriasis from women who are affected. In fact recent endocrinologic reseach to find better methods of contraception and abortion has advanced our understanding of menstruation and identified a biologic basis (prostaglandins) for menstrual cramps.

Pregnancy and childbirth. Although the women's movement is currently calling for recognition of pregnancy and childbirth as normal processes that should not be regarded or preemptively treated as illnesses, this is a relatively new tenet of feminist philosophy. When American feminists were leading social reform efforts in the late 1800s and early 1900s, the nation's maternal and infant mortality rates were high and, except for the wealthy, few pregnant women had access to needed medical, nursing, and hospital care.

In 1908 the Women's City Club of New York established a maternity center that was unique at that time. Its stated objective of providing prenatal and postpartum medical and nursing care to every pregnant woman within a specified district of New York City was a radical departure from the established practice of providing prenatal obstetric care only for women with complications.[54] Feminists supported maternity leave for working women. Establishment of the federal Children's Bureau in 1912 and passage of the 1921 Sheppard-Towner Act, which provided federal support for state health department prenatal clinics, were results of a partnership between women leaders and influential physicians who wanted to make medical (or nurse-midwifery) supervision routine for all pregnant women.[35, 37] Hospitalization for all births was also considered desirable by most people concerned with the welfare of women.

By 1960, hospitalization for childbirth was almost universal in the United States and the experience of childbirth had changed dramatically. Women had left their homes and families to have their babies alone in hospitals for the promises of greater safety and decreased pain. Of the nearly 56,000 pregnancies included in the National Institute of Neurological Diseases and Stroke (NINDS) Collaborative Perinatal Study (1959-1965), only 8% of the white women and 26% of the black women received no anesthesia during delivery.[63] With routine obstetrical anesthesia and analgesia, labor was really no longer "normal" and parturient women found it necessary to assume the "sick patient" role. Groggy and stupified during labor and paralyzed or asleep at delivery, women as individuals were no longer involved in the process of giving birth. Physicians delivered babies and were thanked by grateful fathers. The mother, sleeping off her stupor, had to ask when she woke up whether her baby (now in the nursery) was a boy or a girl. In addition, anesthetized women were helpless in ways that affected the normal processes of labor and birth. They could not support themselves in any position and thus tended to experience labor and delivery flat on their backs—a position in which it is hard to have a bowel movement, much less to push out a baby, especially since the pelvic outlet is tilted *up* when the woman is in the recumbent position. For that reason and because sleeping or paralyzed women could not use their voluntary muscles to help push their babies out, forceps were often needed to actually deliver the babies. In some hospitals, use of forceps became routine. The NINDS Collaborative Perinatal Study found that forceps were used on 57% of the white women who had vaginal deliveries.[54] Episiotomies became routine, primarily because of the use of forceps and concern for vaginal support. In 1977 it was estimated that episiotomies were performed during more than 70% of deliveries in the United States.[19] Eventually it was recognized that systemic painkillers depress not only the mother's but also the baby's respirations and nervous system,[22] and general anesthesia for obstetrics was gradually abandoned. However, epidural anesthesia, which ultimately replaced it, did not usually prevent the need for forceps and episiotomies, and often slowed the normal pace of the first stage of labor, encouraging early artificial rupture of the fetal membranes and the use of oxytocin to hasten labor.

A movement to reduce the use of chemical painkillers and their associated obstetric interventions was started by Grantly Dick-Read, an English obstetrician who had learned from watching his patients that fear during labor leads to tension, which adds to the pain. His book, *Childbirth Without Fear*, started a "natural childbirth movement" in Europe and the United States.

Dick-Read proposed that the cycle of fear, tension, and pain could be broken and the pain of labor reduced or eliminated by educating women in the physiology of labor and training them in muscle relaxation and in exercises to strengthen the voluntary muscles that contribute to the progress of labor. Later a Frenchman, Dr. Fernand Lamaze, expanded on Dick-Read's program, using a method he developed from observing Russian women in what seemed to him to be painless labor. His psychoprophylactic method for childbirth relied on preparing women prenatally with a set of breathing exercises they could use to cope with and control pain during labor. These techniques completely changed the role that hospitalized women could play in labor and delivery. Instead of lying down to be passively delivered by obstetricians, prepared women were active participants who contributed to their own infants' health by avoiding medications, assuming the most advantageous positions during labor, and pushing as required for delivery. Thus they made a conscious and personal contribution to the safe births of their babies, and they could be proud of their strength, self-discipline, and will.

During the 1960s and 1970s, interest and participation in both natural childbirth and breastfeeding increased markedly in the United States, especially among women of the well-educated middle class,[58] (also the main participants of the women's movement). The women's movement no doubt contributed to these trends by priming the women involved with increased self-confidence and assertiveness. But natural childbirth and support for breastfeeding were not specific demands of the women's movement. In *The Female Eunuch*, Germaine Greer, an important theorist of the women's movement, advised women to simply refuse to have children.[32] *Vaginal Politics*[29] was devoted to discussion of self-help clinics, sexism in medicine, the need for women to control abortion, treatment of breast cancer, inadequate screening for gonorrhea, and female sexuality and its mistreatment by psychiatrists. Frankfort's landmark feminist attack on women's health care did not discuss pregnancy and birth. In retrospect, it appears that the movement for equality of women could not focus on the positive aspects of childbirth and motherhood while it was still fighting for the right to avoid them. After the Supreme Court decision on abortion in 1973, a great deal of feminist energy gradually focused on what was happening to women during childbirth.

Some changes concerning childbirth seem to be leading in the direction of more physician "management" and control of childbirth—more cesarean sections, routine use of electronic fetal monitoring during labor, and more mothers forced into large, high technology hospitals because many small community hospitals have had to close their obstetric services as a result of the establishment of regional perinatal centers. However, the net effect has been and will probably continue to be gains for the goals of the women's movement— greater safety for mothers and babies, along with an increased perception of pregnancy and childbirth as essentially normal, healthy processes; an increasingly powerful role for women in the process of childbirth; and greater participation by men in parenting. Although forces other than the women's movement have been the prime movers in these changes, the women's movement was probably a necessary influencing factor.

RAPE

A fourth health-related achievement of the women's movement has been to focus needed attention on the crime of rape, to teach women ways to prevent or defend themselves from rape, and to stimulate improved treatment of raped women by health care personnel.

More than 56,000 forcible rapes were reported to local law enforcement agencies in 1975;[24] criminologists estimate that the actual number of rapes is four to ten times higher than the number reported.[13] Reasons for the vast underreporting of rape are complex but include the expectation on the part of many rape victims that both hospital and police personnel will be unsympathetic and that attempts to seek their help will only cause additional trauma and humiliation.[13] Although there have been significant improvements in recent years, many rape victims' expectations of insensitive hospital treatment are still too often realistic. In many cities, all rape victims are told to go to the emergency room of one specific hospital that has agreed with the municipal authorities to treat all rape victims.[13] In a busy city hospital emergency room, a rape victim without evident physical injury may be seen as having low priority for immediate care. When she is finally seen, she may receive only physical care, with little or no attention to her psychologic trauma. Unless the physician who examines her has been educated to the special needs of rape victims, the pelvic examination may seem to her a "second rape".[16] Unless she has cuts and bruises, she may even be treated hostilely by some physicians and nurses who assume that most rape victims were "asking for it" by provocative appearance or behavior or that they "cry rape" after sex in which they participated willingly.

Care and concern have improved for rape victims only in very recent years; the credit is almost entirely a result of the women's movement. Feminist authors educated the public (including physicians and nurses) about rape through a series of compelling, well-researched, well-written books, especially Burgess' and Holmstrom's *Rape: Victims of Crisis*,[16] and Brownmiller's excellent documentation, *Against Our Will*.[14] Equally or more important were groups of women, some who had been rape victims themselves, who organized women-run rape crisis counseling services in almost every large American city. These services provide sensitive women to be with and support rape victims during their postrape hospital experiences. In addition they provide rape victims with the essential opportunity to talk about their experience and the feelings they have about it both during the immediate postrape period and at later group sessions. Counselors from these services also serve as knowledgeable advocates for rape victims in the hospital, helping them to avoid long waits and ensuring that they receive all the necessary medical care. In the process, they have also served to educate hospital personnel about the deep psychologic trauma and needs of rape victims. Although these services were almost invariably started as volunteer efforts, many hospitals have now incorporated them as a regular hospital service with at least some paid staff.

In 1978 the American College of Obstetricians and Gynecologists published a Technical Bulletin on rape (Alleged Sexual Assault) that reflects progress in the care of rape victims during the past 5 years. A major difference between this bulletin and the 1972 version is new and greatly expanded content on the emotional trauma of rape and the rape victim's needs for immediate and sometimes long-term counseling and support. The 1978 bulletin also includes a new section on *Crisis Intervention Counsel*, which states that "the need for early emotional support and counseling by qualified, sensitive persons in the care of victims of this crime has become quite evident," and recommends appropriate "referral to help victims cope with resultant emotional and social problems." This section also suggests that either "a victim-contact worker of Sexual Assault Care Centers, trusted obstetrician-gynecologist, pediatrician, or the family physician is usually best suited" for active follow-up counseling of the victim after acute crisis intervention. The ACOG technical bulletin on rape is evidence that women's movement concepts and techniques for care of rape victims have been accepted as necessary by authorities in the mainstream of American medicine. In addition it recognizes that other women may often be more effective than physicians (except a physician with a longstanding relationship with the rape victim) at providing certain important aspects of a rape victim's necessary care.

CHANGING WOMEN'S HEALTH CARE BY CHANGING THE CARE PROVIDERS
Effect on the nursing profession

In this country as in others, nursing developed as a female occupation that functioned under the direct or indirect leadership and supervision of primarily male physicians. The nursing skills accorded the most respect were associated with technical tasks related to medical diagnosis and treatment (for example, "giving shots"), which were delegated to nurses by physicians. In addition to carrying out "doctor's orders," nurses tended to the ordinary bodily needs of people unable to do so themselves because of illness, treatment, or hospitalization; provided "tender loving care" to those in physical or emotional pain; coordinated the bureaucratic aspects of hospitalized patients' care (filling out forms and ensuring that patients were moved from place to place at the proper time); managed the hospitals' functional units; and facilitated the work of physicians. Nursing was a women's occupation that provided surrogate mothers (for patients), wife-like supporter-helpers (for physicians), and homemakers (for hospitals). Its status rested on the respect paid to discipline, obedience, orderliness, cleanliness, and self-sacrifice (willingness to work hard for low or no wages—some were nuns); appreciation of sick people's need for the "feminine" characteristics of tenderness, compassion, and supportiveness; and the prestige associated with performance of technical skill tasks that required special training and were highly regarded because they were related to the work of physicians.

Nursing is so thoroughly associated with women's roles that it could not help but be affected by the women's movement. For the past 20 years, nursing in the United States has been struggling to improve its status, pay, and working conditions; to upgrade its educational and scientific basis; and to define its role—its unique contribution to patient care and well-being—independently from that of medicine. Although efforts to upgrade nursing education, stimulate nursing research, and define a unique nursing role antedated the resurgence of the women's movement in the late 1960s, these efforts were essentially confined to university schools and departments of nursing. For many years these goals were either resisted or ignored by the majority of rank and file nurses who believed that the university nurses were "out of touch" with reality. The nursing professors, however, provided the philosophic basis for changes that are occurring now and helped to implement those changes by directing a minority group of nurses (their students) into nursing work places with raised expectations. Except for upgrading nursing education, real implementation of these changes began to occur only when the women's movement started to affect the lives of a broad segment of women, including nurses, by changing their basic assumptions in ways incompatible with their existing "professional" roles.

Recollecting and reading about nursing's struggle to change its role is similar to recollecting and reading about the efforts that millions of individual American women have struggled to make during the past 15 years to evolve more equitable and satisfying relationships with their husbands and to define themselves as complete human beings in their own right, independent of their relationships to men as daughters, lovers, wives, and mothers. The changes many women are trying to make in their marriages are stressful. The stress caused by these changes has broken many marriages and greatly modified many others. Similarly, nursing's struggle for independent professionalization has severely stressed its relationship with medicine. Some components of the medical profession would even like a "divorce," hoping to replace nurses with physicians' assistants, whose relationship to and dependence on physicians is not in question. But for the most part, the marriage of medicine and nursing is intact; the fact remains that the ill and injured need both medical and nursing care concurrently, and cooperation between the professions is necessary. The two professions are natural partners and require each other to function. The marriage will survive, but in a changed form.

Several different kinds of efforts are currently being made by nurses to either change the nursing profession as a whole or to change their own status as individual nurses. They include increased emphasis on education and research, a new willingness to organize for their own benefit and to strike when necessary, increasing encouragement of men to enter nursing (7% of 1975 nursing graduates were male), and the movement of significant numbers of nurses into more independent roles in the management of patients' (or clients') primary health care. This last change is discussed more fully here because it significantly affects the health care options to large numbers of American women.

The nurse-practitioner and nurse-midwife movements. The essence of the nurse-practitioner and nurse-midwife movement is the assumption of responsibility by nurses for management of areas of health care that either do not require medical diagnosis and treatment of disease (for example, normal pregnancy) or within which most of the required medical care can be routinized and is needed by people who also need nursing, that is, education, counseling, assistance, and direct care aimed at health protection and promotion or at meeting the individual's basic physical, emotional, and social needs despite illness, injury, or other alterations in health status.

Nurse-midwifery was introduced into the United States from Great Britian in 1923. It survived but grew slowly in this country until the 1970s, when it became increasingly popular. The nurse-practitioner movement started with a unique program initiated at the University of Colorado in 1965 to train nurses to manage the primary health care required by children. The nurse-practitioner concept has been debated ever since. There is still considerable disagreement within both medicine and nursing about the appropriateness of a more independent role for nurses including management of some medical conditions, the need for such practitioners, the amount of autonomy they should have, and how their roles should be defined.* Nevertheless nurse-midwives and some types of nurse-practitioner are becoming firmly entrenched in the American health care system.

In 1978 the American Nurses Association estimated that about 12,000 nurse-practitioners were practicing in the United States.[41] In addition a study by the American College of Nurse-Midwives found more than 600 nurse-midwives in active clinical practice at the end of 1976; they had delivered more than 1% of all babies born in the United States that year.[50]

The federal government has helped to stimulate development of educational programs for nurse-practitioners,[39] and in 1971 the Department of Health, Education and Welfare published a special committee report entitled *Extending the Scope of Nursing Practice,* which acknowledged the expanding role of professional nurses and stated that the committee (composed of representatives of both medicine and nursing) saw no legal obstacles to such role extension.[23] The committee's statement on lack of legal obstacles was, however, not realistic, as almost all states at that time had laws that prohibited nurses from any acts of diagnosis or therapy. In the early 1970s the American Nurses Association advised state associations to change their state's nurse practice acts to allow diagnosis and treatment by nurses under special rules and regulations, and more than 30 states have now done so.[15]

Nurse-practitioners have found their greatest support and securest niche in providing care to other women, either directly as nurse-midwives or nurse-practitioners functioning in the areas of family planning and/or "well-woman gynecology" or indirectly as pediatric nurse-practitioners. (Children's health care is usually negotiated by their mothers.) The American Academy of Pediatrics supports pediatric nurse-practitioners or "associates" and has formally endorsed the National Association of Pediatric Nurse Associates and Practitioners, which was formed in 1973. The two organizations have jointly published a "Def-

---

*See references 9, 31, 36, 49, and 50.

inition of a Pediatric Nurse Practitioner/ Associate" and "Scope of Practice" statements that define the functions and responsibilities of pediatric nurse-practitioners.[62] The American College of Obstetricians and Gynecologists has been supportive of nurse-midwives and in January 1979 adopted an official statement on the role of obstetric and gynecologic nurse-practitioners.

The popularity and success of nurse-practitioners, as well as the "new" women's movement, have been greatest in the areas of health care that are provided to or through women. The existence of nurse-practitioners provides many women with an important health care option. Although the acceptance of both nurse-midwives and nurse-practitioners was originally based on their service to rural and inner-city populations without adequate access to physician care, their services are now preferred and sought by many middle-class and professional women.

Local medical societies have opposed expansion of the nurse practice acts in many states,[41] and more opposition can be expected as the greatly increased number of medical students graduating in the United States yearly swells that profession. However, women representing nursing and health care consumers are now making institutional changes to support continuation and increase of this health care option for women. A law recently passed in Maryland serves as an example. Because of the efforts and influence of the Maryland Nurses Association, the work of two female Maryland state legislators, and a long history of nurse-midwifery practice and education in Maryland, a recently passed law will require every health insurer in that state to offer the option of providing benefits arising from "care, treatment, or services rendered by a nurse-midwife." This law is a landmark because it also specifies that insurance companies cannot require as a condition for payment that the reimbursed nurse-midwife was employed by or acting under the supervision or orders of a physician.[4]

Effect on the medical profession

American medicine has been as traditionally male as nursing has been female. Until very recently children's books almost invariably portrayed doctors as men and nurses as women. Little girls were encouraged to play nurse instead of doctor. Even excellent female high school and college students were usually counselled to enter the female professions of nursing and teaching rather than the male professions of law and medicine. It was realistic counsel, because they in fact had little chance of admittance to medical or law schools. There were few female physicians to provide role models for girls who might have aspired to medicine. Only 8% of U.S. physicians in 1973 were female.[10] What few women physicians there were practiced mainly as pediatricians (22%). Only 3% of obstetricians-gynecologists were women. Only 10 female thoracic surgeons were known to be practicing in the entire United States.[7] Although female medical students did as well as men academically, more of them dropped out before graduation (16% of the female students as compared with 9% of the males) because of pregnancies and family responsibilities.[38]

The numbers of women admitted to U.S. medical schools increased rapidly and steadily following passage of Title VII of Public Law 92-147 in 1971, which prohibits discrimination in educational opportunities, and passage of Title IX of the Higher Education Act amendments in 1972, which forbids discrimination in educational facilities.[3] The proportion of women among students entering U.S. medical schools increased more than four-fold between 1959 and 1976—from 6% to 25% of the entering class.[48]

What difference will more women physicians make to women's health care? An obvious difference is that more women will have the option of selecting to establish their patient-physician relationship with a female physician. This is especially true in obstetrics and gynecology. The proportion of women entering the first year of ob/gyn residency training programs nearly doubled between 1975 and 1978—from 16% to 30%.[10] To date little objective evidence is available to document the influence of the new female physicians on their professions. Some observers believe that many female students are entering medicine because of a deep personal concern about women's health care and report that they are "extraordinarily sensitive to invasions of the privacy of their patients, unethical professional behavior, and the arrogance of power."[48] One study of personality differences in male and female medical students found that the females were more sensitive to relationship values, were more accepting of feelings, and placed greater value on independence and individuality.[17] Other observers state different views. Navarro reports that female physicians tend to be conservative and identify more with male physicians than they do with other female health workers or female patients.[46] What effect the sexual neutralization of medicine will have on women's health care remains to be seen, but will probably be considerable.

THE FUTURE

What effect is the women's movement likely to have on the future of women's health care? The following predictions seem to be logical:

1. Greater and more sophisticated involvement of feminists in the main stream of health care policy making and administration, leading to institutionalization of desired changes. For example, one of the original members of The Boston Women's Health Book Collective is now also a member of the board of the Health Systems Agency (HSA) for Boston, Massachusetts. That HSA, which is responsible for planning and approving the development of new health care facilities in the Boston area, has as a stated goal that "out-of-hospital alternatives to traditional hospital maternity services should be developed on a pilot project basis for low-risk women in HSA IV" (Boston).

2. Many of the women who created the new women's movement in the late 1960s are now in their late 30s and 40s. Nearly past their childbearing years, they are becoming increasingly interested in different aspects of women's health and health care. Breast cancer, menopause, and the sexuality of older women will probably become the primary targets of their efforts to improve women's health care.

3. In mid-1978, for the first time in history, half of all U.S. females over 15 years of age were in the labor force (either working or looking for work). Women held 42% of the jobs in the United States. It is predictable that the interface between women's work and women's health and health care will receive more attention in the future. The National Institute of Occupational Safety and Health (NIOSH) is currently exploring the problems of protecting women health workers. As more women work while pregnant, the need to protect them and their fetuses from occupational health hazards will become increasingly important and complicated. A recent achievement regarding health care for working women was the passage of a federal law that, as of July 1, 1979, requires employers to com-

pensate their employees for work time missed as a result of illness as well as pregnancy.

REFERENCES

1. American College of Obstetricians and Gynecologists: Standards for obstetric-gynecologic hospital services, Columbus, Ohio, 1965, Charles E. Merrill Publishing Co.
2. American Medical Association, Federal Trade Commission Document No. 9064, Washington, D.C., November 13, 1978.
3. American Medical Association Department of Undergraduate Medical Evaluation and American Association of Medical Colleges Division of Operational Studies: Undergraduate medical education, J.A.M.A. 238:2767-2780, 1977.
4. Anonymous: Landmark Maryland nurse-midwife reimbursement bill passed, J. Nurs.-Midwif. 23:19, 1978.
5. Anonymous: Working women, Parade p. 20, November 12, 1978.
6. Arnold, C. B., and Cogswell, B. E.: A condom distribution program for adolescents: the findings of a feasibility study, Am. J. Public Health 61:739-750, 1971.
7. Baumgartner, L.: Women MDs join the fight, Med. World News 11:22-28, 1970.
8. Bewley, B. R., and Bewley, T. H.: Hospital doctor's career structure and misuse of medical womanpower, Lancet 2:270-272, 1975.
9. Bicknell, W. J., Walsh, D. C., and Tanner, M. M.: Substantial or decorative? Physicians' assistants and nurse practitioners in the U.S., Lancet 2:1241-1244, 1974.
10. Bluestone, N. R.: The future impact of women physicians on American medicine, Am. J. Public Health 68:760-763, 1978.
11. The Boston Women's Health Book Collective: Our bodies, ourselves, ed. 2, New York, 1976, Simon & Schuster, Inc.
12. Breen, J. L., and Greenwald, E.: Rape. In Glass, R. H., editor: Office gynecology, Baltimore, 1976, The Williams & Wilkins Co.
13. Brodyaga, L., and Gates, M.: Rape and its victims: a report for citizens, health facilities, and criminal justice agencies, Washington, D.C., 1975, Center for Women Policy Studies, pp. 58-74.
14. Brownmiller, S.: Against our will, New York, 1975, Simon & Schuster, Inc.
15. Bullough, B.: The law and the expanding nurse role, Am. J. Public Health 66:249-252, 1976.
16. Burgess, A. W., and Holmstrom, L. L.: Rape: victims of crises, Bowie, Md., 1974, Robert J. Brady Co.
17. Cartwright, L. K.: Personality differences in male and female medical students, Psychiatr. Med. 3:313-318, 1972.
18. Center for Disease Control: Abortion surveillance report, Atlanta, 1970, The Center, pp. 3-36.
19. Cogan, R., and Edmunds, E.: The unkindest cut? Contemp. Ob/Gyn 9:55-59, 1977.
20. Collaborative Group for the Study of Stroke in Young Women: Oral contraception and increased risk of cerebral ischemia or thrombosis, New Engl. J. Med. 288:871-878, 1973.
21. Cornell, E. B.: The pill revised. Fam. Plann. Perspect. 7:62-71, 1975.
22. Danforth, D. N., and Moya, F.: Obstetric analgesia and anesthesia. In Danforth, D. N., editor: Obstetrics and gynecology, ed. 3, New York, 1977, Harper & Row, Publishers.
23. Extending the scope of nursing practice, a report of the Secretary's Committee to study extended roles for nurses, Washington, D.C., November, 1971, Department of Health, Education and Welfare.
24. Federal Bureau of Investigation: Crime in the United States, 1975, Washington, D.C., 1976, U.S. Government Printing Office.
25. Federal Register, Vol. 42, No. 90, May 10, 1977.
26. Federal Register, Vol. 42, No. 141, July 22, 1977.
27. Federal Register, Vol. 43, No. 199, October 13, 1978.
28. Flexner, E.: Century of struggle: the women's rights movement in the United States, New York, 1970, Atheneum Publishers.
29. Frankfort, E.: Vaginal politics, New York, 1972, Bantam Books, Inc.
30. Gamble, C. J.: Every child a wanted child, Boston, 1978, Harvard University Press.
31. Golloday, R. L., Smith, K. R., Davenport, E. J., et al.: Policy planning for mid-level health worker: economic potentials and barriers to change, Inquiry 8:80-89, 1976.
32. Greer, G.: The female eunuch, New York, 1971, McGraw-Hill Book Co.
33. Grissum, M., and Spengler, C.: Womanpower and health care, Boston, 1976, Little, Brown and Co.
34. Hatcher, R. A., Stewart, G. K., Stewart, F., et al.: Contrceptive technology, 1978-1979, ed. 9, New York, 1979, John Wiley & Sons, Inc.

35. Hellman, L. M., and Pritchard, J. A.: Williams' Obstetrics, ed. 14, New York, 1971, Appleton-Century-Crofts.
36. Herzog, E. L.: The underutilization of nurse practitioners in ambulatory care, Nurs. Pract. 2:26-29, 1976.
37. Hogan, A.: A tribute to the pioneers, J. Nurs. Midwif. 20:3-6, 1975.
38. Howell, M. C.: What medical schools teach about women, New Engl. J. Med. 291:301-307, 1974.
39. Huggins, G. R., and Manisoff, M.: Using nurse-practitioners in ambulatory gynecology, Contemp. Ob/Gyn 12:109-117, 1978.
40. Kinsey, A. C., Pomeroy, W. B., Martin, C. E., et al.: Sexual behavior in the human female, Philadelphia, 1953, W. B. Saunders Co.
41. Mankish, I. G.: The nurse practitioner movement—where does it go from here? Am. J. Public Health 68:1074-1075, 1978.
42. Mann, J. I., and Inman, W. H. W.: Oral contraceptives and death from myocardial infarction, Br. Med. J. 2:245-248, 1975.
43. Mann, J. I., Vessey, M. P., Thorogood, M., et al.: Myocardial infarction in young women with special reference to oral contraceptive practice, Br. Med. J. 2:241-244, 1975.
44. Martin, H. W., and Prange, A. J.: The stages of illness: psychosocial approach, Nurs. Outlook 10:167-171, 1962.
45. McGuigan, D. G.: A dangerous experiment: 100 years of women at the University of Michigan, Ann Arbor, Michigan, 1970, Center for Continuing Education for Women.
46. Navarro, V.: Medicine under capitalism, New York, 1977, Prodist Publishing Co.
47. Parsons, T.: The sick role and the role of the physician reconsidered, Milbank Mem. Fund Q. 53(3):257-277, 1975.
48. Pearce, W., and Fielden, J.: Manpower planning in obstetrics and gynecology, Chicago, 1978, American College of Obstetricians and Gynecologists.
49. Record, J. C.: The introduction of midwifery in a prepaid group practice, Am. J. Public Health 62:354-360, 1972.
50. Rooks, J. P., Fischman, S., Kaplan, E., et al.: Nurse-midwifery in the United States: 1976-1977, Washington, D. C., 1978, The American College of Nurse-Midwives.
51. Rooks, J. P., Ory, H. W., Ishak, K. G., et al.: The association between oral contraception and hepatocellular adenoma: a preliminary report, Int. J. Obstet. Gynecol. 15:143-144, 1977.
52. Ross, J.: The pill hearings: major side effects, Fam. Plann. Perspect. 2:6-7, 1970.
53. Royal College of General Practitioners: Oral contraception and health, New York, 1974, Pitman Publishing Corp.
54. Speert, H.: Historical highlights. In Danforth, D. N., editor: Obstetrics and gynecology, ed. 3, New York, 1977, Harper & Row, Publishers.
55. Supreme Court of the United States, opinion numbers 70-40 and 70-18, January 22, 1973.
56. Te Linde, R. W.: Operative gynecology, Philadelphia, 1962, J. B. Lippincott Co.
57. U.S. Department of Health, Education and Welfare, Public Health Service: Information for women: your sterilization operation, Washington, D.C., 1978, U.S. Government Printing Office.
58. Watson, J.: Who attends prepared childbirth classes? A demographic study of CEA classes in Rhode Island, J. Obstet. Gynecol. Nurs. 6:36-39, 1977.
59. Webster's Seventh New Collegiate Dictionary, Springfield, Mass., 1969, G. & C. Merriam Co.
60. Westoff, C. F., and Jones, E. F.: Contraception and sterilization in the United States, 1965-1975, Fam. Plann. Perspect. 9:153-157, 1977.
61. Whelan, E. M.: Attitudes toward menstruation, Stud. Fam. Plann. 6:106-108, 1975.
62. William, M. K., Weinbert, E., Burnett, R. D., et al.: The pediatric nurse associate: a model of collaboration between medicine and nursing, New Engl. J. Med. 298:740-741, 1978.
63. The women and their pregnancies: the collaborative perinatal study of the National Institute of Neurological Diseases and Stroke, DHEW Publication No. (NIH) 73-379, 1972, pp. 362-388.

CHAPTER 2

Cultural aspects of health and illness behaviors in childbearing

Velvia M. Garner

INTRODUCTION

Many of the problems nurses experience stem from incongruence of beliefs and value systems between nurse and client. Yet, as a nurse, one will be asked to administer to clients having various sociocultural beliefs, values, and practices. One's nursing capabilities must, therefore, include competence in technical, communicative, interpersonal, and "cultural sensitivity" skills.

When subcultural, racial, or ethnic boundaries are crossed, as when a white, middle-class nurse attempts to administer care to an indigent Black, Hispanic, Asian, or Native American, the nurse is often confronted with a bewildering set of problems. This is not difficult to understand when one considers that both nurse and client belong to subcultures representing diverse lifestyles and beliefs. Each is acting according to a certain set of behaviors that are typical of their respective groups. Thus as nurse and client interact, these special behavioral traits can become barriers to therapeutic interventions, since persons from diverse cultural environments tend to interact at superficial levels. Furthermore, these behavioral patterns are so deeply ingrained at a subconscious level that both the nurse and the client are often unaware of the cause of their interpersonal problems.

OF WHAT SHOULD THE HEALTH PROFESSIONAL BE AWARE?

Many descendants of various ethnic groups adhere to and participate in health practices that appear, to the medically trained, to be unscientific. To provide the best possible support for clients of difficult ethnic and cultural groups, specific areas must be explored.

In many cultures, the childbearing period exposes the expectant mother to powerful ethnic influences, usually traditional and cultural practices that are followed in the expectation of preventing prenatal problems and strengthening the expectant mother. The nurse must determine the nature and extent to which clients from various groups adhere to particular beliefs about dietary habits, sexual practices, rituals, restrictions, or taboos during pregnancy. It is also important to determine how, where, and by whom the delivery is to be handled. Certain groups also maintain age-old practices after delivery. For example, it is customary in some very traditional Asian and Black families to serve ginger soup or ginger tea after delivery and to withhold cold foods. Some groups insist that the placenta be burned or buried in a special place.

To better understand some of these beliefs, it is necessary for the nurse-practitioner to become familiar with the folk practices, health and illness belief systems, and the general cultural characteristics of groups who do not totally subscribe to the health and medical practices of the common culture in this country. It is especially imperative that nurses seeking employment in agencies or areas requiring interactions with members of an unfamiliar subculture group receive orientation and special training to cope with the subtle barriers that arise when persons of different cultures interact.

Assessments of obstetric clients should include special consideration of the clients' cultural value systems and numerous folk beliefs and practices associated with pregnancy and childbearing. Groups continue to practice, in varying degrees, aspects of these traditional and cultural beliefs. The nurse-practitioner must also strive to define *good health* and *illness* as perceived by the client population. Many ethnic and racial minorities in the United States share similar beliefs about pregnancy and childbearing. These beliefs are often in direct conflict with the well-established societal and medical norms.

This chapter will present some of the traditional beliefs and practices of Hispanic, Black, Asian, and Native Americans and their impact on the cultural aspects of health and illness, as well as on pregnancy and childbearing. These cultural considerations will reflect experienced, observed, and reported behaviors. There will be no attempt to judge these behaviors nor to prove that all members of the four groups adhere to them. There will, however, be an attempt to encourage the reader to become more sensitive to the importance that clients attach to their traditional mores.

A review of the literature revealed similarities in some of the traditional health and illness belief systems of many Hispanic, Black, Asian, and Native Americans. These belief systems are not the unique possession of the poor or uneducated but are quite often practiced in varying degrees by middle- and upper-class members of the four groups. Unfortunately, such folk beliefs and practices are rarely included in nursing texts.

HISPANIC, OR SPANISH-SPEAKING, AMERICANS

There are approximately nine million people of Spanish ethnic origin living in the United States.[15] Within the Spanish-speaking population there are various subgroups: Puerto Ricans, Cubans, Central and South Americans, Mexican Americans, Mexicans, and Spanish Americans. They are not easily differentiated. Many are United States citizens by birth, while others are Mexican nationalists who have become naturalized citizens of the United States. Still others are immigrants who have decided not to renounce their native citizenship.

Physically, they share features in common with their Spanish, Mexican, and Indian ancestors. Sociologically, language and cultural traits link them with the Spanish and Mexican nations. These similar ancestral and physical characteristics probably account for their feeling of identity with one another. Nevertheless, their differing historical, political, social, and economic backgrounds tend to disrupt their sense of unity.[13]

Saunders categorizes three of the major subgroups: (1) Spanish Americans, (2) Mexicans, and (3) Mexican Americans.[13] These groupings are identified rather loosely throughout the Southwest, where the term *Hispanic* is often used to designate all groups inclusively.

Brief historical perspective

Spanish Americans, never legally Mexicans except for the brief time when Mexico won its independence from Spain, are genetic descendants of sixteenth and seventeenth century Spain and the Indian population. *Mexicans,* on the other hand, migrated from the interior of Mexico. They represent a large percentage of the "wetback" population that illegally crosses the border from Mexico into the United States to seek employment. Many are uneducated, agrarian, and speak only Spanish.[13]

Mexican Americans have genetic backgrounds similar to those of the Spanish Americans. Physical characteristics typically mirror their Indian ancestors. Many migrated from Mexico and some were born in the United States. Some five million of the Spanish-speaking are Mexican Americans, who make up one of the largest subgroups. Large numbers have found themselves unable to participate in the wider communities because job and educational opportunities have not been readily available to them.[12]

Early in this country's development, Mexican Americans represented a large percentage of the agriculture population. More recently, many of them formed the backbone of the migrant labor force. Today, the majority of Mexican Americans live in the five western states of Texas, Colorado, Arizona, New Mexico, and California. The greatest urban populations are recorded in Los Angeles, San Antonio, El Paso, and San Francisco.[13,15]

These three subgroups—Spanish Americans, Mexicans, and Mexican Americans—have cultural beliefs, values, and histories unique to each group. They also exhibit major similarities, particularly in their health practices. Therefore, to keep the following discussion within necessary constraints, the observations and recorded behaviors of the Mexican Americans will be described as representative of all three subgroups.

Characteristic cultural features

Cultural traditions of various Mexican Americans still reflect the influence of Mexico and Spain. There appears to be a strong orientation toward the present and the immediate past. According to Martinez "material objects are seen as necessities and not an end in themselves."[11] He further states that work is viewed as a necessity for survival but not as a value in itself. Martinez also states that Mexican Americans believe that it is more valuable to experience things directly through intellectual awareness and emotional experiences rather than indirectly and through past accomplishments and accumulation of wealth.

Traditional patterns of family life

Mexican Americans are a proud people with a strong sense of family identity. Because the family unit is considered the most important social unit, the family is considered first and individual needs tend to be of secondary importance.[13] The Mexican American concept of family defines the husband, wife, and children as the nuclear family. The grandparents, uncles, aunts, and cousins are included in the extended family. A special subset is that of the *compadres* (godparents). There is a great deal of communicating, advising, and sharing between these groups. Children are taught respect for the elderly and for the father, who assumes leadership of the household. Very few decisions are made without his input or consent. He is warm and loving, but he is also the major disciplinarian.[4] The wife supports her husband's actions and decisions, and it is through her efforts that close relationships among family members are nourished and maintained. Although family needs have highest priorities, our changing society is making an impact on the traditional family. Women and children are now less willing to accept the traditional passive roles assigned to them by their ancestors.

Beliefs about health and illness

There is a strong religious orientation among Spanish-speaking peoples. Closely allied with the religious values is the belief in witchcraft and *curranderisma*. *Curranderisma* is a belief that folk illnesses can be cured by a *curandero* (lay healer) who has been given certain powers by God. Witchcraft is the belief that a person or thing harms another through the use of magic. The combination of these two beliefs by some Mexican Americans probably accounts for their belief that they have limited control over nature. Many also believe that God both gives health and sends illness. Illnesses are defined in relation to pain or the inability to perform daily activities. Since the concept of health and illness is directly related to one's soul one must be in compliance with God's will.

Beliefs about diseases

Ideas concerning the cause of diseases are as diverse as the subgroups represented in the Spanish-speaking population. Many diseases are considered punishment for transgressions, and others are believed to be caused by demons or witches.[1,4,13] This section will discuss (1) diseases of hot and cold imbalance, (2) diseases of dislocation of internal organs, (3) diseases of magical origin, (4) diseases of folk origin, and (5) standard medical diseases.[4]

Diseases of hot and cold imbalance. The hot and cold concept in relation to disease is believed by some to have originated in India and spread to the western parts of the world with the Spanish explorers. Others believe this concept was derived from the Hippocratic theory, which postulated that health was determined by a balance in blood, phlegm, black bile, and yellow bile.[4,7] Some of these four humors are thought to be hot, while others are thought to be cold. Food is also categorized as hot or cold, and dietary regulation is viewed as being vital to good health. Cold diseases are treated with "hot" foods, and hot diseases are treated with "cold" foods. (However, these disease classifications have nothing to do with absence or presence of fever.)

Diseases of dislocation of internal organs. This category includes diseases or illnesses caused by the shifting of real or imaginary body parts from their normal positions. For example, Clark describes a condition called *mollera caida* (fallen fontanelle) in which "parts of the head" directly under the anterior fontanelle of an infant "drop" or shift position.[4]

Diseases of magical and folk origin. Diseases of magical origin can be caused by someone or some supernatural power. Many believe that someone, especially a female, can admire a child without touching him and the child may then fall ill of *mal ojo* (evil eye). It is characterized by much crying, restless sleep, unexplained fever, vomiting, and diarrhea.[6]

Clark describes two folk disorders called *latido* and *empacho*. With *latido* (palpitation), severe pains develop in the stomach and the victim becomes increasingly unable to eat. After several days, pulsations can be felt in the stomach. Severe forms can produce extreme weight loss and become quite serious and sometimes fatal. *Empacho* (surfeit) is a disorder characterized by a large ball in the stomach that causes the stomach to swell. It is believed to be caused by overeating.[4]

Diseases of emotional origin. Severe emotional experiences such as fright (*susto* or *espanto*) or anger (*bilis*, or bile) can cause illnesses. *Bilis* results when an adult becomes so angry that he or she exhibits acute physical symptoms such as nervous tension, fatigue, and malaise.[4]

Standard medical diseases. This category refers to diseases that are recognized by both medical personnel and barrio people. Some of these include *sarampion* (measles), *pulmonia* (pneumonia or bronchitis), and *tos ferina* (whooping cough).[4]

Beliefs about childbearing

Beliefs about pregnancy are related to beliefs about religion, the hot and cold phenomena, witchcraft, and other folk theories. Some believe that a pregnant woman has an unusually warm body during pregnancy. This necessitates the avoidance of "cold" foods during pregnancy to maintain a balance.[11] The belief further directs expectant mothers to protect themselves from natural cold forces such as air and water. It is believed that air can enter the body and cause illness and that water intake should be decreased because it might cause excessive growth of the baby's head.[13] Pregnancy is not considered an illness in itself. However, the pregnant state is thought to predispose a woman to problems.

Although many women are now seeking hospital deliveries, many others seem to dislike hospital deliveries because American obstetrical procedures differ drastically from traditional Mexican childbirth procedures. Many Mexican American women employ a *partera* (midwife). The *parteras* encourage walking until moments before the delivery. Immediately after the delivery, the mother's legs are placed close together to prevent air from entering the womb.[3]

The new mother is expected to stay in bed for a minimum of 3 days. Once she is up and around, a *faja* (cloth binder) is applied to the abdomen to prevent cold from entering the reproductive organs and to facilitate the process of uterine involution—"to help the organs go back to where they belong."[3,4] The ensuing postpartum period, which may be as long as 40 days after delivery, requires special care and instruction.[4] Relatives, neighbors, and friends voluntarily assist the new mother with household chores, bring gifts, and provide strong emotional support.

Beliefs about specific dietary restrictions and taboos. These beliefs vary from region to region, but most Mexican American and other Hispanic women agree that some restrictions after delivery are necessary. Hot chiles, pickles, and foods prepared in vinegar are some of the forbidden foods.[4] Pork and citrus fruits are considered either cold or too acid and therefore contributive to illness.[4] Postpartum diets should include foods to facilitate lactation. Many mothers believe that it is unnatural to feed their babies with a bottle. Furthermore, breastfeeding is believed to be a form of birth control. Some of the required foods are chicken, eggs, cooked cereals, milk, and bread. Mothers are encouraged to adhere to the dietary restrictions for 40 days and often until the child is weaned.[4]

In many instances, newborn males are not circumcised. Many believe that it disfigures the baby and makes him look "ugly."[3,4] The ears of infant girls are usually pierced. Fingernails and hair are not cut until the infant is at least 6 weeks old, since it is believed that these practices will make the infant weak and retard the ability to learn.[4]

BLACK AMERICANS
Brief historical perspective

Black Americans had a stormy beginning in this country. Alex Haley's historic novel about his family's struggles presented a vivid picture of the forceful importation of Blacks into the United States. Blacks were uprooted from their culture, families, friends, and homeland. Once settled in this country, Blacks even found themselves without a common language, enslaved, and deprived of support systems. They have consistently been subjected to systematic exclusion from participation and influence in the major institutions in this society.[12]

More than 100 years ago, 90% of all Blacks lived in the rural South. This pattern of residence has changed continuously over the years. Since World War I, the Black population in the South has decreased. The urbanization of the Black population varies region by region, with the greatest concentration at present in the large urban areas of both the North and the South.[2]

Black Americans, for many years, were embarrassed by their African background. However, careful analysis of historical and ethnographic data has revealed numerous, highly civilized, varied, and complex African cultural systems. Families and their lifestyles were rich in rituals, customs, and tradition.[2]

Traditional patterns of family life

Western African traditions stressed recognition of the nuclear and extended family. Kinship ties were ascribed in some groups to the father's or mother's side of the family. In the southern portion of Africa, double descent was recognized.[2] Marriage joined husband, wife, and extended families. Household organization included nuclear and extended families with rigidly prescribed roles for all family members.

When the Africans were transported to this country, slavery had a definite negative impact on these family traditions. Slaves worked long hours and children were cared for by older or disabled slaves. The children learned to assume responsibility for themselves at an early age and families were often separated through the slave trade. Today's families, however, are close and large. A large family has historically been advantageous for economic reasons, and parents often depend on children for support, especially as they grow older.

Beliefs about health and illness

There are many beliefs about health and illness as they relate to pregnancy and childbearing. The Black folk medicine belief system is similar to that of the Spanish-speaking groups. It is based on the division of the universe into natural and unnatural phenomena. Those events that have to do with the world as God made it are "natural" events. "Unnatural" events, implying the exact opposite, upset the natural events intended by God; therefore, they represent the work of the devil.[11,21]

Natural and unnatural illnesses. Just as there are natural and unnatural events, there are also natural and unnatural illnesses. Natural illnesses are those produced by natural agents such as air, which may enter the body orifices, or impurities in the air or food. On the other hand, unnatural illness is sometimes considered punishment sent by God for a sin. Others are believed to be caused by individuals who can mobilize unnatural or evil powers. Blacks will say "I'm a victim of rootwork," or "I'm fixed." These beliefs derive from voodoo.[17] This type of unnatural illness, because of its origin, cannot be controlled by medical doctors. Lay practitioners are employed to relieve unnatural disorders.[14,21]

Harmony and balance. Excess in anything is not good for you. The results might not be visible immediately, but the practice will contribute to poor health. For example, strength and weakness or susceptibility to illness is related to age and sex. The young and the elderly are considered weak and susceptible. Women are weaker than men. The unborn infant is the weakest.[11,14,21] Even emotional states can affect the unborn infant. Many believe that if an expectant mother hates an individual, the baby might be born resembling the hated one; or if the mother worries about a particular problem, the baby will develop the disorder. These beliefs have been validated by direct questions asked of my extended family and a convenient sample of 20 Blacks from a community in rural, southern Texas. In addition, there is evidence of a strong belief in witchcraft as it relates to animal intrusion. An evil person "fixes" another by introducing a lizard or snake into the body through magic.[14]

If illness is caused by supernatural powers, treatment and care must be performed by a lay healer. The maintenance of good health is based on harmony, which requires that the rules of nature be adhered to.[14,21]

Beliefs about childbearing

Since the infant and the female are considered the most susceptible to illness, many precautions must be observed during pregnancy. As with the Spanish-speaking people, emotional states must be kept uneventful. Many Blacks believe that severe emotional states such as anger, hate, fear, and worry can adversely affect the unborn child.[14] Again, as with the Mexican Americans, there is some reflection of the importance of the four body humors. Cold is associated with phlegm and upper respiratory conditions. Warm is associated with blood disorders, fevers, and rashes.[14] However, it has been my experience that pregnancy is considered a natural occurrence. Craving during pregnancy is also considered natural, including craving for items other than food. Many crave laundry starch (Argo), clay, or dirt. The ingestion of these items is called *pica*.[3]

Black American women, in my experience, appear to be stoical during labor and delivery. Many of them prefer to have a female in attendance, while others refuse medications because they believe that pain is necessary to culminate a natural phenomenon. The grandmother often served as a granny (midwife) and would encourage walking until just before delivery. They also prepared ginger or black pepper tea for the expectant mother during labor and talked to her while rubbing and massaging her abdomen. This practice was comforting, reassuring, and supportive. Following delivery, special care was taken to bury the afterbirth very deeply in a secluded area. The abdomens of both mother and infant were bound with a cloth to provide support for the mother as well as to "push the organs back into place." The baby's umbilicus was lubricated with castor oil and bound to protect the cord and prevent an umbilical hernia.

Cold foods were avoided, especially fresh citrus fruit. Soups, cereals, breads, and meats were encouraged. Activities were restricted for a minimum of 2 weeks. Other relatives would volunteer to care for the baby to allow the new mother to recuperate. Care was taken to protect both baby and mother from "natural forces." A confinement period of up to 1 month was rigidly enforced. Hygiene did not include immersion baths; rather, a daily sponge bath for as long as 1 month was recommended. Visitors were restricted for several weeks as a precautionary measure for mother and infant. The infants were kept very warm and fully clothed. Daily care included careful shaping of the head and nose. For 2 to 6 weeks, the new baby was confined to the house. Breastfeeding was highly recommended; cereal and other solid food were begun the second or third week of life.

ASIAN AMERICANS
Brief historical perspective

The Asian population in this country comprises two major subgroups: Chinese Americans and Japanese Americans. Although the Chinese and the Japanese have distinct cultural traditions, certain beliefs are sufficiently similar that a discussion focused on the Chinese American culture will also be applicable to the Japanese.

There are about 435,000 Chinese Americans in the United States. It is estimated that by 1980 there will be nearly 750,000. The Chinese tend to reside in large cities such as New York, Los Angeles, San Francisco, and Honolulu. The smallest recorded groups are in the central states.[16]

It is recorded that many Chinese were among the first settlers in the American West during the gold rush, which occurred in 1848. Many came in search of a better life. Many mined for gold, while others were merchants. The transcontinental railroads were completed almost exclusively by Chinese laborers. However, discrimination, heavy taxes, and rigid immigration laws served to halt the increase in Chinese immigrants to this country; and for many years they were not allowed to apply for citizenship.[16]

"Chinatowns" developed because Chinese immigrants experienced the need to make themselves as inconspicuous as possible. Jobs were limited and housing was almost nonexistent. These community arrangements provided protection and helped to maintain their rich cultural traditions.[16]

Traditional patterns of family life

The Chinese, like the Mexican Americans, imbue the concept of the extended family with a great deal of pride and tradition. The traditional extended family includes grandparents, uncles, aunts, cousins, brothers, sisters, and immediate family members. The father is the head of the household and the mother assumes a subordinate role. Her status is always enhanced by the birth of a son, particularly because the son will carry on the family name. Family members must conduct themselves to avoid bringing shame and disgrace on the family. In Chinese tradition, maintenance of respect for the well-being of the family or group is of primary importance. Individual needs are of secondary importance. Furthermore, respect for elders is one of the most important ancient traditions.[3]

Preservation of ancient cultural practices, which include religion, folklore, customs, foods, and lifestyles, is encouraged. For many generations, marriage was not a personal matter between male and female. Parents selected mates for their children. The selection was carefully made so that family traditions were preserved.[16] Religion is a major part of the lifestyles, since beliefs are built around a body of knowledge that tells people how to live a good and moral life. Preservation of cultural practices is further evidenced by the continued use of the Chinese calendar, which is based on revolutions of the moon around the earth. This places the Chinese New Year somewhere between the latter part of January and the first part of February.[16] Rose describes the ancient custom of considering a child 1 year old at birth. Since a child celebrates a birthday every New Year's Day, the child born in November would be considered 2 years old on New Year's Day.[3]

Beliefs about health and illness

The Chinese, like the Spanish-speaking people, believe in harmony and moderation to maintain good health.[3] Diseases are caused by the imbalance between Yin and Yang. Yin and Yang as defined by Wallnofer are "the twin potencies that regulate the universe."[20] They are also responsible for the powers that are given unto all "ten thousand things" within the universe.[7,18,20] Yang, which represents the male, is positive energy responsible for producing light, warmth, and fullness.[7,20] Yin, which represents the female, is negative energy producing the forces of darkness, coldness, and emptiness.[7,20] Health, then, is a state of balance between the Yin and Yang forces within the body, and illness is a result of their imbalance.[7,18,20]

Another belief the Chinese share with Hispanics and Blacks is that blood loss will weaken the body. Thus, a very sensitive problem is posed by surgery. Many Chinese believe that to open the body will release energy and cause weakness. Still others believe that somatic complaints will occur as a result of being exposed to the "wind" *(fang)*. This belief is related to the hot and cold theory. The hot and cold elements dominate social occasions, religious rituals, and childbirth.[7]

Beliefs about childbearing

The Chinese have few taboos during pregnancy. Mutton (lamb), believed to cause the child to have seizures, is forbidden.[7] Foods listed as "cold" foods are also to be eaten in moderation or not at all. A Chinese nurse colleague in the San Francisco area related the following observations about dietary restrictions for pregnant women: many women refused to eat sea foods, especially shell fish, because they believe it causes skin eruptions; turkey, because it releases toxins harmful to the child; and melons (cold), because they cause respiratory syndromes. A pervasive belief seems to be that overindulgence predisposes to disharmony, which eventually leads to illness.[9]

Childbirth is not considered an illness. It is a very happy occasion. Maintaining warmth and decreasing possible exposure to natural forces is stressed. Immediately after delivery, precautions are taken to protect the mother and child from natural forces such as drafts and other cold elements.[7] Dietary restrictions are also enforced. "Hot" foods are encouraged.[9] The same Chinese nurse colleague in the San Francisco area confirmed these beliefs with her observations that new mothers are encouraged to consume ginger, chicken, and whiskey, which are believed to get rid of a wind; pig's feet in ginger and vinegar, which are believed to aid lactating mothers through the effects of the vinegar in abstracting calcium from bones; and salted chicken and rice, a "hot" food that has protein for mending. She further stated that many women will abstain from sex up to 100 days after delivery. Another practice observed in the San Francisco area is abstention from full baths or shampoos for a month or longer. These practices are probably related to a combination of the hot and cold and Yin and Yang theories.

NATIVE AMERICANS
Brief historical perspective

The Native American population represents such a diverse group that it is difficult to define specifically who is considered a Native American and who is not. They are people with a variety of body types. Their complexions range through dark brown, red, yellow, and white hues.[5] According to Highwater, anthropologic data suggest that the Native American population is so racially distinct that some anthropologists believe they represent a unique fourth race. For example, Native Americans have several similar racial traits, such as low occurrence of baldness, grey hair, red-green color blindness, and the presence of hair on the middle segments of fingers.[5]

Legislative definitions have not produced an acceptable definition of a Native American, although Native American communities use family linkages to determine their own classifications of individuals.[5] Highwater, an impressive Native American writer, further reveals that the standard determination is based on whether or not an individual's family is known to other Native Americans and lives among Native Americans on a reservation or in a Native American community. He further states that to be eligible for basic Bureau of Indian Affairs (B.I.A.) services, an individual must live on or near trust or restricted land under the Bureau's jurisdiction and must also be a member of a tribe, band, or group recognized by the federal government.[5]

The original definition of tribe, according to Highwater, meant a group of peoples bound together by ties of blood, speaking a common language, and possessing similar social, religious, and political aspirations in a defined territory. Now, membership is accomplished through birth, adoption, or by meeting membership requirements in other ways. Most Native Americans today speak English. Many Southwestern Native Americans also speak Spanish, and the Northeastern groups also speak French. From approximately 300 distinct Native American languages spoken in 1492, the number has dwindled to between 50 and 100 languages.[5]

Reservation living and the assistance of the B.I.A. have altered traditional meanings. The B.I.A.'s groupings define 263 Native American tribes that are eligible for federal aid. There are also 300 Native Alaskans defined by the B.I.A. who are eligible for services and 160 Native American communities that are not recognized by the B.I.A. but are recognized by city, county, and state agencies.[5]

Reservations provide arbitrary boundaries designated by the federal government.[5] Many Native Americans believe that reservation living is necessary to provide some sense of security. Tribal government controls matters within the reservation boundaries. However, reservation living, contrary to many beliefs, is not tax free, because individual taxes must be paid.[3,10] There is no land tax, however.

It is doubtful that census figures for the Native American population are correct. The B.I.A., however, estimates that there are some 800,000 to 1,000,000 Native Americans in the United States.[5] Most of them reside in Arizona, Oklahoma, New Mexico, and Alaska.[3]

The Native American groups are descendants of a rich culture with well-defined norms and expectations. This makes it more difficult to speak of them in generalities. I will not group them all together, but will attempt to speak to the specific areas where there seem to be similar beliefs and practices, especially those necessary for the preservation of their personal identities.

Traditional patterns of family life

The Native American family has survived years of turmoil, prejudice, and other disruptions. It continues to be one of the most basic units in the Native American society. The father is the head of the household. The mother assumes the responsibility for maintaining the family unit. The extended family is a basic subconcept and family members have rigidly prescribed roles. The Crow, Navajo, Mohawk, Seneca, Creek, and Seminole continue to practice the custom of assigning the children to the mother's clan. Children are treated with respect and admiration. A permissive upbringing in which physical punishment is rare still prevails among many groups.[3] Children are allowed to toilet train themselves. There appears to be more respect for individual differences.

A variety of practices surround marriage. In the Navajo culture, a man who marries must leave his family and move to his wife's residence. If there is a divorce, the wife automatically retains her household goods and the rights to the children. Cherokee girls are believed to be ready for marriage as soon as they reach puberty, which could be as young as 12 or 13 years of age. Boys are encouraged to wait until they are 20 years of age. The residence is established at the girl's home since Cherokees are traditionally matrilineal.[3]

Beliefs about health and illness

Most Native Americans, such as the Navajo, are very concerned about their health.[1] Many believe that health is directly related to a person's relationship with the total environment. The Navajos believe that health is symptomatic of a correct relationship between man, his supernatural environment, the world around him, and his fellow man.[1,19] Health is associated with positive values in life, such as beauty and blessings.[1] Illness means that an individual has fallen out of balance with nature. Illness is also related to witchcraft or a breaking of the taboos.[8,19] Disease–object intrusion (snake, insect, or other animal has entered the body), spirit intrusion (possessed by the devil), soul loss (the soul leaving the body during a dream and traveling about), and taboo violations appear in Southwestern as well as other tribes.[19]

Healing, then, is practiced by a medicine man, or Shaman. Various tribes have different descriptions and expectations of these practitioners. A variety of treatments and practices are observable among the tribes.[8,19]

Beliefs about childbearing

Many tribes consider pregnancy a normal event. Childbearing, on the other hand, is not likely to be considered in the same light. The Laguna tribe, for example, cautions the mother to be careful with her physical activity during pregnancy. She should walk slowly and refrain from sewing with bone or needle while she is pregnant.

During labor the mother is given a belt that has been blessed so that she can hang onto it to help with the labor pains. This is done to discourage the use of painkillers. The number four is sacred with this group because it represents the four seasons, the directions, and the four colors in the rainbow.[3] Four days of confinement are suggested. After 4 days the baby is named.

The Navaho tribe considers pregnancy a normal, blessed event. The expectant mother is protected from excessive mental stimulation and from exposure to illness and death. Expectant mothers and fathers are warned not to participate in braiding or tying a rope, which is believed to cause difficult labor.[3]

The Seneca tribe believe drinking, gossiping, quarreling, and evil activities will have an undue effect on the expectant mother. Religious preferences teach husband, wife, and family to love one another and to be kind to all children.[3]

These examples are representative of the diverse beliefs and practices among some of the Native American groups. There are more than 300 Native American tribes in the United States. Many of the very traditional practices are not easily shared with persons outside the group. Similarities seem to be associated with family structures and roles, customs related to lifestyle and religion, and beliefs about their socialization networks.

IMPLICATIONS OF CROSS-CULTURAL NURSING

The foregoing discussion has sketched some beliefs and practices of traditional Hispanics, Blacks, Asians, and Native Americans. There are many alternatives within the boundaries of any culture. People always have choices. All traditional women of the same status will not manifest all elements of their culture all the time.

Culture is not static: many individuals will alter some of their traditional cultural habits over time. The commitment to traditional practices will be determined by numerous variables. Education, socioeconomic status, and the close linkage to third- and fourth-generation family members often determine the degree of participation in the more traditional cultural practices, especially those that are different from the practices of the common culture in our society.

All women will not adhere totally to all the aforementioned cultural beliefs. Many will not even be aware of some of them. There will be varying degrees of adherence observable at any one time and in specific regional areas. The important challenge for nurses is to identify those beliefs and practices that, at times, are in distinct conflict with well-established scientific, medical, and nursing interventions. Take your cues directly from the individual client.

Nurses must discontinue their tendency to judge the behaviors of others solely by their own standards. Culture is a complex phenomenon. Geographic location, racial and ethnic factors, and socioeconomic conditions will affect an individual's response to a given situation.

Nurses must not overlook the impact of religious practices, since there is a tendency for many to be very dependent on belief in God. Closely connected to this response is the belief in magic, witchcraft, and supernatural beings. Nurses must respect these beliefs and give special consideration to their effect on their clients. The involvement of local lay practitioners whenever possible is strongly recommended. Because these four groups seem to share beliefs in balance and harmony in all aspects of their lifestyles, it is imperative that the nurse become familiar with and supportive of their need to participate in various rituals. Many of the rituals are both preventive and indeed necessary to maintain health.

A variety of areas need special consideration. In childbirth itself, culture and custom tend to dictate where and in what position a mother delivers. She might squat, kneel, or lie down. She might be supported by female relatives rather than by her husband. The important thing to remember is that there might be variations desired that do not coincide with well-established routines. To prevent undue anxiety in such clients, be ready to help make adaptations.

The postnatal phase is also laden with beliefs that often require adaptations in nursing interventions. Client need for rituals, dietary restrictions, and other practices continue to direct a flexible interpretation of traditional hospital routines. Beliefs and practices about sexual intercourse and sexual modesty, an area surrounded by a great deal of emotion, vary widely. Because of this variance, nurses should approach the subject of birth control and client/infant care with special tact. Most importantly, nurses must keep open minds. Be inquisitive, explore some of the areas mentioned, ask questions, and be observant. The more informed a nurse becomes, the easier it will be to make adjustments in prescribed interventions if needed.

If you are unfamiliar with persons from a specific group, get to know your client. Casual interviews about beliefs and practices pertaining to both family and childbearing can provide invaluable data. It will give a better understanding of the client, a basic awareness that will enhance empathy and promote appropriate nursing care for all involved.

REFERENCES

1. Adair, J., et al.: Patterns of health and disease among the Navahos, Ann. Am. Acad. Polit. Sci. Soc. Sci. **311**, 80-94, 1957.
2. Billingsley, A.: Black families in white America,

Englewood Cliffs, N.J., 1978, Prentice-Hall, Inc.
3. Clark, A.: Culture, childbearing, health professionals, Chapters 2, 3, 4, and 6, Philadelphia, 1978, F. A. Davis Co.
4. Clark, M.: Health in the Mexican American culture, Berkeley, 1959, University of California Press.
5. Highwater, J.: Indian America. New York, 1961, David McKay Co., Inc.
6. Ingham, J. M.: On Mexican folk medicine, Am. Anthropol. **72,** (1):76-77, 1970.
7. Kleinman, A., and Kunstàdter, P.: Medicine in Chinese cultures, Chapters 8, 10, 20, and 21, Washington, D. C., 1975, Department of Health, Education and Welfare.
8. Kluckbohn, C.: Navaho witchcraft, Boston, 1944, Beacon Press.
9. Leslie, C.: Asian medical systems: a comparative study, Berkeley, 1976, University of California Press.
10. Levitan, S., and Hetrich, B.: Big brother's Indian programs: with reservations, New York, 1971, McGraw-Hill Book Co.
11. Martinez, R.: Hispanic culture and health care, St. Louis, 1978, The C. V. Mosby Co.
12. Popenol, D.: Sociology, ed. 2, Chapter 4, Englewood Cliffs, N. J., 1974, Prentice-Hall, Inc.
13. Saunders, L.: Cultural difference and medical care, New York, 1954, Sage Publications, Inc.
14. Snow, L.: Folk medical beliefs and their implications for care of patients, Ann. Intern. Med. **81:** 82-96, 1974.
15. Stoddard, E.: Mexican Americans, New York, 1973, Random House, Inc.
16. Sung, B. L.: Chinese Americans, New York, 1977, Franklin Watts, Inc.
17. Tingling, D.: Vodoo, rootwork and medicine, Psychosom. Med. **29:**483-492, 1967.
18. Tseng, W. S.: The development of psychiatric concepts in traditional Chinese medicine, Arch. Gen. Psychiatry **29:**569-575, 1965.
19. Vogel, V.: American Indian medicine, Norman, Ok., 1970, University of Oklahoma Press.
20. Wallnofer, H., et al.: Chinese folk medicine, New York, 1965, Crown Publishers, Inc.
21. Whitten, N.: Comtemporary patterns of malign occultism among Negroes in North Carolina, J. Am. Folklore **75:** 311-325, 1962.

CHAPTER 3

Psychophysical preparations for childbirth

Colleen Conway

INTRODUCTION

Women enter their childbearing years anticipating great change, sometimes frightening change. Their bodies, their relationships, and their responsibilities are dramatically and irreversibly altered. The developmental crisis of childbearing can be either growth producing or growth inhibiting. The result depends on a complex of previous experiences, "old wives tales," the woman's comfort level with her own body and her own sexuality, and the type of formal and/or informal input and teaching she has received in preparation for her labor experience. When we started hospitalizing normal women for normal deliveries, we also became interested in reducing their discomfort. Since the pain phenomena was complex and pharmacologic agents plentiful for analgesia, teaching and conditioning women and their families for the childbearing experience was considered superfluous.[3] However, women became increasingly disenchanted with this type of childbearing environment as well as with the high perinatal morbidity and mortality rates and began to question whether it was desirable, or even safe, to be "knocked out" while having a baby. At the same time, they acknowledged the pain of childbirth and the need to control that pain in some manner—thus the beginnings of the "natural childbirth" movement.

METHODOLOGIES OF PAIN RELIEF

The *natural childbirth* movement is somewhat of a misnomer. Today the term *natural childbirth* is sometimes applied indiscriminately to any kind of activities that purport to prepare women and their families for the childbirth experience. In fact, there are essentially three "schools" of childbirth preparation currently practiced in the United States and most share certain commonalities such as (1) an educational component to teach the physiology of labor, (2) an exercise component to improve muscle tone, and (3) a breathing component to assist in relaxation and control. These major methods are (1) the Read method, (2) the Lamaze method, and (3) hypnosis. Each will be discussed in this chapter, and a detailed guide for implementing each technique is presented at the end of the chapter.

The Read method

This method most appropriately claims the title of "natural childbirth" since the term was coined by Dr. Grantly Dick-Read[9] in the 1930s in England. Proponents of the method in the United States are Buxton,[4] Bradley,[2] and Thoms,[33] who further emphasizes the role of the father during labor and delivery. Natural childbirth is a broad concept that supports the need for educating the pregnant women and her family about the physiologic and psychologic aspects of pregnancy and delivery so that fears and anxieties are reduced.

Another synonym for "natural childbirth" might be "physiologic childbirth."[14] Read saw childbirth as a beautiful, natural, normal, physiologic experience that was not pain related.[23] Read believed that culturally induced anxiety and fear had somehow become part of our expectations for childbirth and that the pain of labor and delivery was psychologic in origin. These fears caused tension that interfered with cervical dilatation and stimulated nerve endings in the uterus and therefore caused pain. He refered to this as the *fear-tension-pain syndrome*. He advocated replacing this syndrome with a calm, welcoming attitude. To decrease fear, he educated women about labor and delivery, corrected false information, insisted that they relax and accept motherhood as a joyous event, and took them on a tour of the hospital before delivery. To decrease tension, he developed a technique of slow abdominal breathing coupled with some chest breathing called *abdominal-costal breathing*. He postulated that abdominal breathing (lifting the abdominal musculature off the contracting uterus) would decrease discomfort created by two opposing forces and promote general relaxation. Costal breathing (high-chest breathing) was to be used in late active labor during transition to prevent pushing.

The Read method eventually incorporated education, psychologic training, and physical conditioning of abdominal and perineal muscles to foster relaxation. Read strongly believed that weak musculature contributed to fear and pain and that learning to relax would contribute to a painless labor. Exercises during pregnancy would improve posture and body balance, increase muscle strength and flexibility used in childbirth and postpartum restoration, increase the elasticity of perineal muscles, and improve circulation in the pelvic area. He believed that analgesia was induced by provision of information that reassures the expectant mother and her family and by relaxation that reduces tension. He could not explain the precise physiology of this mechanism although he related it to the absence of anxiety.[5]

Read attempted to answer the questions "Is labor easy because a woman is calm, or is a woman calm because labor is easy?"; and "Is a woman pained and frightened because her labor is difficult, or is her labor difficult and painful because she is frightened?" He concluded that fear is in some way the chief pain-producing agent in otherwise normal labor and that fear probably has a deleterious effect on the quality of uterine contractions and on cervical dilatation.[14]

Moore[23] identifies the major problem with the Read method as the tendency to deny the possibility of pain completely rather than teaching the woman to increase her ability to cope with pain. In his original works, Read did not rule out the use of analgesics but suggests that if his method is properly used, they will not be needed. This area of vagueness has led some of his followers to expect a painless labor if they have prepared for it, and they are unpleasantly shocked and frightened when painful sensations begin in spite of their best efforts. However, Read was a forerunner in establishing credibility to the fact that psychologic concerns were also part of the childbearing process and that a woman needed some tools besides medication to

Table 3-1. Read method of childbirth preparation

	Stage of labor			
	Early and mid first stage	Late first stage	Late first stage – second stage	Third stage
Quality of contraction	2-5 min apart for 60-90 sec	1½-2 min apart for 60-90 sec	1½-2 min apart for 60-90 sec	1½-2 min apart for 60-90 sec
Extent of dilatation	Up to 7 cm	8-10 cm	8-10 cm	10 cm
Type of breathing	Effacement and dilatation breathing	Transition breathing		Expulsion breathing
Pattern of breathing	Abdominal breathing	Costal breathing (diaphragmatic)	Panting	Bearing down
Description of breathing	Lie on back with knees bent. Place both hands on abdomen under umbilicus so fingertips meet. Breathe in through nose and lift abdomen wall up off the irritated uterus, keeping chest still. Exhale and allow wall to sink back down. Observe rise and fall of hands with each breath.	Lie on back with knees bent. Place hands at sides of ribs. Inspire through nose; feel ribs move sideways against hands. Exhale, feel ribs move away from hands.	Lie on back with knees bent. Let head sink into pillow. place fingers of one hand over sternum. Breathe in and out rapidly using top part of chest. Sternum should rise up and fall down. Similar to dog's panting.	Lie on back with head and shoulders elevated. Draw legs up against abdomen in squatting position. Hold legs with hands. Raise head – take deep breath – hold it and push. (This breath "fixes" diaphragm so abdominal wall exerts more pressure on uterus and baby.) Take short "catch-up" breaths as needed.
Rate	6 breaths per 30 sec (12-18 per contraction)	6 breaths per 30 sec (12-18 per contraction)	Consecutively during urge to push before cervix is completely dilated.	2-3 breaths each 60 sec of breathing

carry her through it. One advantage of the Read technique is that it can be quickly taught to an "unprepared" woman in labor (Table 3-1).

The Lamaze method

The psychoprophylactic method (neo-Pavlovian or Nicolaiev method) was a precursor of the Lamaze psychoprophylaxis practiced in the United States today.[35] The neo-Pavlovian method reflects the Russian interest in nervous reflexes and behavior patterns of the 1920s and 1930s. The original psychoprophylactic breathing techniques grew out of original research in the 1920s on the effects of hypnosis on women in childbirth by their physicians – Drs. Nicolaiev, Velvolski, and Platnov. They were attempting to render childbirth painless. Since hypnosis was time-consuming and usually demanded a one-to-one relationship, they began to look at other methods of pain control based on the ideas of Pavlov.[34] They developed a breathing routine during labor that they believed was psychoprophylactic (psychoprophylaxis literally translates into mind prevention). Its theoretical basis is drawn from Pavlov's theory of conditioned reflexes (the substitution of a favorable conditioned reflex for an unfavorable one). Through stimulus-response conditioning during labor, women could learn specific behaviors that they would automatically use during labor and delivery to eliminate pain associated with childbirth.[6] They also believed that exercises during pregnancy would strengthen abdominal muscles and relax the perineum. By 1949, Nicolaiev was prepared to say that the pain of childbirth depended on the nervous system and relationships between the cortex and subcortex (this has yet to be proved). He called the system "Psychoprophylaxis" and presented it at the 1949 Karkov Conference. By 1951, the Russian government ordered it to be used throughout the country for analgesia during childbirth.

A French physician, Dr. Fernand Lamaze, had attended the Karkov Conference and introduced the method, with some adaptations, into France, where it was well received. He went to Leningrad in 1951 to further observe the method and devised some improvements in the original respiratory technique. His adaptations consisted primarily of rapid, shallow breathing during the latter part of the first stage of labor and forced exhalation during transition. This was designed to raise the threshold of cerebral sensitivity by creating a high level of respiratory activity (rapid, shallow breathing) that could further inhibit the woman's perception of painful stimuli from the uterus.[35] This respiratory activity characterizes the Lamaze method of psychoprophylaxis as contrasted with the Nicolaiev method of psychoprophylaxis.

Interestingly, Lamaze techniques were supported in France by both the leftists and the Catholic church. Chertok[5] discusses the fact that Lamaze techniques were originally practiced by French leftists who had a powerful ideologic motivation regarding the uselessness of suffering, faith in science and its techniques, demystification of sex, and freedom for women. Conversely, Pope Pius XII studied the Pavlovian principles and also supported the use of Lamaze techniques. Therefore, Catholic women who used the Lamaze method did so in the name of personalistic Christian moral values—the humanization of natural functions, the emphasis of the importance of motherhood and female nature, the dignity of effort, and the value of self-mastery.

In the United States, the Lamaze method was championed by Elizabeth Bing,[1] a British-trained physical therapist, and Marjorie Karmel,[17] an American who delivered her baby in France under Dr. Lamaze's care. Her book, *Thank You, Dr. Lamaze*, further publicized the method. Bing and Karmel joined with Dr. Alan Guttmacher to form a Childbirth Education Program at Mt. Sinai Hospital in New York City, from where the Lamaze technique was promulgated. In 1960, the American Society for Prophylaxis in Obstetrics was formed by these people and others.[21]

The Lamaze method consists of techniques in relaxing, exercising, and breathing. The relaxing component has as its goal the achievement of neuromuscular control. "Neuromuscular exercises are intended to develop muscle control, giving the woman the ability to isolate muscle groups"[6] by learning to actively use one set of muscles while relaxing others. This prepares her to control and relax her entire body during contractions. As pregnancy progresses, she can practice this with Braxton-Hicks contractions. "The woman is conditioned to respond with . . . dissociation (or relaxation) of the uninvolved muscles."[25] This allows her to control her perception of stimuli associated with labor. The first technique of pain management represented here is focal-point visualization. Stone[32] defines this as a relaxation procedure in which the laboring woman concentrates her attention on a particular object to the exclusion of all else in the visual field while consciously relaxing all voluntary muscles and using various breathing patterns.

The exercising (body building) component has as its goal helping the body to achieve its optimal level of functioning to reduce muscle strain during pregnancy and prepare for the stresses and movements of labor.

The breathing component, as Lamaze developed it, consisted of specific breathing patterns that changed as labor progressed. They represent the second technique of pain management during labor and consist of three different breathing cycles applied sequentially to corresponding increases in distress associated with labor contractions.[32] These cycles include (1) effacement breathing (slow and deep), (2) dilatation breathing (shallow, accelerated, decelerated), (3) transition breathing (shallow and forced blowing out), and (4) expulsion breathing. The specific Lamaze breathing regimen is outlined on pages 46 and 47. All breathing episodes involve (1) focusing on a significant object with intense concentration and (2) taking a deep cleansing breath before and after each breathing episode. (This cleansing breath also signals to the labor support person that a contraction is about to begin). In addition to focusing, the woman may also use effleurage in an effort to provide another "focus for concentration and help relieve abdominal tension during contractions."[6] Effleurage is gentle massage of the abdomen, a light stroking action that is not irritating to the uterus. The mother's hands move in contrasting circular motions up from the pubis on the midline, outward toward the pelvis, and down to the pubis. About 15 effleurage movements occur during a contraction. It is performed in conjunction with breathing— as respiration exercises increase, effleurage movements increase.

Critics of educated childbirth techniques express concern about hyperventilation, excessive fatigue, and corpopedal spasm, along with maternal respiratory alkalosis and fetal acidosis. These problems are not restricted to women using special breathing techniques, however; hyperventilation can occur just as easily when an unprepared woman undergoes labor. It is essential to continuously assist the woman in evaluating the possibility of hyperventilation; if first symptoms appear (numbness of lips, tingling of fingers), rebreathing in a paper bag is an effective antidote along with extra vigilance.[25]

The Lamaze breathing techniques have undergone periodic review and clarification. New adaptations in breathing, with greater emphasis on slow chest breathing throughout the first stage and accelerated-decelerated shallow breathing as necessary, extend the time the more efficient respiratory pattern of slow chest breathing is used. This reduces the possibility of hyperventilation and eliminates the "panting" image.[26] A current, detailed description of Lamaze relaxing, exercising, and breathing techniques is presented in Table 3-2.

Today's Lamaze couple has much more freedom to personalize their labor and delivery experience than did couples a generation ago when techniques were rigorously followed as originally developed. The couple, not the teacher, nurse, or physician, is encouraged to set their own realistic, flexible goals, and not to predetermine criteria that must be met if "success" is to be achieved. Today there is more emphasis on the childbearing team—the couple, the physician, the nurse, and the teacher—and couples generally meet a receptive environment in the labor and delivery area as they go in to have their "Lamaze" baby.

Table 3-2. Lamaze psychoprophylaxis method for childbirth

	Stage of labor				
	Early part of first stage (preliminary phase)	Middle of first stage (accelerated phase)	End of first stage	Second stage	Third stage
Quality of contraction	30-60 sec contractions with 5-20 min interval	2-4 min apart for 45-60 sec	1-1½ min contraction with 30-60 sec interval	1-1½ min apart for 30-60 sec	1-1½ min apart for 30-60 sec
Extent of dilatation	Up to 5 cm	5-8 cm	8-10 cm	10 cm	10 cm
Type of breathing*	Effacement breathing	Dilatation breathing	Transition breathing	Expulsion breathing	Expulsion breathing
Pattern of breathing	Slow chest breathing	Shallow, light chest breathing	Combination of light, shallow chest breathing with puffs at height of contraction	Breath holding and pushing	Continuation of second stage breathing, may occasionally pant at physician's request to slow down the speed of delivery of the head
Description of breathing	Place fingers on ribs, feel them spread during slow, deep inspiration	Quiet and low	Quiet and low with 4:1 to 8:1 breath: puff ratio; at height of contraction, 6-8 puffs may occur as urge to bear down increases	Take breath—hold—tighten abdominal muscles—relax vagina—push—take another breath—push again	
Rate	10 breaths per min increasing to 12-18 breaths per min as labor intensifies	1 breath per sec—may have a "hee-hee" sound	1 breath per sec	2-3 breaths per contraction	

*All breathing episodes are started and ended by a "cleansing breath"—a deep breath that is blown out—that is also a signal to the support person that a contraction is about to begin or end.

Similarities and differences between the Lamaze method and the Read method

The Lamaze method and the Read method are similar in that they both emphasize education and exercise. In fact, they both recognize the value of "deconditioning" the woman and use similar body-building exercises. However, the Lamaze method is referred to as "prepared childbirth," while the Read method is referred to as "natural childbirth." While Read emphasizes the naturalness and painlessness of the experience and the need to approach it in a calm, relaxed manner, Lamaze emphasizes the "unnaturalness" in that it requires a high degree of involvement, commitment, preparation, time, and energy. He views pregnancy as a time of vigorous mental and physical conditioning and training to avoid the perceptions of pain in labor where the woman will respond to uterine contractions with actively controlled relaxation and respiratory activity capable of inhibiting painful stimuli.[35] Lamaze goes beyond Read in that he believed that with an active approach, women could be positively conditioned to avoid the perception of pain. "A uterine contraction was made the signal for the initiation of a new, precise, repetitive, acquired reflex."[35] This new reflex required intense mental and physical concentration and thus somehow

---

LAMAZE PSYCHOPROPHYLAXIS PREPARATORY EXERCISES

practice every day with support person beginning at 7 month's gestation

Neuromuscular control exercises
to teach concentration, relaxation, and voluntary control of muscle groups

Lie on your back with one pillow under your head. If desired, place one pillow under knees. Rest arms on floor a little distance from your body. Take a deep, cleansing breath.

1. Contract right arm. Release.
   Contract left arm. Release.
2. Contract right leg. Release.
   Contract left leg. Release.
3. Contract right arm and right leg. Release.
   Contract left arm and left leg. Release.
4. Contract right arm and left leg. Release.
   Contract left arm and right leg. Release.

Pay particular attention to contracting strongly when indicated while absolutely relaxing the rest of the body. Practice daily, with coach giving commands and checking relaxation.

Body-building exercises

All exercises must be practiced evey day on a hard surface (not in bed) without pillows. Repeat Exercises 1 through 5 three to five times.

1. Sit cross-legged for pelvic stretch, stretching of thigh muscles and strengthening of pelvic floor muscles.
2. Sit on floor. Pull feet as near body as comfortable. Put hands under knees, knees gently toward floor.
3. Lie down, arms at side, inhale through nose, raise right leg slowly, point toes. Exhale through lips, flex foot, lower right leg slowly. (Repeat with left leg.)
4. Lie down, spread out arms, inhale through nose, raise right leg, point toes. Exhale through lips while lowering leg to right as far as comfortable. Inhale through nose, raise leg sideways, up, flex foot, and lower leg while exhaling. (Repeat with left leg.)
5. Pelvic rocking: Lie on back with legs bent, feet firmly on ground. Press back and shoulders firmly against floor, while contracting abdominal muscles, Release. With breathing, flatten back while *exhaling,* release back while *inhaling.* (Repeat 10 times.)
6. To rise from lying position: bend knees, turn from back to side, push up with help of both arms.

First stage of labor: breathing exercises (focus on an object)

1. Early labor: Slow, rhythmic chest breathing, inhalation through nose, exhalation through lips. Preceded and followed by deep, cleansing breath. To be practiced with massage (effleurage). Practice for 1 minute three times daily. Use 6-9 breaths per minute.
Early labor

20-45 seconds
5-20 minutes

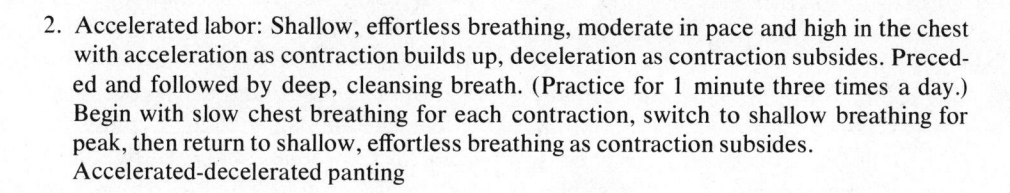

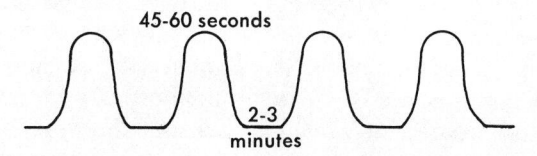

2. Accelerated labor: Shallow, effortless breathing, moderate in pace and high in the chest with acceleration as contraction builds up, deceleration as contraction subsides. Preceded and followed by deep, cleansing breath. (Practice for 1 minute three times a day.) Begin with slow chest breathing for each contraction, switch to shallow breathing for peak, then return to shallow, effortless breathing as contraction subsides.
Accelerated-decelerated panting

45-60 seconds
2-3 minutes

3. Transition: Support abdomen with both hands from below. Take 4-6-8 fast shallow breaths, followed by 1 short blow. Repeat. Preceded and followed by deep inhalation-exhalation. (Practice for 60-90 seconds, three times daily.)
Practice blowing only to avoid pushing when permission to push has not yet been given.

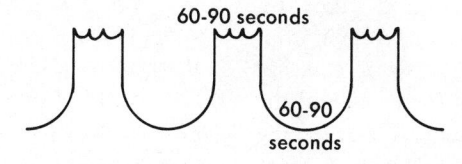

60-90 seconds
60-90 seconds

Second stage of labor: expulsion exercises

1. Pelvic floor contractions and relaxation: contract sphincter, vagina, and urethra, hold to a count of six, then release. (Practice as often as possible, at least 20-30 times daily.)
2. Pushing for delivery: Assume 75-degree angle position with feet flat and knees bent, elbows out, hands under knees: inhale-exhale, inhale-exhale, inhale, exhale a little, hold breath, bend head forward, lean on diaphragm, push to count of 10. Exhale. Inhale quickly, exhale a little — hold and push, exhale. Repeat. Release breath when contraction is over and take deep, cleansing breath. (Practice one a day without pushing.) When asked in delivery room not to push, use transition breathing or blow if urge to push is very strong.

modified or eliminated the awareness of the undesirable stimulus of labor pains. The Lamaze method emphasized (even more than the original Read method) the crucial need for a labor-support person, who hopefully is the baby's father.

The hypnosuggestive method

Hypnosuggestive is derived from the Greek "hypnos" meaning sleep. But the hypnotic state is not a sleep state. It has been described as a state of altered awareness or altered consciousness during which the subject is especially suggestible to whatever the hynotist says with a corresponding reduction in the awareness of surroundings. There is no special breathing program or exercise program attached to hypnosis. Women are instructed in either a one-to-one setting or small group classes by the hypnotist at the end of the second trimester. Instruction in self-hypnosis is also given so women can practice between lessons. The goal is to have each woman to be able to enter a trance-like state easily and quickly at a level where she is virtually free from painful stimuli and yet can readily respond to directions and questions.[13]

Hypnosis during childbirth was originally investigated by Nicolaiev and other researchers and influenced by Pavlov's principles of conditioned response. It was not attractive as a labor support because of the one-to-one relationship needed between the hypnotist and the patient, whereas these men were searching for a method that could be easily taught to large groups of people. United States advocates of hypnosis during childbearing include Kroger,[18] DeLee and Greenhill,[8] and Gross and Posner.[12] Posner studied 73 hypnotized and 73 unhypnotized primigravidas, with the hypnotized primigravidas having 50% shorter first stage of labor, and 126 hypnotized and 127 unhypnotized multigravidas, with the hypnotized multigravidas having a 33% shorter first stage.

Perchard[24] has written extensively on hypnosis during the childbearing cycle. He believes that three factors must be present to have a successful hypnotic experience: (1) the woman must be anxious to cooperate, (2) the hypnotist must exude poise and confidence, and (3) the woman must be essentially normal psychologically and physically with a relatively high degree of intelligence. Hypnosis is contraindicated for women who have a history of psychiatric illness or bizarre behavior or who seek hypnosis for the wrong reasons, such as fear of the entire childbearing process.

The mechanism behind hypnosis is still unclear, but the technique of hypnosis uses two behavior states: the attention state and the habituation state.[24] Parts of the nervous system, whose functions were previously unknown, are now thought to provide a monitoring system that regulates all the sensory impressions streaming into the body, allowing some to reach consciousness and suppressing others at a lower level. This mechanism is believed to be responsible for the attention state and the habituation state in animals. In the attention state, the attention of the animal becomes fixed on one important object, so that it remains for the time being totally unaware of anything else (as in a cat watching a bird). The habituation state presents the opposite picture. If a stimulus is applied to an animal, it will, at first, be aware of it, but if it is repeated monotonously, it becomes blocked from the animal's conscious mind. Further continuation of the stimulus appears to lead to a spread of the blocking effect so that the animal notices less and less of its surroundings and eventually goes to sleep. "The theoretical framework underlying hypnosis suggests that when all voluntary musculature is relaxed, the uterus works at peak efficiency since there are no opposing forces,"[25] and the fear-tension-pain syndrome has been virtually eliminated.

Perchard[24] documented the effects produced by hypnosis. He believed that suggestibility (an idea planted in the mind with supporting evidence to substantiate it) is greatly increased as the patient's attention becomes fixed on the words of the hypnotist. Explaining to the patient how the suggestions will help her will increase their effectiveness. Posthypnotic suggestions (an extension of the phenomenon) can also produce a response. It is therefore likely that suggestions given during pregnancy can have an effect on labor.

Perchard also observed the effects of hypnosis in relation to anesthesia. He found that a decreased sensitivity to touch and pain may occur to some degree in 50% of all hypnotized women. In 10% to 15% of these women, a marked degree of anesthesia may occur. It seems likely that for these women, hypnosis might augment or replace pain medication during labor.

He believed that amnesia, even after deep hypnosis (somnambulism), was a rare, transient occurrence and events that occurred under hypnosis are usually recalled later without prompting. Amnesia does occur in light hypnosis, which is usually the level used in obstetrics. Somnambulism (the ability to open one's eyes, walk about, and converse while in a trance) occurs in about 10% of hypnotized women who are highly suggestible and is a deeper level than necessary for labor and delivery. There is no danger, however, of a woman being made to do something contrary to usual norms of behavior—she would either ignore the command or come out of hypnosis.

Altered muscular behavior can occur during hypnosis as relaxed or cataleptic behavior (the second level of hypnosis). To produce relaxation, suggestions are given to the woman to remain relaxed and sleepy throughout labor, allowing her to conserve energy, relax her abdominal wall and pelvic muscles, and decrease nervous inhibition of uterine contractions. It seems likely, therefore, that altering muscular behavior to a relaxed state might increase resistance to fatigue by suggestion. Furthermore, time perception may be accelerated or retarded by means of suggestion and is often used during the first stage of labor.

Hypnosis can be used during pregnancy to control nausea and vomiting, food binges, and sleep disturbances. It can be used during labor and delivery to alter pain and time perception and facilitate expulsion and relaxation of the perineum during expulsion. The woman's increased suggestibility can also be used to give general reassurance and allay fears. It can be used during the postpartum period as analgesia for engorgement, to assist the woman in early voiding, to render the perineum numb for several days, and to assist the woman in having a bowel movement on the third day postpartum.

When a woman uses hypnosis as a labor analgesic, she is even more vulnerable, since hypnosis drastically alters pain perception, a major body defense mechanism. Severe, startling, or untoward pain is often a danger symptom, heralding an emergency. Women who are hypnotized during labor still need support people with them; quiet, warm, continuous reassurance; and the usual comfort measures (backrubs, mouthwash, and the like). A hypnotized woman in labor does not need absolute silence, but does need a quiet environment with low-pitched, nonstartling commands and reassurance.

THEORETICAL FRAMEWORK OF PAIN RELIEF IN LABOR

While the various methods of psychophysical pain relief do vary, they all share some degree of three elements: (1) a *didac-*

tic element, in which instruction is given about the anatomy, physiology, and psychology of the childbearing process in an effort to control and reduce the fear-tension-pain syndrome; (2) a *physiotherapeutic* element, in which the woman is taught various types of body-building exercises, breathing exercises, and relaxation exercises; and (3) a *psychotherapeutic* element, which is the quality of the relationship between/among the woman and those who have been involved in her preparation for labor as support persons.[5] The body-building exercises are equally important and similar in the two major methods used in the United States today—the Lamaze method of psychoprophylaxis and the Read method of natural childbirth. The breathing exercises are quite different. The relaxation exercises are also quite specific to each method. Read sees them as promoting both a passive kind of relaxation called "mental relaxation" and an active kind called "conscious" or "voluntary" relaxation. Lamaze sees them as more of a training program whereby conscious relaxation of specific muscle groups is under voluntary control; overall passive relaxation is not part of his technique since he believes that this kind of relaxation may result in a harmful lowering of attention focusing and deter a woman from her specific, learned tasks. A detailed outline of these elements in each of the major methodologies of pain relief is presented in Table 3-3.

There are two possible theories as to how pain relief during labor is achieved. Analgesia under hypnosuggestion probably results from cortical inhibition and is of a passive nature, while analgesia under the Lamaze method (and partly the Read method) results from cortical excitation and thus is facilitated by various forms of activity—acquisition of knowledge, breathing exercises, relaxation exercises, and so forth.[5]

Much controversy exists as to the physiologic mechanism by which the Lamaze method reduces the perception of pain. Clausen et al.[6] believes that distraction plays an important role in reducing the perception of pain. People intensely absorbed in a task are less aware of painful stimuli. It is possible that the cortex will only respond to the strongest stimuli sent to it. If a woman carries out a series of tasks during a contraction, the cortex may concentrate on completing the tasks and the perception of "pain" with a contraction may be diminished.

A woman's concern about pain in labor is very realistic. Childbirth does cause tissue damage, which is sensed and transmitted by pain receptors. However, how this transmission is received and perceived is greatly influenced by the woman's mental state. Her mental state, in turn, depends on higher brain centers that are influenced by the woman's history, culture, present state of attention focusing and anxiety, and type and intensity of pain stimulus.

Steven's research[29-31] has contributed a great deal to our knowledge about the interrelationships between labor pain and various modalities of control and intervention. He acknowledges that while breathing and relaxing exercises do not relieve pain, the five psychologic strategies that reduce pain perception are present in various techniques.

1. *Systematic relaxation* is a phenomenon that reduces anxiety and increases pain tolerance by tightening and relaxing selected muscle groups while the woman concentrates on the feeling of relaxation. The goal is to be able to voluntarily relax specific muscle groups to produce a relaxed mental state of minimal anxiety. Lamaze added a feedback technique to this strategy by having a support person actually move the woman's arms, legs, and neck during train-

Table 3-3. Body-building exercises used in all childbirth preparation methodologies

Specific exercise	Purpose	Frequency	Description
Good posture	The center of gravity shifts as pregnancy progresses and an increased level of hormones causes a softening of the ligaments and pelvic joints, which causes low back pain.	At all times	
Kegel	Improves muscle tone of the pubococcygeal muscle (vaginal sphincter) surrounding the vagina. Good tone allows this muscle to stretch during delivery and also to alternately contract and relax around the penis during intercourse. This exercise is also recommended for women with orgasmic difficulties since they become sensitive to different "feelings" of stimulation in the vaginal area and begin to take responsibility for initiating, controlling, and then enjoying those feelings.	50 times twice a day	Start and stop urine flow when voiding to first learn which muscles to contract, then relax the flow, hold for a moment, then repeat. (Do not contract inner thigh muscles while doing this.)
Pelvic rock	Relieves low back pain.	10 times twice a day	The pelvic rock is done either lying on the floor or standing. It should not be done while kneeling since this can stretch the sacrolumbar ligaments already stretched in pregnancy. Lying: Lie on back, knees bent, feet flat on floor, small pillow under head. A. Tighten lower abdomen and buttocks. This will elevate coccyx and press small of back into floor. Do not lift buttocks off floor. Your back should become a straight line. B. Relax, arch back as high as possible. C. Do 5-6 times daily. Standing: Standing two feet from chair that is level with hips: A. Bend slightly forward from hips, placing hands on chair back, elbows straight. B. Rotate hips backward and sag with your abdominal muscles creating a real swayback. C. Unlock knees, flexing them slightly. D. Slowly rotate hips forward, tucking buttocks under as if someone were pushing your buttocks from behind. E. Do 3-4 times daily.
Tailor sit	Firms muscles of pelvic floor, relieves pain, stretches thigh muscles.	As often as possible	Sit on floor with soles of feet together. Place hands under knees and exert downward pressure on hands by thigh muscles. Do not push knees to floor with hands; this simply jerks muscles and does not allow them to strengthen.

ing to determine completeness of relaxation and communicate such to the woman. This relaxed, physical state promotes a mental state of decreased anxiety and makes the woman less fearful of painful stimulus. Therefore, the mind has less awareness of painful sensations, and tolerance and endurance are enhanced.

2. With *cognitive control*, the mind is involved in mental activities other than awareness of incoming pain sensations (for example, staring at a fixed object). Two major forms of cognitive control used in methodologies of labor pain relief are dissociation and interference. In *dissociation*, the mind focuses on a nonpainful characteristic of the painful stimulus. It then dissociates one of the other characteristics of the stimulus from the painful stimulus (for example, ice cold water is not felt as icy and painful, but rather as cool and refreshing). This strategy can increase the pain threshold and increase the endurance time. A woman in labor can view the uterus as having muscular contractions rather than labor pains. *Interference* uses two additional forms of cognitive control: distraction and attention focusing. *Distraction* (a passive process of competition between two sensory stimuli—one painful and the other distracting—for the attention of the woman) involves passive, perceptual interference by using such distractors as noise, music, pictures, and the like. It is most effective in increasing endurance to pain when the onset is slow with a steady, maximum, predictable peak intensity.[22] Thus, it may provide effective pain relief during early labor, but will lose its effectiveness when contractions become stronger, more frequent, and peak rapidly. *Attention focusing* (a more effective form of interference than distraction) is an active, intentional, purposeful mental activity that involves focusing on another phenomenon within the room. The combination of attention focusing and feedback relaxation (the support person tests the woman for muscle relaxation by moving her arms and legs when relaxed and giving verbal encouragements) is the most successful of the psychologic strategies.[30] It is exemplified in psychophysical childbirth techniques by the use of breathing exercises, relaxation exercises, and effleurage. It increases the woman's pain endurance by decreasing its intensity. Repeated use of these strategies also increases their effectiveness,[30] thus the repeated practice sessions used in childbirth preparation techniques.

3. *Cognitive rehearsal* is defined by Stevens[30] as providing the woman with a clear, sequential explanation of the upcoming event and allows the woman to rehearse specific fear images and diffuse them to reduce anxiety and therefore increase pain tolerance. The woman must be provided with enough information to allow her to go through some mental practice exercises of the upcoming events. Both subjective information (what she can expect to feel) and objective information (what will be going on around her, where she will be, tour of the labor and delivery area) are needed for effective cognitive rehearsal as well as verification of the accuracy of the subjective information by the woman's ongoing experiences during labor.[28] Here the need for collaboration between the physician, who is the usual provider of objective information, and the nurse, who is the usual provider of subjective information, is obvious. Childbirth preparation classes contribute much more additional objective information than that provided by the physician since women need additional objective and subjective information about a wide range of possible, although unanticipated, experiences. (For example, the possibility of cesarean section). If a woman's subjective information

does not approximate the reality of her experience, she will lose confidence and her anxiety will rise.[28]

4. The *Hawthorne effect* is familiar to most researchers. The more time and attention that is devoted to a person, the better that person will perform. The obvious implication for the childbearing family is that the woman needs special attention from everyone since this can contribute to the success of the experience. Conversely, the omission of attention during pregnancy, and particularly during labor, may cause unnecessary requests for medication as a subconscious bid for attention and reassurance.

5. *Systematic desensitization* is a psychologic procedure that combines systematic relaxation, cognitive rehearsal, cognitive dissociation, and the Hawthorne effect to decrease certain patient anxieties that may be incapacitating. Stevens[29] describes the technique as involving a complete state of mental and physical relaxation (systematic relaxation), confidence in the therapist (Hawthorne effect), weekly discussions of selected aspects of the fear (cognitive dissociation), and alleviation of anxiety about selected aspects of the feared stimulus (cognitive rehearsal). The relationship between this type of approach and childbirth education classes is clear, as they both provide an informal type of systematic desensitization of labor pain. Any successful childbirth education course must include these multiple approaches. Stevens[29] believes that the success of attention focusing and feedback relaxation alone provides a rationale for breathing strategies increasing the level of psychoanalgesia.

Helping the mother to consciously and effectively prepare herself and her family for a major life cycle event, such as a birth, emphasizes the normalcy and growth potential of the childbearing year's. A woman's attitude toward her delivery is a major influence on the ease, and perhaps the length and outcome, of that labor. While an unprepared woman's natural reaction to pain is an uncontrolled flight response that manifests itself in extreme restlessness, crying out, or panic, the prepared mother has an increased level of awareness and ability to cope with the physical and emotional demands of cnildbirth.[10]

LEBOYER'S INFLUENCE

While Charles Leboyer,[20] a French obstetrician, focused more on providing the newborn with a gentle, pleasant introduction into the world outside the womb, his emphasis on abstinence from unnecessary intervention encompasses a philosophy of having a prepared, controlled mother participating in the process. His interest in a gentle delivery came from his recall, through psychoanalysis, of the emotional trauma of his own birth.[11]

There are four aspects of Leboyer's approach to delivery: (1) gentle, controlled delivery, (2) not stressing the craniosacral axis, (3) not overstimulating the infant's sensorium or breathing, and (4) importance of maternal-infant bond. His theoretical framework grows from Janov's psychoanalytic theory of primal pain, which states that human neuroses begin when human needs go unfulfilled for any length of time.[16] Leboyer seeks to minimize the trauma of unmet needs surrounding the shock of birth.

During a Leboyer delivery, great caution is taken not to stress the craniosacral axis. The infant is eased, not tugged, out into a quiet, dimly lit room; he is placed belly down on the mother's abdomen and given a back massage as the cord stops pulsating; he remains thus for an extended period while delivery technologies (for example, footprinting) are delayed and is then placed in a large warm tub of water (usually held by the father) to reassure him that his extrauterine environment is not so strange. He then is wrapped and returned to his mother for cuddling, stroking, and nursing.

THE NURSE-PRACTITIONER'S ROLE

The nurse-practitioner working with pregnant women needs to plan intervention with two goals in mind: (1) to maintain the safety of mother and infant and (2) to meet the woman's emotional need to make the most of the childbearing experience. The nurse-practitioner has the unique opportunity to clarify the objective information supplied by the physician (or to supply it personally) as well as to expand and interpret the subjective experience of pregnancy, labor, and delivery with the woman.

The nurse-practitioner and the woman (and family) should set clear objectives of care at the first visit so that all involved can cooperate in meeting those objectives. The woman should be seen as a member of the birth team and needs to be appraised of her progress in meeting those objectives. The nurse-practitioner should also interpret variations of response to pregnancy that are still within normal range.

CONCLUSION

Clinical studies[7,15,27,35] have shown that prepared childbirth techniques are effective in decreasing subjective pain perception and increasing pain endurance. Prepared mothers successfully handle childbirth pain, cooperate with the physician, use fewer analgesics and anesthetics, express great satisfaction with the childbirth experience, and experience less postpartum depression. But the question of whether these techniques, particularly attention focusing and feedback relaxation, actually alter or decrease the subjective pain experience remains unanswered and debated.[31]

RESOURCES FOR CHILDBIRTH PREPARATION MATERIALS

American Academy of Husband-Coached Childbirth, Box 5224, Sherman Oaks, California, 91413.
American Society for Psychoprophylaxis in Labor (ASPO), 1523 L St. N.W., Washington, D.C., 20005.
Birth and Family Journal (ICEA & ASPO), 110 El Camino Real, Berkeley, California, 94705.
International Childbirth Education Association (ICEA), Box 5852, Milwaukee, Wisconsin, 53220.
Maternal Child Nursing, The American Journal of Maternal Child Nursing, 10 College Circle, New York, New York, 10019.
Maternity Center Association (MCA), 48 E. 92nd St., New York, New York, 10028.

REFERENCES

1. Bing, E.: Six practical lessons for an easier childbirth, New York, 1969. Bantam Books, Inc.
2. Bradley, R.: Husband-coached childbirth, New York, 1965, Harper & Row, Publishers.
3. Broadribb, V., and Corliss, C.: Maternal-child nursing, Philadelphia, 1973, J. B. Lippincott Co.
4. Buxton, C.: Study of psychophysical methods for relief of childbirth pain, Philadelphia, 1962, W. B. Saunders Co.
5. Chertok, L.: Psychosomatic methods of preparation for childbirth, Am. J. Obstet. Gynecol. **98:** 698-707, 1967.
6. Clausen, J., Flook, M., and Ford, B.: Maternity nursing today, New York, 1979, McGraw-Hill Book Co.
7. Davis, C., and Curi, J.: A comparative clinical study of a prepared childbirth program, Conn. Med. **32:**113-121, 1968.
8. DeLee, J., and Greenhill, J., editors: Year book of obstetrics and gynecology, Chicago, 1939, New York, 1959, Harper & Row, Publishers.
9. Dick-Read, G.: Childbirth without fear, ed. 2, New York, 1959, Harper & Row, Publishers.
10. Doening, S., and Entwisle, D.: Preparation during pregnancy and ability to cope with labor and delivery, Am. J. Orthopsychiatry **45:**825-837, 1975.
11. Gimbel, J.: and Nocon, G.: The physiological basis for the Leboyer approach to childbirth, J. Obstet. Gynecol. Nurs. **6:**11-15, 1977.
12. Gross, H., and Posner, N.: An evaluation of hypnosis for obstetric delivery, Am. J. Obstet. Gynecol. **87:**912, 1963.
13. Hamilton, P.: Basic maternity nursing, ed. 3, St. Louis, 1975, The C. V. Mosby Co.
14. Hellman, L., and Pritchard, J.: Williams' Obstet-

rics, ed. 14, New York, 1971, Appleton-Century-Crofts.
15. Huttel, F., Mitchell L., Fischer, W., et al.: A quantitative evaluation of psychoprophylaxis in childbirth, J. Psychosom. Res. **16**:81-91, 1972.
16. Janov. A.: The primal scream, New York, 1971, Dell Publishing Co., Inc.
17. Karmel, M.: Thank you, Dr. Lamaze, Philadelphia, 1959, J. B. Lippincott Co.
18. Kroger, W.: Childbirth with hypnosis, New York, 1961, Doubleday & Co., Inc.
19. Lamaze, F.: Painless childbirth: the Lamaze method, New York, 1972, Pocket Books.
20. Leboyer, F.: Birth without violence, New York, 1975, Alfred A. Knopf, Inc.
21. Maternity Center Association: Preparation for childbearing, ed. 4, New York, 1972, The Association.
22. Melzack, R., Weisz, A., and Sprague, L.: Strategems for controlling pain, contributions of auditory stimulation and suggestion, Exp. Neurol. **8**:239-247, 1963.
23. Moore, M. L.: Realities in childbearing, Philadelphia, 1978, W. B. Saunders Co.
24. Perchard, S.: Hypnosis and the pregnant woman, Nurs. Mirror **124**:1-5, 1967.
25. Reeder, S., Mastrianni, L., Martin, L., et al.: Maternity nursing, ed. 13, Philadelphia, 1976, J. B. Lippincott Co.
26. Sasmore, J., Castor, C., and Hassid, P.: The childbirth team during labor, Am. J. Nurs. **73**:444-447, 1973.
27. Scott, J., and Rose, N.: Effects of psychoprophylaxis (Lamaze preparation) on labor and delivery in primiparas, New Engl. J. Med. **294**:1205-1207, 1976.
28. Staub, E., and Kellet, D.: Increasing pain tolerance by information about adverse stimuli, J. Pers. Soc. Psychol. **21**(2):198-203, 1972.
29. Stevens, R.: Psychological strategies for management of pain in prepared childbirth, Birth Fam. J. **3**:157-164, 1976.
30. Stevens, R.: Psychological strategies for management of pain in prepared childbirth, Birth Fam. J. **4**:4-9, 1977.
31. Stevens, R., and Heide, F.: Analgesic characteristics of prepared childbirth techniques; attention focusing and systematic relaxation, J. Psychosom. Res. **21**(6):429-438, 1977.
32. Stone, C., Demchik-Stone, D., and Horan, J.: Coping with pain; a component analysis of Lamaze and cognitive-behavioral procedures, J. Psychosom. Res. **21**(6):451-456, 1977.
33. Thoms, H.: Childbirth with understanding, Springfield, Ill., 1962, Charles C Thomas, Publishers.
34. Vellay, P.: Childbirth with confidence, New York, 1969, The Macmillan Co.
35. Yahia, C., and Ulin, P.: Preliminary experience with a psychophysical program of preparation for childbirth, Am. J. Obstet. Gynecol. **93**:942-949, 1965.

BIBLIOGRAPHY

Anderson, J.: A clarification of the Lamaze method, J. Obstet. Gynecol. Nurs. **6**:53-54, 1977.
Bonstein, I.: Psychoprophylactic preparation for painless childbirth: its theory and practical approach, London, 1958, Heinemann.
Bowers, P.: Natural childbirth, Med. Clin. North Am. **39**:1789-1799, 1955.
Brenner, S.: Childbirth education research, Prof. Med. Assist. **10**:12-13, 1977.
Chabon, I.: Awake and aware, New York, 1966, Dell Publishing Co., Inc.
Davis, C., and Morsone, F.: An objective evaluation of a prepared childbirth program. Am. J. Obstet. Gynecol. **84**:1196, 1962.
Ewy, D., and Ewy, R.: Preparation for childbirth, New York, 1972, The New American Library Inc.
Fielding, W., and Benjamin, L.: The childbirth challenge: common sense versus natural methods, New York, 1962, The Viking Press, Inc.
Flapan, M., and Schoenfeld, H.: Procedures for exploring women's childbearing motivations, alleviating childbearing conflicts and enhancing maternal role development, Am. J. Orthopsychiatry **42**:38-39, 1972.
Fyalkowski, W.: New ways of psychophysical preparation for childbirth, Am. J. Obstet. Gynecol. **92**:1018-1022, 1978.
Goodrich, F.: Preparing for childbirth, Englewood Cliffs, N. J., 1966, Prentice-Hall, Inc.
Harlow, H.: Fundamental principles, J. Psychol. **55**(2):893-896, 1962.
Ingalls, A., and Salerno, M.: Maternal and child nursing, St. Louis, 1975, The C. V. Mosby Co.
Iorio, J.: Principles of obstetrics and gynecology for nurses, ed. 2, St. Louis, 1971, The C. V. Mosby Co.
Jensen, M., Benson, R., and Bobak, I.: Maternity care, St. Louis, 1977, The C. V. Mosby Co.
Kitzinger, S., and Litt, B.: A fresh look at antenatal exercises, Nurs. Mirror **129**:14, 1969.
Kopp, L.: Ordeal or ideal—the second stage of labor, Am. J. Nurs. **71**:1140-1143, 1971.
Kroger, W., and DeLee, S.: The use of the hypnoidal state as an amnesic analgesic, and anesthetic agent in obstetrics, Am. J. Obstet. Gynecol. **46**:655, 1943.
Kroger, W., and Freed, C.: Psychosomatic gynecology, Los Angeles, 1962, Wilshire Book Co.

Laird, M., and Hogan, M.: An elective program on preparation for childbirth at the Sloane Hospital for Women, Am. J. Obstet. Gynecol. **72:**641, 1956.

Leonard, R.: Evaluation of selection tendencies of patients preferring prepared childbirth, Obstet. Gynecol. **42**(3):371-377, 1973.

Lipkin, G.: Psycho-social aspects of maternal child nursing, St. Louis, 1974, The C. V. Mosby Co.

McDonald, R.: Current programs for childbirth, Child Fam. **2:**4-6, 1963.

Moore, P.: Prepared childbirth: the pregnant couple and their marriage, J. Nurs. Midwif. **22:**18-26, 1977.

Mulcahy, R., and Jonz, N.: Effectiveness of raising pain perception threshold in males and females using a psychoprophylactic childbirth technique during indured pain, Nurs. Res. **22:**423, 1973.

Newton, N.: New methods for easing childbirth, Child Fam. **5:**17, 1966.

Rothenstein, L.: Prepared childbirth, J. Pract. Nurs. **27:**20-25, 1977.

Sasmore, J.: Stress adaptation, a theory for childbirth education, J. Obstet. Gynecol. Neonat. Nurs. **2:**48-50, 1973.

Shearer, M.: Obstetrical acupuncture, Birth Fam. J. **1:**14-18, 1974.

Strunk, K., and White, E.: The elements of style, ed. 2, New York, 1972, The MacMillan Co.

Thomas, H., and Wyatt, R.: One thousand consecutive deliveries under a training for childbirth program, Am. J. Obstet. Gynecol. **61:**205, 1951.

Ulin, P.: Changing techniques in psychoprophylactic preparation for childbirth, Am. J. Nurs. **63:**60-67, 1963.

Windiver, C.: Relationship among prospective parents locus of control, social desirability, and choice of psychoprophylaxis, Nurs. Res. **26**(2):96-99, 1977.

Wonnel, E. B.: The education of the expectant father on childbirth, Nurs. Clin. North Am. **6:**591-603, 1971.

PART TWO

Fetal and neonatal development

Accurate estimations of fetal size and growth have remained elusive clinical goals, goals that are important in determining fetal well-being and making decisions regarding appropriate interventions. Gabbe discusses the problems associated with the assessment of fetal size and growth and presents tools and suggestions for the practitioner to use in performing an assessment and carrying out appropriate interventions.

Buerger focuses on the early assessment of neonatal behaviors and its significance in terms of facilitating bonding and preventing the development of learning and behavioral problems. Concepts and screening tools are presented to aid the practitioner in assessing neonatal behavior and identifying potential problems.

Visintine and Nahmias present the findings of their work pertaining to the TORCH syndrome, including the significance of careful clinical and epidemiologic observations, the potential of different methods of diagnosis, and the possibilities for prevention and therapy. Tables illustrating routes of transmission of TORCH agents to the fetus and newborn and a summary of outcomes and clinical findings associated with TORCH agent infections are included.

CHAPTER 4

Assessment of fetal size and growth

Steven G. Gabbe

INTRODUCTION

Normal fetal growth has long been accepted as a reassuring sign for the pregnant woman and her health care provider: the nurse-practitioner, nurse-midwife, or obstetrician. Yet, an accurate evaluation of fetal growth and the precise determination of fetal size have remained elusive clinical goals. This chapter will review the practical techniques that have been used to estimate fetal size in the past and introduce data generated using new ultrasonographic methods.

Accurate assessment of fetal growth and size has great importance in clinical practice. Fetal growth depends on both the intrinsic growth potential of the fetus and the supply of nutrients received from the mother.[16] A fetus that achieves a gestational age of 37 weeks or more and birth weight of 2500 gm is at a low risk for perinatal mortality. A favorable outcome is less likely in low–birth weight or macrosomatic infants. The former group includes those babies less than 2500 gm. One third of these infants are growth retarded and susceptible to an eightfold increase in perinatal mortality and a four-fold increase in intrapartum asphyxia.[20] The clinician fails to detect two thirds of these fetuses during routine antepartum evaluation.[4] Fetal macrosomatia increases the likelihood of traumatic vaginal delivery, which could be prevented by accurate estimation of fetal weight and elective cesarean section.

The interrelationships between gestational age, fetal size, and fetal maturity are often difficult to predict for a given patient. In general, one expects a fetus of known gestational age to have achieved a specified weight and degree of functional maturity. However, Yerushalmy has pointed out that more than 60% of infants of less than 37 weeks gestation may weigh over 2500 gm, while 45% of low–birth weight infants may be 37 weeks gestational age or more.[45] Gould and co-workers have emphasized the advanced pulmonary and neurologic function that may be observed in the growth-retarded infant.[15]

Accurate evaluation of fetal size and maturity is essential prior to elective induction of labor or cesarean section. Goldenberg and Nelson concluded that untimely or unwarranted intervention was responsible for 15% of their cases of respiratory distress syndrome (RDS).[12] Hack and co-workers found that 12% of all infants with RDS in their neonatal intensive care unit were born after elective intervention.[17]

None of these infants had had documentation of pulmonary maturity prior to delivery. In 11 of their 19 cases, obstetric dating was 3 or more weeks greater than subsequent pediatric assessment of gestational age. Eighteen of the infants weighed at least 2000 gm. The mean hospital stay for these babies was 23 days, and two deaths were recorded. Maisels and co-workers have recently reported their experience with 18 cases of RDS caused by elective obstetric intervention.[27] Analysis of amniotic fluid for the lecithin/sphingomyelin (L/S) ratio was used in only one case and ultrasound dating in just three. Seven infants did weigh less than 2500 gm. All the patients in Maisel's study were under the care of private obstetricians, had received adequate prenatal care, and would be expected to have reliable menstrual histories. It would appear that the available clinical tools used by many nurse-practitioners and obstetricians are inadequate for accurate prediction of fetal size and maturity.

ASSESSMENT OF FETAL SIZE AND GROWTH
Abdominal palpation

Most clinicians rely on a carefully taken menstrual history and serial assessment of uterine growth for their calculation of the patient's gestational age (Table 4-1). The reported last menstrual period (LMP) is reliable in most cases.[45] It is essential that the regularity of the menses, their interval, and the time of the previous menstrual period also be obtained. If the patient has recently used oral contraceptives, her menstrual history may be difficult to interpret.

Having calculated the fetal gestational age, the clinician may predict the expected uterine size and subsequent growth pattern. A pelvic examination during the first trimester is most useful and correlates well with early ultrasound dating of the pregnancy.[1] Uterine size may be larger than expected if a multiple gestation or hydatidiform mole is present. Other causes of apparent uterine enlargement include a thick abdominal wall, full bladder and/or rectum, ovarian cysts, and uterine myomata.[43] The uterine fundus is usually midway between the symphysis pubis and umbilicus at 16 weeks gestation. The fundus of the uterus lies at or just below the umbilicus at 20 weeks and just above at 24 weeks gestation. Thereafter, the fundal height increases two finger breadths every 4 weeks, reaching the xiphisternum at 36 weeks gestation.[43] Serial measurements of fundal growth may be made using a tape measure or pelvimeter. MacDonald's measurements are made with a tape placed along the surface of the abdomen from the symphysis to the top of the fundus. MacDonald's rule states that, after the sixth month of pregnancy, the distance

Table 4-1. Assessment of fetal size and growth

Determination	Information obtained	Information inferred
Menstrual history	Gestational age	Fetal age and viability
Early bimanual exam	Uterine size	Gestational age
Fundal height	Uterine size	Fetal weight
Radiologic methods	Bone length; ossification centers	Gestational age
Ultrasound		
Crown-rump length	Fetal size	Gestational age
Biparietal diameter	Fetal head size	Gestational age

Adapted from Lind, T.: The estimation of fetal growth and development, Br. J. Hosp. Med. **3:**501-507, 1970.

recorded in centimeters divided by 3.5 equals the lunar month of pregnancy. According to Ahlfeld's rule, the distance measured from the presenting part to the top of the fundus with a pelvimeter equals half of the fetal crown-rump length.[30]

Wide variations in the length of the maternal abdomen and position of the umbilicus place significant limitations on the use of the measurements described above. Beazley and Underhill found the position of the umbilicus varied from 11.5 to 19 cm above the symphysis in 233 patients.[1] They concluded that, before 28 weeks gestation, it was impossible to gauge fetal maturity from fundal height more accurately than within 8 weeks. Because the maternal abdomen varied 17.5 cm in length, a range of 8 to 12 weeks was reported in assessing gestational age after 28 weeks. They concluded that clinical detection of a large-for-gestational-age or small-for-gestational-age fetus required at least a 4- to 6-week difference between the expected level of the uterine fundus and the fundal height observed.

Determinations of fetal weight by abdominal palpation have also been fraught with large errors. Johnson and Toshach derived an arbitrary formula for predicting weight based on measurement of the fundal height and the station of the fetal head.[22] Using this approach, 50% of newborns weighed within ± 240 gm of actual birth weight. Loeffler evaluated the accuracy of 2868 predictions of birth weight made by 106 observers on 585 patients in labor.[26] Almost 80% of these estimates were within 1 pound of the actual birth weight. Loeffler points out that, if one simply guessed a birth weight of 7½ pounds, one would be within 1 pound of actual weight in 70% of normal term infants. The greatest inaccuracies in determining fetal weight arise when the infant weighs less than 2500 gm or over 4000 gm. Several studies have demonstrated that the clinician often underestimates the weight of the large infant but overestimates that of the small infant.[2,26,33] The accuracy does not appear to be related to the physician's clinical experience or even the use of abdominal measurements. Simmons has recently reported that weights of fetuses between 500 and 1500 gm are usually *underestimated* by 250 gm.[38] This error may have crucial impact on the therapeutic decisions made during the intrapartum management of the low-birth weight infant.

Radiologic evaluation

Many attempts have been made to predict fetal gestational age and weight with radiologic methods.[29,39] Measurements of the length of fetal bones, such as the lumbar vertebrae, or detection of a specific ossification center, such as the distal femoral epiphysis, are of limited value.[28] Fetal bones are often difficult to visualize if they overlie the maternal pelvis. The hazards of radiation for both mother and infant must also be considered. Finally, there may be wide variation in the timing of bone ossification, and these changes are unrelated to functional maturity.[34] While almost all infants demonstrate ossification of the distal femoral epiphyses by 37 weeks gestation, 40% of these infants may still have an immature L/S ratio.[10] On the other hand, close to 40% of infants without visible distal femoral epiphyses have a mature L/S ratio. Ultrasound techniques have replaced these radiologic methods in current practice.

Ultrasonography

The practical application of ultrasound scanning to obstetrics has revolutionized the clinical assessment of fetal growth and development. The technique is noninvasive, repeatable, and can be performed at bedside. Short pulses of low-intensity, high-frequency sound are directed toward the fetus. The returning reflected echoes may then be converted into a visible picture.[4]*

Crown-rump length measurement

During the first trimester, ultrasonic measurement of fetal crown-rump length provides an excellent index of gestational age. Crown-rump length increases from 10 mm at 7 weeks to 70 mm at 13 weeks gestation.[36] Robinson has successfully predicted the onset of spontaneous labor to within 3 days using this method. Hobbins and Winsberg have determined the size of the gestational sac, which increases from approximately 2 cm at 6 weeks to 5 cm at 10 weeks gestation.[20]

Biparietal diameter

Ultrasound cephalometry has had the greatest application for the evaluation of gestational age and fetal growth. The individual performing the examination must locate the widest transcoronal or biparietal diameter (BPD), which contains the midline or falx. This determination is easiest to obtain with the head in the occiput transverse position, but almost impossible to assess with the head directly occiput anterior or posterior. During the second trimester, there is an excellent correlation between the BPD and gestational age. The BPD increases rapidly in an almost linear pattern from 14 to 30 weeks gestational age, growing at 3.3 mm per week. Between 30 and 36 weeks gestation, the growth rate slows to 2.0 mm per week and by term is 1.2 mm per week.[4,7] Measurements of BPD by ultrasound are within 2 mm of postnatal caliper determinations.[6] The standard error of measurement of the BPD is about 2 mm.[20] Thus, BPD determinations made before 30 weeks gestation, when the head is growing rapidly, will be of the most value in accurately dating a pregnancy. Campbell evaluated the accuracy of BPD determinations in 313 patients evaluated between 13 and 30 weeks gestation.[4] Ninety-three percent of those studied went into spontaneous labor within 14 days of the ultrasound-predicted delivery date. This figure represented a 7% improvement in predicting the date of delivery over that obtained from the patient's menstrual history and a 20% improvement over estimates made from clinical examination.

Serial measurements are required to determine fetal growth rate. Before 36 weeks gestation, determinations made at 2-week intervals should show significant growth. As noted above, the growth rate after 36 weeks gestation is reduced and approaches the error of the method itself. Campbell, as well as Hobbins and Winsberg, have emphasized that, while there is a close correlation between gestational age and BPD when the latter is measured during the second trimester, the more advanced the pregnancy, the less reliable the information obtained.[4,20]

A BPD of 8.5 cm or greater does not correlate well with gestational age and may be a misleading index of maturity. Goldstein and co-workers have observed that 34.5% of babies with a BPD of 8.7 cm or greater will have an immature L/S ratio.[13] For infants with a BPD of 9.0 cm or more, this figure was a surprising 29.5%.

Normal fetuses appear to grow at their own characteristic rates. Sabbagha and co-workers have found that three cephalic growth patterns may be differentiated: large (BPD ≥ 75th percentile), average (BPD in 25th to 75th percentile), and small (BPD ≤

---

*See Afriat, C. L., and Schifrin, B. S.: Antepartum fetal evaluation. In McNall, L. K., and Galeener, J. T., editors: Current practice in obstetric and gynecologic nursing, vol. II, St. Louis, 1978, The C. V. Mosby Co.

25th percentile).[37] Two BPD determinations are necessary to distinguish these groups, one before 26 weeks gestation and a second between 30 and 33 weeks gestation. This approach will permit a better prediction of gestational age. There are no differences in BPD growth between the fetuses of diabetic and normal women between 30 and 37 weeks gestation.[32] Thereafter, the BPD in diabetic women is significantly larger. Accurate detection of the large-for-dates infant may depend on measurement of the fetal chest area. In macrosomatic babies, the chest area is larger, while the head to chest ratio may be significantly lower.[44]

Fetal weight

Initial attempts to predict fetal weight using BPD measurements alone were disappointing. Ianniruberto and Gibbons reported an absolute mean error of 368 gm and concluded that the wide variation in neonatal weight for a given BPD was too great for clinical application.[21] Gonzalez and co-workers have also reported that a single random BPD is of little value in predicting birth weight.[14] It has been established that virtually all infants with a BPD of 8.7 or more will weight over 2500 grams (Table 4-2).[40]

In an effort to improve their estimations of fetal birth weight, investigators have included other body dimensions in their calculations. Thompson and Makowski, measuring both the BPD and anteroposterior chest diameter, achieved an accuracy of ± 290 gm.[41] They noted that their estimations were no more accurate than those made from a history of the last menstrual period. Considerably greater accuracy has been achieved using the fetal abdominal circumference as an index of fetal weight. These measurements are usually made at the level of the ductus venosus. Kearny and co-workers have reported that 82% of infants were found to be within 15% of their actual birth weight using this approach.[23] Higginbottom and co-workers predicted 94% of birth weights within 145 gm, although their study included few very small or large infants.[19] Combining both the BPD and abdominal circumference, Warsof and co-workers have achieved an accuracy of 106 gm per kg of body weight.[42] This approach is well suited to clinical practice and would be especially valuable in the low–birth weight infant.

Methods have also been devised to calculate fetal volumes and relate them to birth weight. Morrison and McLennan have predicted fetal weight with an accura-

Table 4-2. Prediction of fetal weight

Author	Measurement	Accuracy	Standard deviation (gm)
Ianniruberto and Gibbons[21]	BPD		368
Thompson and Makowski[41]	BPD, AP chest diameter		290
Kearney and co-workers[23]	Abdominal circumference	82% within 15% of birth weight	
Higginbottom and co-workers[19]	Abdominal circumference	94% within 145 gm of birth weight	
Warsof and co-workers[42]	BPD, abdominal circumference		106/kg
Morrison and McLennan[31]	Fetal volume		106
Picker and Saunders[35]	Trunk volume plus limb volume	64% within 200 gm of birth weight	

cy of 106 gm by taking multiple cross-sectional measurements of the fetus and determining fetal volume.[31] Picker and Saunders have estimated 64% of birth weights to within 200 gm, calculating the contributions of fetal body and limbs as if they were cylinders.[35] These techniques would be difficult to apply to routine patient management.

Growth retardation

As noted earlier in this chapter, the growth-retarded infant will contribute significantly to perinatal morbidity and mortality. These poor outcomes could be avoided if earlier detection of fetal deprivation were possible. A growth-retarded infant is one whose birth weight falls on or below the fifth percentile or two standard deviations below the mean for gestational age.[4] Serial assessment of BPD alone will not adequately define this population, because, in many cases, fetal brain and skull growth is normal. Campbell has described two types of growth retardation that are of great diagnostic importance.[3] In approximately 70% to 80% of cases, a *late flattening* pattern is observed with normal BPD growth until late in gestation, when growth slows. This pattern may be seen in hypertension and is associated with perinatal asphyxia. Late flattening growth retardation may be produced in rats by decreasing uterine blood flow.[20] These rat offspring, like growth-retarded human newborns, exhibit significant reduction in liver size, but their brain is relatively spared. The second type of growth retardation that may be seen has been called the *low profile* pattern. A low growth rate of both BPD and body size are observed throughout the second and third trimester. The brain to liver ratio is usually normal, resembling the pattern seen in newborn rats whose mothers have been nutritionally deprived. Many of these infants will have chromosomal abnormalities.

Techniques that compare head and abdominal circumference have improved the detection of growth retardation.[24] In normal pregnancies, the head circumference to abdominal circumference ratio exceeds 1 through 30 weeks gestation. Between 32 and 36 weeks gestation, the ratio equals 1. As the liver increases in size and the abdominal circumference expands, the ratio falls below 1 at term.[20] Campbell has applied this principle in cases of suspected growth retardation and found that infants with a late flattening pattern whose brain is spared will maintain an abnormally high head to abdominal circumference ratio.[8] In patients with low profile growth retardation, a normal ratio is observed but BPD measurements remain small.

Gohari and co-workers have devised a unique method for predicting growth retardation.[11] Because growth retardation is often associated with not only a smaller fetus but also a reduction in placental size and amniotic fluid volume, they have determined the total intrauterine volume (TIUV). The anteroposterior, transverse, and longitudinal dimensions of the uterus are measured, and the TIUV is calculated using the formula for the volume of an ellipsoid. If the TIUV falls below 1.5 standard deviations for dates, the fetus will be growth retarded. The volume of the fetal bladder can be determined in a similar fashion. Hourly fetal urine production rates are decreased in the growth-retarded fetus and have been measured as a research tool to identify these infants.[9]

CLINICAL GUIDELINES
First trimester

Assessment of fetal size and growth begins with a careful menstrual history and ideally a pelvic examination during the first trimester.

CORRELATION OF DATA IN DETERMINING FETAL
GESTATIONAL AGE

Menstrual history

LNMP: Date_____ Duration_____ Amount_____

LMP: Date_____ Duration_____ Amount_____

PMP: Date_____ Duration_____ Amount_____

Menarche_____ Interval_____ Duration_____

Hx of menstrual irregularity _____

Contraceptive history

Type of contraceptive _____

When stopped _____

Pregnancy test

Date _____ Type _____ Result _____

Clinical evaluation

First uterine size estimate: Date _____ Size _____

FHT's first heard: Date _____ Doptone _____ Fetoscope _____

Date of quickening _____

Current fundal height _____ EFW _____

Current weeks gestation _____

Ultrasound: Date _____ Weeks' gestation _____ BPD _____

Reliability of dates _____

Impression

EDC _____ Estimated gestational age _____

Estimation based on _____

Comments _____

Signature _____ Date _____

Fig. 4-1. Correlation of data in determining fetal gestational age. (Modified and adapted by McNall, L. Developed by Department of Obstetrics, Women's Hospital, University of Southern California Medical Center, Los Angeles, California.)

Second trimester

If the patient is not seen until the second trimester, a baseline ultrasound may be obtained. This approach is especially important in patients whose infants are at risk for growth retardation or who may require elective delivery. A baseline BPD will be of great value in women with hypertension, diabetes mellitus, and renal disease or those scheduled for elective repeat cesarean section. Serial measurements of fundal growth by a single examiner will prove useful during the second and third trimester. Errors caused by hydramnios, abnormal fetal position or presentation, or maternal obesity must be considered. Hertz and co-workers have evaluated the role of menstrual history, first unamplified audible fetal heart tones, and quickening in predicting gestational age.[18] They found these parameters to be of great clinical importance. Patients should be asked prospectively to note the date of quickening. In Hertz's series, quickening occurred at 18.6 weeks in nulliparas and 18.4 weeks in multiparas. Patients should be seen every 1 to 2 weeks after 17 to 18 weeks gestation for early detection of fetal heart tones. To be 90% certain that an infant will be at least 38 weeks gestational age at delivery, one must have heard fetal heart tones for 21 weeks, noted quickening for 25 weeks, or have a reliable LMP recorded 42 weeks prior to birth.

Third trimester

Campbell has suggested that all patients have a repeat ultrasound in the third trimester to evaluate fetal growth.[5] This approach may be difficult to apply in many clinics. Certainly all patients at high risk for growth retardation would warrant a second evaluation. One may also see a patient for the first time during the third trimester whose uterine size is less than expected for the given menstrual history. An initial BPD determination at this time could be compatible with growth retardation or an error in dating. However, a repeat measurement in 1 to 2 weeks should show rapid growth if an error in dating has been made because smaller fetal heads grow more quickly. If minimal growth in the BPD is observed during the 1- to 2-week interval, growth retardation must be considered.

CONCLUSION

While accurate evaluation of fetal growth and the precise determination of fetal size are elusive clinical goals, observation and assessment of all evaluative parameters continue to be important in the identification and management of actual or potential problems and the reduction of fetal/neonatal morbidity and mortality rates.

REFERENCES

1. Beazley, J. M., Underhill, R. A.: Fallacy of the fundal height, Br. Med. J. **4:**404-406, 1970.
2. Bossak, W. S., and Spellacy, W. N.: Accuracy of estimating fetal weight by abdominal palpation, J. Reprod. Med. **9:**58-60, 1972.
3. Campbell, S.: Fetal growth, Clin. Obstet. Gynecol. **1:**41-65, 1974.
4. Campbell, S.: Fetal growth. In Beard, R. W., and Nathaniels, P. W., editors: Fetal physiology and medicine, Philadelphia, 1976, W. B. Saunders Co.
5. Campbell, S.: Physical methods of assessing size at birth. In Ciba Foundation Symposium: Size at birth, North Holland, 1974, Elsevier, Excerpta Medica.
6. Campbell, S.: Ultrasonic fetal cephalometry during the second trimester of pregnancy, Br. J. Obstet. Gynaecol. **77:**1057-1063, 1970.
7. Campbell, S., and Newman, G. B.: Growth of the fetal biparietal diameter during normal pregnancy, Br. J. Obstet. Gynaecol. **78:**513-519, 1971.
8. Campbell, S., and Thoms, A.: Ultrasound measurement of the fetal head to abdomen circumference ratio in the assessment of growth retardation, Br. J. Obstet. Gynaecol. **84:**165-174, 1977.
9. Campbell, S., Wladimiroff, J. W., and Dewhurst, D. J.: The antenatal measurement of fetal urine

production, Br. J. Obstet. Gynaecol. **80:**680-686, 1973.
10. Cruz, A. C., Buhi, W. C., and Spellacy, W. N.: Comparison of the fetogram and L/S ratio for fetal maturity, Obstet. Gynecol. **45:**147-149, 1975.
11. Gohari, P., Berkowitz, R. L., and Hobbins, J. C.: Prediction of intrauterine growth retardation by determination of total intrauterine volume, Am. J. Obstet. Gynecol. **127:**255-260, 1977.
12. Goldenberg, R. L., and Nelson, K.: Iatrogenic respiratory distress syndrome, Am. J. Obstet. Gynecol. **123:**617-620, 1975.
13. Goldstein, P., Gershenson, D., and Hobbins, J. C.: Fetal biparietal diameter as a predictor of a mature lecithin/sphingomyelin ratio, Obstet. Gynecol. **48:**667-669, 1976.
14. Gonzalez, A. C., Dale, E., Byers, R. H., et al.: Limitations in prediction of gestational age and birthweight by ultrasonographic methods, J. Clin. Ultrasound, **6:**233-238, 1978.
15. Gould, J. B., Gluck, L., Kulovich, M. V.: The relationship between accelerated pulmonary maturity and accelerated neurologic maturity in certain chronically stressed pregnancies, Am. J. Obstet. Gynecol. **127:**181-186, 1977.
16. Gruenwald, P.: Growth of the human fetus, 1. Normal growth and its variation, Am. J. Obstet. Gynecol. **94:**1112-1119, 1966.
17. Hack, M., Fanaroff, A. A., Klaus, M. H., et al.: Neonatal respiratory distress following elective delivery. A preventable disease? Am. J. Obstet. Gynecol. **126:**43-47, 1976.
18. Hertz, R. H., Sokol, R. J., Knoke, J. D., et al.: Clinical estimation of gestational age: rules for avoiding preterm delivery, Am. J. Obstet. Gynecol. **131:**395-402, 1978.
19. Higginbottom, J., Slater, J., Porter, G., et al.: Estimation of fetal weight from ultrasonic measurement of trunk circumference, Br. J. Obstet. Gynaecol. **82:**698-701, 1975.
20. Hobbins, J. C. and Winsberg, F.: Ultrasonography in obstetrics and gynecology, Baltimore, 1977, Williams & Wilkins Co.
21. Ianniruberto, A., and Gibbons, J. M., Jr.: Predicting fetal weight by ultrasonic B-scan cephalometry, Obstet. Gynecol. **37:**689-694, 1971.
22. Johnson, R. W., and Toshach, C. E.: Estimation of fetal weight using longitudinal mensuration, Am. J. Obstet. Gynecol. **68:**891-896, 1954.
23. Kearney, K., Vigneron, N., Frischman, P., et al.: Fetal weight estimation by ultrasonic measurement of abdominal circumference, Obstet. Gynecol. **51:**156-162, 1978.
24. Kurjak, A., and Breyer, B.: Estimation of fetal weight by ultrasonic abdominometry, Am. J. Obstet. Gynecol. **125:**962-965, 1976.
25. Lind, T.: The estimation of fetal growth and development, Br. J. Hosp. Med. **3:**501-507, 1970.
26. Loeffler, F. E.: Clinical foetal weight prediction, Br. J. Obstet. Gynaecol. **74:**675-677, 1967.
27. Maisels, M. J., Rees, R., Marks, K., et al. Elective delivery of the "term" fetus—an obstetrical hazard. J.A.M.A. **238:**2036-2039, 1977.
28. Margolis, A. J. and Voss, R. G.: A method for radiologic detection of fetal maturity, Am. J. Obstet. Gynecol. **101:**383-389, 1968.
29. Martin, R. H., and Higginbottom, J.: A clinical and radiological assessment of fetal age, Br. J. Obstet. Gynaecol. **78:**155-162, 1971.
30. McLennan, C. E., and Sandberg, E. C.: Synopsis of obstetrics, St. Louis, 1970, The C. V. Mosby Co.
31. Morrison, J., and McLennan, M. J.: The theory, feasibility and accuracy of an ultrasonic method of estimating fetal weight, Br. J. Obstet. Gynaecol. **83:**833-837, 1976.
32. Murata, J., and Martin, C. B., Jr.: Growth of the biparietal diameter of the fetal head in diabetic pregnancy, Am. J. Obstet. Gynecol. **115:**252-256, 1973.
33. Ong. H. C., and Sen, D. K.: Clinical estimation of fetal weight, Am. J. Obstet. Gynecol. **112:** 877-880, 1972.
34. Perkins, R. P.: Antenatal assessment of fetal maturity, Obstet. Gynecol. Surv. **29:**369-384, 1974.
35. Picker, R. H., and Saunders, D. M.: A simple geometric method for determining fetal weight in utero with the compound gray scale ultrasonic scan, Am. J. Obstet. Gynecol. **124:**493-494, 1976.
36. Robinson, H. P.: Sonar measurement of fetal crown-rump length as means of assessing maturity in first trimester of pregnancy, Br. Med. J. **4:** 28-31, 1973.
37. Sabbagha, R. E., Hughey, M., and Depp, R.: Growth adjusted sonographic age, a simplified method, Obstet. Gynecol. **51:**383-386, 1978.
38. Simmons, M. A.: Personal communication.
39. Southworth, J. D.: Fetal age as determined by x-ray, J. Maine Med. Assoc. **55:**212-213, 1963.
40. Stocker, J., Mawad, R., Deleon, A., et al.: Ultrasonic cephalometry, its use in estimating fetal weight, Obstet. Gynecol. **45:**275-278, 1975.
41. Thompson, H. E., and Makowski, E. L.: Esti-

mation of birth weight and gestational age, Obstet. Gynecol. **37:**44-47, 1971.
42. Warsof, S. L., Gohari, P., Berkowitz, R. L., et al.: The estimation of fetal weight by computer-assisted analysis, Am. J. Obstet. Gynecol. **128:** 881-892, 1977.
43. Wilson Clyne, D. G.: A textbook of gynecology and obstetrics, London, 1963, Spottiswoode, Ballantyne.
44. Wladimiroff, J. W., Bloemsma, C. A., and Wallenburg, H. C. S.: Ultrasonic diagnosis of the large-for-dates infant, Obstet. Gynecol. **52:**285-288, 1978.
45. Yerushalmy, J.: Relation of birthweight, gestational age, and the rate of intrauterine growth to perinatal mortality, Clin. Obstet. Gynecol. **1:** 107-129, 1970.

CHAPTER 5

Developmental profile of the neonate

Ede Marie Buerger

The early identification of neurologically at-risk infants is essential to prevention of disabled children and to development of intervention strategies. Fundamental to early identification is a growing appreciation for the remarkable behavioral repertoire of the neonate and the plasticity of the maturing central nervous system.

In previous years, there was much controversy in the predictive value of neonatal examinations. Confluence of data suggests that maturational, environmental, and psychosocial factors have profound influence on emerging interactional behavior of infants. It is doubtful that behaviors assessed during a single examination of the newborn are valid predictors because they depend largely on existing and emerging capacities of neuroanatomic structures. Single-examination data may be modified temporarily by existing health/illness status, conceptual age, and sleep/wake state of the infant. While considerable variability is normal, variability may be further altered by previous interactional experience with the environment, environmental stimulation, handling episodes, and posturing. Moreover, individual and innate variables such as excitability and autonomic activity constitute additional influential factors.

Furthermore, insults to the central nervous system (CNS) are frequently not manifested until months and sometimes years after the precipitating cause occurred. Emergence of unusual motor and sensory patterns is correlated with the maturation of an injured CNS. All too often difficulties of at-risk infants are compounded by disorganized and/or inappropriate environmental factors that alter integration of CNS mechanisms.

It is well recognized by developmental specialists that examinations conducted on a regular and periodic basis provide relevant data that may allow for the development of appropriate intervention strategies. Hence, skill in testing, knowledge of the orderly, sequential progression of neurobehavioral development in premature infants, and utilization of age-specific tests are of paramount importance to nurse-practitioners working with mothers and newborns. For instance, specific primitive reflexes such as rooting, suck, moro, flexor withdrawal, and neck righting should emerge between the viable gestational ages of 26 weeks and 40 weeks. Other reactions such as body righting, landau, amphibian, parachute, and protective extension occur at later ages and are thought to be precursors of new behaviors such as crawling and walking.

PRONENESS AND ASSESSMENT

Early identification requires two activities: proneness and assessment. Proneness screening is identifying an implied increased probability of handicapping behaviors in childhood. Hence, in screening, the process is that of separating those infants who have experienced events that are associated with later developmental problems. (This process must take into account the dynamic state of the maturing nervous system.) Thus, the nurse-practitioner moves beyond identifying existing problems to anticipating problems. This involves two levels of perception. First, one identifies elements or conditions that interfere with or alter the health status of the neonate. One becomes sensitive to indicators that give reliable estimates of proneness for unfavorable developmental outcomes. Second, one assesses existing developmental patterns. One observes, records, and identifies the behavioral profile of an infant and compares it with known patterns of behavior in large groups of infants of similar age and cultural background. This is also the second activity of early identification.

A proneness (screening) profile includes many factors since no one variable gives a complete answer. Interactions of characteristics and events are examined closely. In a study of over 189 infants, Bernard[2] found that the following variables are significant in screening:
1. Perinatal health status of mother and infant, including complications of pregnancy, delivery, and neonatal period
2. Characteristics of the care-giver, including temperament, educational level, perception of life situation, and perception of infant
3. Characteristics of the infant, including alertness, activity pattern, and sensory threshold level
4. Behaviors of care-giver and infant interacting with one another

Thus, it is apparent that nurse-practitioners are engaging not only in preventing learning and behavior problems of infants but also in facilitating the acquaintance process (maternal-infant familiarization) and the adaptation process (maternal-infant adjustment to each other).

Screening is initiated no later than when infant and care-giver interact with one health care system. This may be in family-planning clinics as a woman prepares for pregnancy, in prenatal clinics as a woman proceeds through pregnancy, and in the labor, delivery, and postbirth settings. A proneness screening may be initiated no later than in the newborn nursery. Such a health care delivery service thereby requires improved professional and agency linkage between community resources and acute care institutions.

In the assessment process, a developmental profile is collected by the nurse-practitioner. The following should be considered:
1. Characteristics of the infant, including adaptation and response to environment, ability to give interpretable cues, and developmental progress as compared with established norms
2. Characteristics of the care-giver, including adaptation to a new infant, sensitivity to infant cues, methods of alleviating distress, and provisions for growth
3. Home health status, including environmental health, safety, comfort, and stimulation

The assessment process establishes a regular and periodic program of examination and intervention. It is initiated no later than when proneness screening suggests the presence of elements or conditions that may interfere with or alter the health status of the neonate. At Loma Linda University, we have found that quarterly visits by nurse-practitioners to homes of at-risk infants are most beneficial and involve such basic nursing activities as: (1) counselling of care-giver, (2) teaching of normal developmental progress, (3) evaluating nutrition of infancy and early childhood, (4) devising infant activity programs, and (5) introducing community resources on parenting. Thus, a comprehensive program of activities, unique to nursing but often neglected or poorly understood by other professions, has been introduced into our system of health care. If this is not available in other communities, assessment and case-finding can be initiated in well-baby clinics and in already operational immunization programs for children.

TOOLS AND IMPLICATIONS
Perinatal health states

Perinatal health states are frequently discussed in the medical history. Screening data include Apgar scores and maternal and/or infant health/illness status. Avery's *Neonatology: Physiology and Management of the Newborn* provides a thorough survey of perinatal care with reference to the newborn.[23]

Characteristics of the care-giver

Care-giver characteristics take into account the influence of the parents' view of infant behavior on developmental outcomes. It is becoming evident that parental perceptions[7] and education levels[26] are major determinants in shaping environmental response to infants. Temperament and personality play key roles in parental emotional orientation and annoyance levels.[7] A description of tools and implications of these factors may be found in Currie and Pepper's *Mental Retardation*.[8]

Characteristics of the infant

Infant characteristics can be evaluated by using a behavioral profile. At Loma Linda University, a developmental profile format has been devised for premature infants. It has been used since 1974. The categories for evaluation include: (1) gross motor and reflex maturation, (2) fine motor skills, (3) adaptive and cognitive abilities, (4) language, (5) socialization, (6) self-control and self-help skills, (7) body symmetry and movement, and (8) muscle tone and range of motion limitations. Through this developmental profile, other professionals and parents are provided with information regarding the premature infant's developmental/gestational age in each category, CNS organization, integration, and adaptability at time of testing. This profile is performed serially and supplemented with data collected from other age-appropriate examinations until the infant is 1 year of age.

During hospitalization, these profiles are used as guidelines for a program of therapeutic interventions such as activity schedules, care-giver education, behavior modification interventions, parental values clarification, grief counselling, and data base for interdisciplinary case management at the time of discharge. The results of these profiles may be used for determining need for referral to community resources such as occupational therapy programs in Crippled Children Services, follow-up-in-normal-development programs in Developmental Disabilities (Regional) Centers, special education programs, and/or private therapy services.

The *developmental profile* is a product of three specific examinations: gestational age inventory,[1,6,11] neurologic examination,[3,13,18,19] and Neonatal Behavioral

Assessment Scale.[5] Each examination is performed in its entirety by individuals trained in application of test tools, with intertester reliability in scoring results when appropriate.

The *gestational age inventory* is a somewhat reliable estimation of the physical age of a premature infant. It uses two sets of observations: physical findings and neuromuscular development. It is most useful as a frame of reference for initial and progressive evaluations. Fig. 5-1 demonstrates the findings of gestational age that are appropriate for examination immediately after birth. Fig. 5-2 contains signs that are delayed until after the infant is physiologically stable. We have revised Fig. 5-2 from its original form[6] to include more current information.[1] While the data in Fig. 5-1 require almost no manipulation, the data in Fig. 5-2 require handling that may stress unstable infants.

The physical findings on the gestational age inventory are self-explanatory. However, the neuromuscular findings require further comment. In premature infants, development of muscular tone begins in the lower extremities and proceeds in a caudocephalad direction.[10] Furthermore, younger premature infants are flaccid and emerge into flexor hypertoxicity. For example, there is a generalized decrease in flexor and extensor tone in an infant of 28 weeks gestation, whereas an infant of 32 weeks gestation has improved tone in the lower extremities. At 40 weeks gestation, the infant is somewhat hypertonic. Various limb angles represent passive tone and decrease as muscle tone matures.

The *neurologic examination* has long been an accepted method of CNS assessment.[18] The integrity of selected neuropathways can be most easily demonstrated by testing of reflexes. Patterns of emergence and disappearance of selected reflexes are significant in defining functional neuromuscular status and motor development in childhood. Table 5-1 lists the reflexes that are considered useful in developmental profiles; however, this list is not complete.

The *Neonatal Behavioral Assessment (Brazelton) Scale* provides common descriptors of behavioral responses.[5] It is particularly sensitive to variances in alertness, motor activity, sensory threshold levels, and selective discrimination. The influence of state and self-control on infant behavior is apparent. Hence, individual infant disposition is subject to definition and description. With some revision it is easily adaptable to the premature infant. Endurance, fatigue, stability of responses, control of input, CNS organization, and infant's ability to use stimulation and robustness can then be observed.

The Brazelton Scale deviates further from the other two exams. Sensitivity and attentiveness to new and graded stimuli are evaluated through a series of visual, auditory, and tactile experiences. The infant's responses are evaluated as to: (1) how information is obtained, integrated, and acted on, (2) what assists are needed for an action, and (3) what influences infant participation. Primary exploratory behaviors, curiosity, discriminator skills, patterns of motor communication, tolerance levels, and socializing skills are thus subject to examiner scrutiny. These data are particularly valuable to nurses as one considers interactional adaptation, acquaintance process, and mothering needs of clients.

The Brazelton Scale provides insight about the influence of an individual's state and self-control on neuromuscular and reflex findings. Hence, testing for gestational age–related data and neurologic data is integrated into the process of Brazelton Scale testing. Reliability in identify-

PHYSICAL FINDINGS		20	21	22	23	24	25	26	27	28	29	30	31	32	33	34	35	36	37	38	39	40	41	42	43	44	45	46	47	48
		WEEKS GESTATION																												
VERNIX		APPEARS				COVERS BODY, THICK LAYER														ON BACK, SCALP, IN CREASES		SCANT, IN CREASES		NO VERNIX						
BREAST TISSUE AND AREOLA		AREOLA & NIPPLE BARELY VISIBLE NO PALPABLE BREAST TISSUE														AREOLA RAISED		1-2 MM NODULE		3-5 MM	5-6 MM	7-10 MM				?12 MM				
EAR	FORM	FLAT, SHAPELESS														BEGINNING INCURVING SUPERIOR		INCURVING UPPER 2/3 PINNAE			WELL-DEFINED INCURVING TO LOBE									
	CARTILAGE	PINNA SOFT, STAYS FOLDED												CARTILAGE SCANT RETURNS SLOWLY FROM FOLDING				THIN CARTILAGE SPRINGS BACK FROM FOLDING				PINNA FIRM, REMAINS ERECT FROM HEAD								
SOLE CREASES		SMOOTH SOLES ꞇ CREASES												1-2 ANTERIOR CREASES			2-3 ANTERIOR CREASES	CREASES ANTERIOR 2/3 SOLE		CREASES INVOLVING HEEL				DEEPER CREASES OVER ENTIRE SOLE						
SKIN	THICKNESS & APPEARANCE	THIN, TRANSLUCENT SKIN, PLETHORIC, VENULES OVER ABDOMEN EDEMA												SMOOTH THICKER NO EDEMA				PINK		FEW VESSELS		SOME DESQUAMATION PALE PINK		THICK, PALE, DESQUAMATION OVER ENTIRE BODY						
	NAIL PLATES	AP-PEAR												NAILS TO FINGER TIPS										NAILS EXTEND WELL BEYOND FINGER TIPS						
HAIR		APPEARS ON HEAD			EYE BROWS & LASHES					FINE, WOOLLY, BUNCHES OUT FROM HEAD									SILKY, SINGLE STRANDS LAYS FLAT					?RECEDING HAIRLINE OR LOSS OF BABY HAIR SHORT, FINE UNDERNEATH						
LANUGO		AP-PEARS	COVERS ENTIRE BODY												VANISHES FROM FACE					PRESENT ON SHOULDERS				NO LANUGO						
GENITALIA	TESTES									TESTES PALPABLE IN INGUINAL CANAL								IN UPPER SCROTUM				IN LOWER SCROTUM								
	SCROTUM									FEW RUGAE								RUGAE, ANTERIOR PORTION				RUGAE COVER		PENDULOUS						
	LABIA & CLITORIS											PROMINENT CLITORIS LABIA MAJORA SMALL WIDELY SEPARATED						LABIA MAJORA LARGER NEARLY COVERED CLITORIS				LABIA MINORA & CLITORIS COVERED								
SKULL FIRMNESS		BONES ARE SOFT								SOFT TO 1" FROM ANTERIOR FONTANELLE							SPONGY AT EDGES OF FONTANELLE CENTER FIRM			BONES HARD SUTURES EASILY DISPLACED				BONES HARD, CANNOT BE DISPLACED						

Fig. 5-1. Gestation age inventory: examination first hours. (Adapted approximation based on Brazie, J. V., and Lubchenco, L. O.: Current pediatric diagnosis and treatment, ed. 3, Lange Medical Publications, 1974, Los Altos, Calif.; Amiel-Tison, C.: Modern perinatal medicine, Chicago, 1975, Year Book Medical Publishers, Inc.)

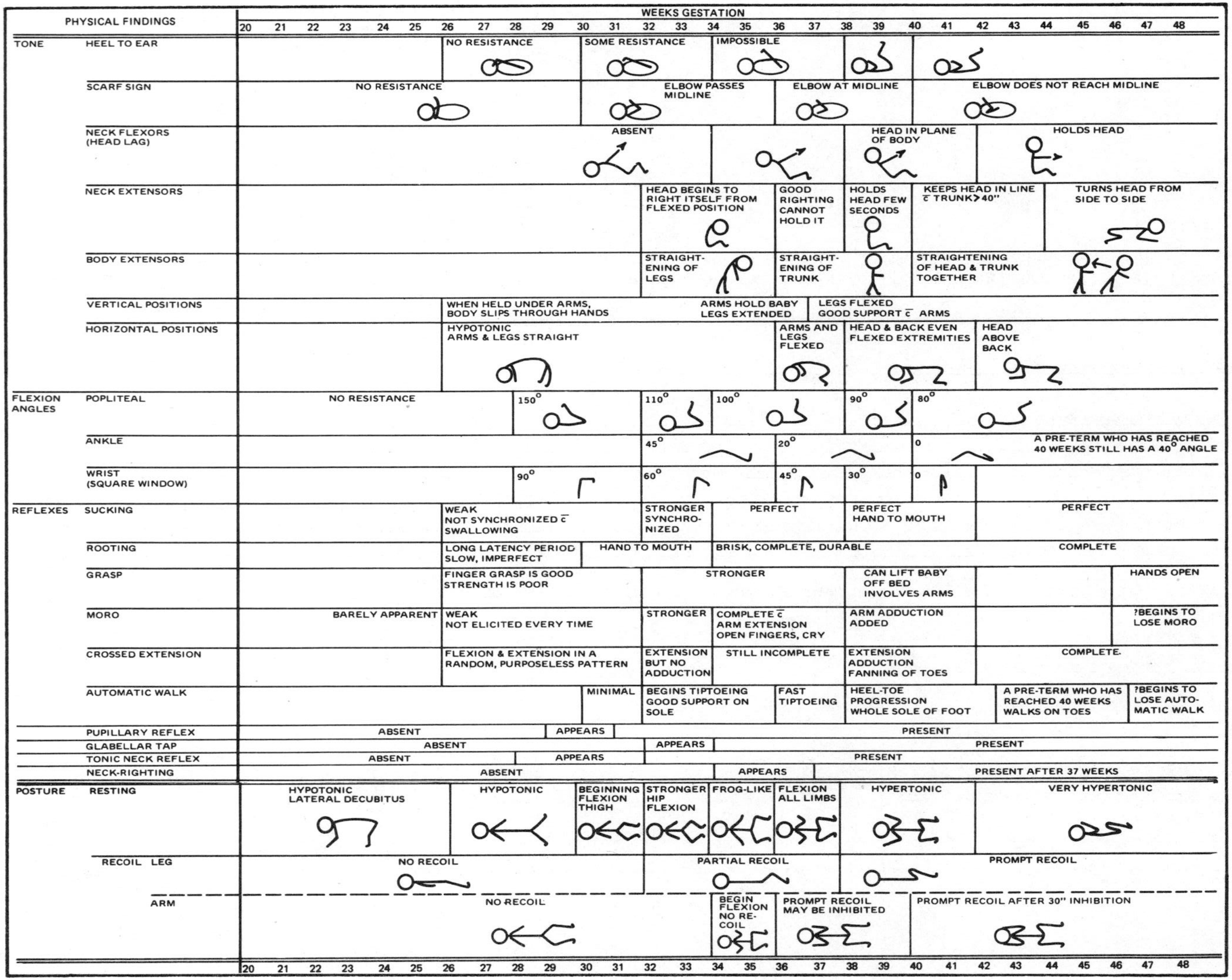

74 Fetal and neonatal development

Fig. 5-2. Gestation age inventory: examination first hours. (Adapted approximation based on Brazie, J. V., and Lubchenco, L. O.: Current pediatric diagnosis and treatment, ed. 3, Lange Medical Publications, 1974, Los Altos, Calif.; Amiel-Tison, C.: Modern perinatal medicine, Chicago, 1975, Year Book Medical Publishers, Inc.)

Table 5-1. Neonatal reflexes*

Reflex	Stimulus technique	Normal response	Significance
Chvostek's (5th and 7th cranial nerves)	Tap briskly over parotid gland (in front of ear). Test when baby is drowsy or alert.	Slight twitch on stimulated side.	Repetitive facial twitching may indicate tetany, hypoglycemia, or IDM.
Corneal (3rd and 5th cranial nerves)	Touch cornea lightly with wisp of cotton.	Eyes close.	Absence of response may indicate 5th cranial nerve paralysis.
Glabellar (3rd and 5th cranial nerves)	Tap briskly on bridge of nose. Test when baby is drowsy or alert.	Eyes blink and/or close.	Lack of symmetry may indicate paralysis. Low threshold may indicate hyperexcitability.
Optical blink (2nd and 5th cranial nerves)	Turn off lights in room. Shine light suddenly at open eyes of baby. Test when baby is awake or drowsy.	Dorsal flexion of head with eye closure occurs as early as 28 weeks gestation.	Lack of response may indicate poor light perception. The frequency of blinking is decreased in meningitis. Frequent rhythmic blinking may be seizure activity.
Pupil (2nd cranial nerve)	Shine light in open eyes.	Size: 2-3 mm. Pupil may react at 29 weeks gestation. Pupil constriction is consistent by 32 weeks gestation.	Assymetry in pupil may suggest neurologic dysfunction.
Rooting (5th and 7th cranial nerves)	Gently stroke lip from midline to cheek. Test when awake, drowsy, or active.	Head should turn direction of stroking. Younger premature infants and satiated infants may turn opposite direction.	Lack of response may indicate hyposensitive face or CNS depression.
Suck (5th, 6th, and 12th cranial nerves; swallowing requires 9th and 10th cranial nerves)	With examiner's littlest finger, gently stroke upper palate inside infant's mouth. Test in drowsy, awake, active, or crying states.	Tongue midline with intermittent, rhythmic lifting. Lips curve around stimulus source. Premature cycle is 4-6 bursts of sucking; mature cycle is 8-12 bursts. Premature will not obtain good lip closure. Good strength is present in mature infant. Suck/swallow coordination occurs between 32 and 34 weeks gestation.	Lack of adequate bursts per cycles may cause feeding problems. Too strong bite reflex will interfere with feeding. Poor lip closure in older infants may be caused by CNS depression, damage, fatigue in premature infants, IDM, and asphyxia. Asymmetries of lip closure in older infants may indicate paralysis. Lack of coordination between suck/swallow activity may result in aspiration. Easy gagging may indicate hypersensitivity in the mouth. Easy fatigue with feeding may result in congenital heart failure, bronchopulmonary dysplasia, and tachypnea. Frequent, rhythmic smacking of lips may be seizure activity.
Masseter (5th cranial nerve)	Place one finger on chin. Tap sharply with index finger. Test in drowsy or alert state.	Examiner should feel chin-lift. Present first 10 days of life.	Absence may mean brainstem lesion or lesions of 5th cranial nerve.

*Adapted from Dargassies (11), Netter (17), Peiper (18), Prechtl and Beintema (19), and Volpe (24).

Continued.

Table 5-1. Neonatal reflexes—cont'd

Reflex	Stimulus technique	Normal response	Significance
Palmar grasp	Gentle stroking of palm, particularly from ulnar side. Head should be midline. Sucking will facilitate response.	Fingers curl. Strength improves with gestational age. Much hand opening is appropriate in younger, premature infants. Palmar grasp is present at 28 weeks, strong at 32 weeks, and of sufficient power at 36 weeks gestation to lift infant from bed.	Absence may indicate peripheral nerve lesion, hypotonia in older infants, and drug depression. Asymmetries occur in Erb's paresis and sometimes after clavicular fracture.
Galant	Put infant in ventral suspension, tap/ stroke finger parallel to spinal column from pelvis to shoulder. Test in drowsy, awake, or active state.	Infant's body will curve toward stimuli.	Constant, spontaneous posturing may indicate gluteal abscess or sciatic nerve plexis paralysis. Asymmetrical responses may not be significant. Lack of any response may indicate paralysis or hypotonia.
Perez	In ventral suspension, tap finger along spine from caudal to cephalad. Do not test infant in active or crying states.	Head and tail should elevate as stimulated. Infant should also void.	Strength of response improves with gestational age. Lack of head lift may indicate poor neck flexor and extensor tone. This is commonly seen in IDM and asphyxia. Lack of tail-life may indicate hypotonia or paralysis.
Deep tendon	Support leg at thigh. When relaxed, tap briskly just below knee cap. Head must be midline. Do not test infant in active or crying state.	Quick extension of leg may be felt or seen.	Testing procedure greatly influences response. Lack of response may indicate neuronal fatigue during testing, poor testing technique, or spinal cord depression. Exaggeration may be seen in hyperactive infants.
Plantar grasp	Light pressure is applied to balls of feet. Test in quiet state.	Toes curl in plantar flexion.	Lack of response may mean spinal cord depression or lesion.
Babinski	Stroke side of sole of foot from heel to ball of foot and across from little toe to big toe.	Dorsal flexion of big toe and fanning of other toes. (Normal in premature and term infants, caused by immature pyramidal tracts.)	May indicate lesions of pyramidal tract or lesions in motor neurons. (Fanning should not occur until infant begins to walk.)
Ankle clonus	Suspend leg at thigh and relax. Sharply press against soles of feet, dorsiflexing entire foot. Then release quickly. Test in quiet, awake, or drowsy state.	Foot returns to pretest position. Fast, involuntary, irregular contractions are normal. Spontaneous clonus may occur in young, premature and in older, premature infants when positioned in hyperextension supine position.	Slow, sustained contractions are suspicious. Easily elicited clonus in the presence of other abnormal neurologic signs is suspicious.
Cross extension	Extend one leg by holding knee, stroke foot for Babinski response. Test infant when awake or drowsy.	Opposite leg should extend and adduct slightly, depending on gestational age. In young, premature infant, nonspecific random flexion and extension may be seen.	Lack of response may indicate voluntary override by stretching activity of baby, spinal cord lesion, or, if weak, peripheral nerve damage.

Table 5-1. Neonatal reflexes—cont'd

Reflex	Stimulus technique	Normal response	Significance
Placing	While baby is upright, stroke dorsum of foot gently. Test in alert and quiet states.	Fanning of toes and stepping action. Stepping action is not present in young, premature infant.	Lack of response may indicate paralysis.
Automatic walk	While baby is upright, let soles of feet rest on solid surface. Test in alert state.	Stepping action, dependent on gestational age. Minimal with tiptoeing is expected in young, premature infant.	Lack of leg muscle tone may be seen in IDM, asphyxia, paralysis, drug depression, and breech delivery. Any scissoring of legs and hyperextension is suspicious.
Vestibular (8th cranial nerve)	Slowly turn head from side to side or hold infant upright and spin slowly. Test in quiet or alert states.	Nystagmus or duration of eyes toward turn and then countermove. This reflex is best shown on seventh day of life in term infant. Nystagmus may occur spontaneously. It should be present by 32 weeks gestation.	Asymmetry may indicate abducens paresis. Lack of response may indicate brainstem lesion. It is also possible to obtain proprioceptive eye opening in these infants by raising the infant to an upright position. *Sustained* nystagmus after slight movement of head is suspicious. (Constant strabismus is abnormal and may indicate abducens paresis.)
Crawling	Place baby prone with arms and legs flexed and head face down. Pressure is applied to soles of feet or gentle pushing of buttocks. Test in quiet or alert states.	Head should move from side to side; alternately adducts legs and flexes arms in crawling fashion. Components and vigorousness of response is age related.	Lack of response in extremities should be correlated with the lack of response of reflexes in same extremities. In hypotonic infant, head movement component of this reflex may be poor because of poor neck flexor and extensor tone.
Acoustic blink (3rd and 8th cranial nerves)	When environment is quiet and infant is resting, examiner should slap hands together loudly. Test when infant is quiet or alert.	Blink and/or startle response by 28 weeks gestation.	Lack of response is usually related to high auditory levels in environment or sleep. This reflex is not a reliable test for hearing.
Moro	Hold baby on back with one hand supporting trunk and the other hand supporting head. As soon as infant relaxes, drop head a few centimeters. Test when infant is not active or crying.	This reflex has four components: 1. Extension (opening up) movement of arms with a "C" formation of first finger and thumb. This occurs by 28 weeks gestation. 2. Cry. This occurs by 32 weeks gestation. 3. Embrace of arms. This occurs after 34 to 36 weeks gestation. 4. Legs may draw up.	Lack of response may indicate drug depression, asphyxia, and/or hypotonia. Asymmetrical movement responses should be correlated with lack of or poor responses to reflex or testing of same extremities.

ing gross behavioral discrepancies is enhanced.[21]

In recent years many myths have been identified about term infants and premature infants. A detailed discussion of all findings, normal and abnormal, would detract from the objectives of this chapter and will not be attempted. However, selected data collection items will be discussed in relation to infants who have experienced certain events.

Alertness. Levels and qualities of alertness vary according to numerous factors. An infant of 28 weeks gestation has brief alert states that frequently have delayed onset, much variability in quality, and may occur spontaneously.[11] There appears to be a unique state in the infant of 28 to 31 weeks gestation—a "transition state." The infant is bright and glassy-eyed and will respond to orienting stimuli repeatedly. Once fully open-eyed with active limb movement, the infant will continue to respond and be spontaneously active for a prolonged period. It is as though in this infant there is no ability to habituate or limit intake of stimuli. In relatively healthy premature infants of this age, we have not observed significant autonomic changes in this state. However, in the chronically ill premature infant of this age, we have observed apnea and/or bradycardia in response to stimulation on occasion. By 32 weeks gestation, premature infants demonstrate more definitive sleep/wake cycles and more consistent and improved quality of alertness. By 36 to 37 weeks gestation, infants are vigorous and have good quality alertness.

Optimal level and quality of alertness can be reached by premature infants if the examiner uses graded stimuli to awaken infants and specific handling techniques. We have observed longer periods of high activity and crying behavior as well as disorganized motor activity when the examiner attempts to awaken the infant (1) from a deep sleep state,[12] (2) by presenting most aversive stimuli first, (3) by fast handling, (4) by supine posturing without supporting arms and legs, (5) by hyperpronation posturing, and (6) by attempting an examination shortly before an infant-cycled feeding time.

Low-level behaviors may be the result of inadequate stimuli, deep sleeping, and/or attempting examination shortly after an infant-cycled feeding time. Obtunded and coma states are accompanied by other abnormal neurologic findings.

Vision. An infant of 28 weeks gestation will blink persistently to light.[11] We have been able to document following of head with delayed eye following the examiner's face and/or voice in infants of 27 to 28 weeks gestation (Fig. 5-3). We have also found that infants of 31 to 35 weeks gestation will follow visual and auditory animate stimuli. The older the infant, the more consistent the response. Even infants of 36 weeks gestation will inconsistently follow red circles and selected other inanimate auditory and visual stimuli.

The premature infant, who is recovering from a long illness, will make eye-to-eye contact with (1) a primary care-giver and/or (2) only the most persistent and skilled examiner. Some authors have suggested that long-term hospitalization may be a factor.[4]

Hearing. Loud noises will startle infants of 28 weeks gestation.[11] A decrease in motor activity, regular respirations, and widening of the eyes will become more apparent and more consistent as this infant matures.[18] The chronically ill infant tends to respond to auditory and visual experiences more appropriately than to tactile experiences. Hence, animate auditory and visual stimuli can be effective consoling interventions for the distressed, intubated infant who has apnea or bradycardia to touch.

Motor. A common suspicious finding of

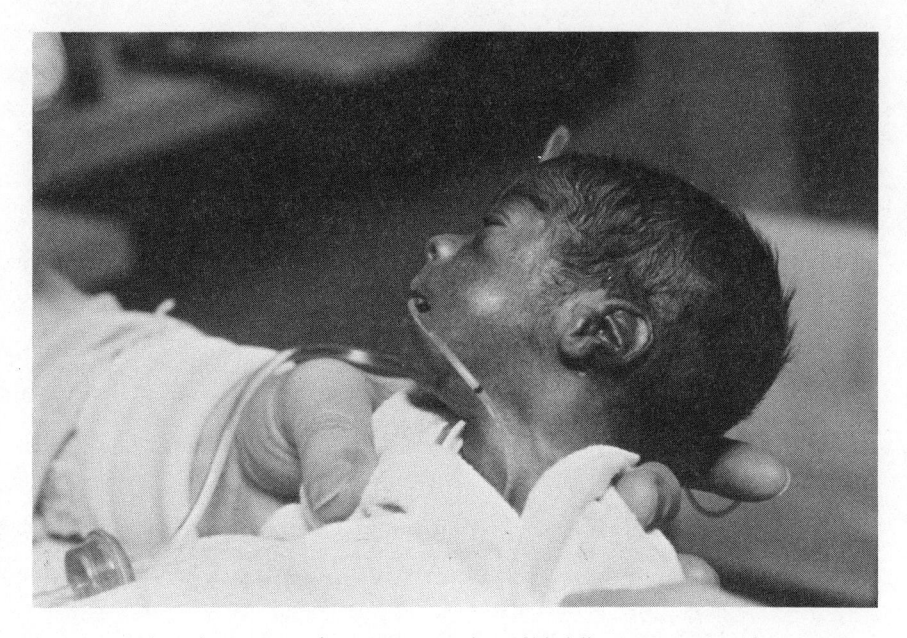

Fig. 5-3. An infant of 27 to 28 weeks gestation at 2 days of life following examiner's face and voice.

major CNS disturbance is generalized hypotonia. Frequently, the medical history will demonstrate hypoxic-ischemic episode, intracranial hemorrhage, meningitis, or recurrent hypoglycemia. Hypotonia of a secondary nature may be seen in congestive heart failure and sepsis. In these latter cases, improved tone may be obtained with manipulation. When hypotonia is marked on one side more than another, deep tendon reflexes may be absent and ankle clonus may be present.

The evolution of motor motility and maturity is interesting. In infants of 26 to 28 weeks gestation, limb jitteriness is commonly seen in the supine extended position as movement is attempted. Hand-to-face activity and sudden extension are common. Movements tend to be cogwheel-like and jerky with overshooting of target. Uncoordination between arm and leg movements is obvious. As maturity progresses, cogwheel-like movements and overshooting decrease. Smooth movements with small arc angles appear more frequently. Sudden tonus changes decrease. Disorganized mobility is apparent primarily in active and crying states, sometimes in sleep states, and when positioned in supine, extended positions. Arm-leg coordination in alert states and froglike posture in sleep is present.

By 36 weeks gestation, many premature infants have spontaneous, organized postures with flexion, arm-leg coordination with manipulation, and smooth movements with 45- to 60-degree arcs much of the time. These infants can often maintain smooth movements in supine, extended positions. Modulated tonus changes are apparent. If any disorganized, jerky movements occur, they are usually isolated to upper extremities.

The small premature infant who has had prolonged respiratory illness frequently is delayed or uneven in motor progression.

Table 5-2. Categories of adaptive and maladaptive mothering behaviors*

	Adaptive	Maladaptive
Feeding behaviors	Offers appropriate amounts and/or types of food to infant.	Provides inadequate types or amounts of food for infant.
	Holds infant in comfortable position during feeding.	Does not hold infant, or holds in uncomfortable position during feeding.
	Burps baby during and/or after feeding.	Does not burp infant.
	Prepares food appropriately.	Prepares food inappropriately.
	Offers food at comfortable pace for infant.	Offers food at pace too rapid or slow for infant's comfort.
Infant stimulation	Provides appropriate verbal stimulation for infant during visit.	Provides no or only aggressive verbal stimulation for infant during visit.
	Provides tactile stimulation for infant at times other than during feeding or moving infant away from danger.	Does not provide tactile stimulation or only that of aggressive handling of infant.
	Provides age-appropriate toys.	No evidence of age-appropriate toys.
	Interacts with infant in a way that provides for infant's satisfaction.	Frustrates infant during interactions.
Infant rest	Provides quiet or relaxed environment for infant's rest, including scheduled rest periods.	Does not provide quiet environment or consistent schedule for rest periods.
	Ensures that infant's needs for food, warmth, and/or dryness are met before sleep.	Does not attend to infant's needs for food, warmth, and/or dryness before sleep.
Perception	Demonstrates realistic perception of infant's condition in accordance with medical and/or nursing diagnosis.	Shows unrealistic perception of infant's condition.
	Has realistic expectations of infant.	Demonstrates unrealistic expectations of infant.
	Recognizes infant's unfolding skills or behavior.	Has no awareness of infant's development.
	Shows realistic perception of own mothering behavior.	Shows unrealistic perception of own mothering.
Initiative	Shows initiative in attempts to manage infant's problems, including actively seeking information about infants.	Shows no initiative in attempts to meet infant's needs or to manage problems. Does not follow through with plans.
Recreation	Provides positive outlets for own recreation or relaxation.	Does not provide positive outlets for own recreation or relaxation.
Interaction with other children	Demonstrates positive interaction with other children in home.	Demonstrates hostile-aggressive interaction with other children in home.
Mothering role	Expresses satisfaction with mothering.	Expresses dissatisfaction with mothering.

*Adapted from Harrison, L.: Nursing intervention with the failure-to-thrive family, Am. J. Maternal Child Nurs. 1:111, 1976. Copyright March/April 1976, the American Journal of Nursing Company. Reproduced with permission from MCN, The American Journal of Maternal Child Nursing, vol. 1, No. 2.

Usually the disappearance of tremors, jitteriness, and sudden startles is prolonged. Hypertonia appears to progress rapidly, and the infant gives the impression of being hypertonic at rest. We have found that this hypertonia/hypertensive responsiveness becomes less evident as a warm, loving care-giver assumes 24-hour care. This transient state has been observed in premature infants by others.[24] Although the etiology is unclear, we are investigating the effects of repetitive, long-term vestibular stimulation on its occurrence. In these infants, it should be remembered that carefully controlled and not intense stimulus is most effective. Response characteristics to such stimuli depend in considerable part on parameters and sequence of stimuli as well as posturing state of the infant.[14]

Rhythms. Sleep/wake cycles, spontaneous cry, and spontaneous suck behaviors are part of the infant's rhythmic pattern and are often overlooked during assessment. In severely injured infants, these basic rhythms may be significantly altered and may be a cue to possible adaptation problems after discharge. We have found that behavior modification and environmental controls can facilitate and enhance such an infant's adaptation to new situations. Such interventions have been particularly useful at discharge from hospital to home.

Care-giver–infant interaction. Feeding is an excellent source of data collection for care-giver–infant behavioral interactions (Table 5-2). Sensitivity to stress, infant satiation and distress cues, fostering of growth through visual, tactile, auditory, and kinesthetic stimulation, and alleviation of distress techniques can be evaluated. Reciprocal infant behaviors are also easily evaluated (Table 5-3). They include pre-

Table 5-3. Categories of adaptive and maladaptive infant behaviors*

	Adaptive	Maladaptive
Sleeping behavior	Receives adequate sleep for normal growth—at least 16 hours per day—without restless sleep patterns or prolonged crying at nap or bedtime after other needs have been met.	Receives inadequate sleep for normal growth—less than 16 hours per day. Shows restless sleep patterns and/or prolonged crying at nap or bedtime.
Feeding behavior	Actively seeks food offered. Effectively sucks and swallows food. Demonstrates pleasurable relief after eating.	Resists food offered. Does not suck effectively. Remains fussy after adequate amount of feeding—no pleasurable relief.
Response to environment	Demonstrates active response to environment by exploring or reaching-out behavior.	Seems apathetic to environment.
Vocalizing	Demonstrates vocalizations when alert, if developmentally ready.	Makes infrequent or no vocalizations during visit although developmentally ready.
Smiling	Demonstrates smiling behavior if older than 2 months.	Does not demonstrate smiling behavior during visit.
Cuddling	Cuddles when held.	Resists being held or stiffens when held.

*Adapted from Harrison, L.: Nursing intervention with the failure-to-thrive family, Am. J. Maternal Child Nurs. **1:**111, 1976. Copyright March/April 1976, the American Journal of Nursing Company. Reproduced with permission from MCN, The American Journal of Maternal Child Nursing, vol. 1, No. 2.

feeding arousal level, approach and attachment behaviors, cues to satiation or distress, responses to mother, and success in achieving task. Attention should be paid to how mother and infant "read" each other and who is in charge.

NURSING INTERVENTIONS: PRINCIPLES

While it is not my intent to explore the topic of interventions, specific principles merit comment. Any therapeutic program of interventions must be developed with the care-giver. Success can be enhanced by recognizing:

1. The family is the most economical and effective agent for fostering and sustaining an infant's neuromotor development.
2. Care-givers (the family) are effective motivators. Their responsiveness provides the infant with an incentive to achieve goals.
3. Enduring effects are most evident when parental involvement occurs in early infancy.
4. Promoting parental understanding of their infant's uniqueness and enhancing interactional processes are valuable by-products of parental participation in the setting of goals and planning of interventions. Parental roles in facilitating infant development have been ignored by health care professionals for too long.

Interventions should be based on the physiologic and developmental status of the infant. Piaget demonstrated that each stage of development is the basis for the next level.[26] The nurse-practitioner uses behavioral continuums in conjunction with existing infant behaviors to reinforce appropriate responses, to inhibit inappropriate responses, and to facilitate new behaviors. For instance, infants of 28 weeks gestation benefit from vestibular stimulation. It enhances CNS integration, neuromuscular coordination, and limbic system maturation; thus fostering the infant's ability to deal with the earth's gravitational pull.[16]

Infant activity programs have four basic objectives:

1. To inhibit abnormal response patterns, such as inversion until relaxation and fetal/flexion posturing for the hypertonic infant.
2. To enhance development of neuroassociation circuits, such as stimulating sucking activities during gavage feeding.
3. To facilitate appropriate responses, such as alerting and toning exercises for hypotonic infants.
4. To foster an appropriate sensory environment, such as waking premature infants only when they are in active sleep and not in quiet sleep[12] and reducing random light touch experiences for premature infants by providing repetitive, gentle firm touch experiences.

Successful activity programs utilize a variety of interventions. In neonatal nurseries, stimulation programs consist of temporally regulated, low-frequency, repetitive movements[16] and sounds,[21] age-appropriate visual configurations and colors,[15] and sensorimotor exercises.[9]

Finally, interventions should demonstrate complete learning loops. The infant is prepared for success, actively participates in the response, and is positively reinforced for the accomplishment. An example is the premature infant who is alerted before responsiveness to visual stimulation; the stimuli is placed within visual range and responds to the infant's gaze (Fig. 5-4). This activity is one that, when paired with auditory stimuli, is effective with even the youngest, viable age, infant.

Developmental profile of the neonate 83

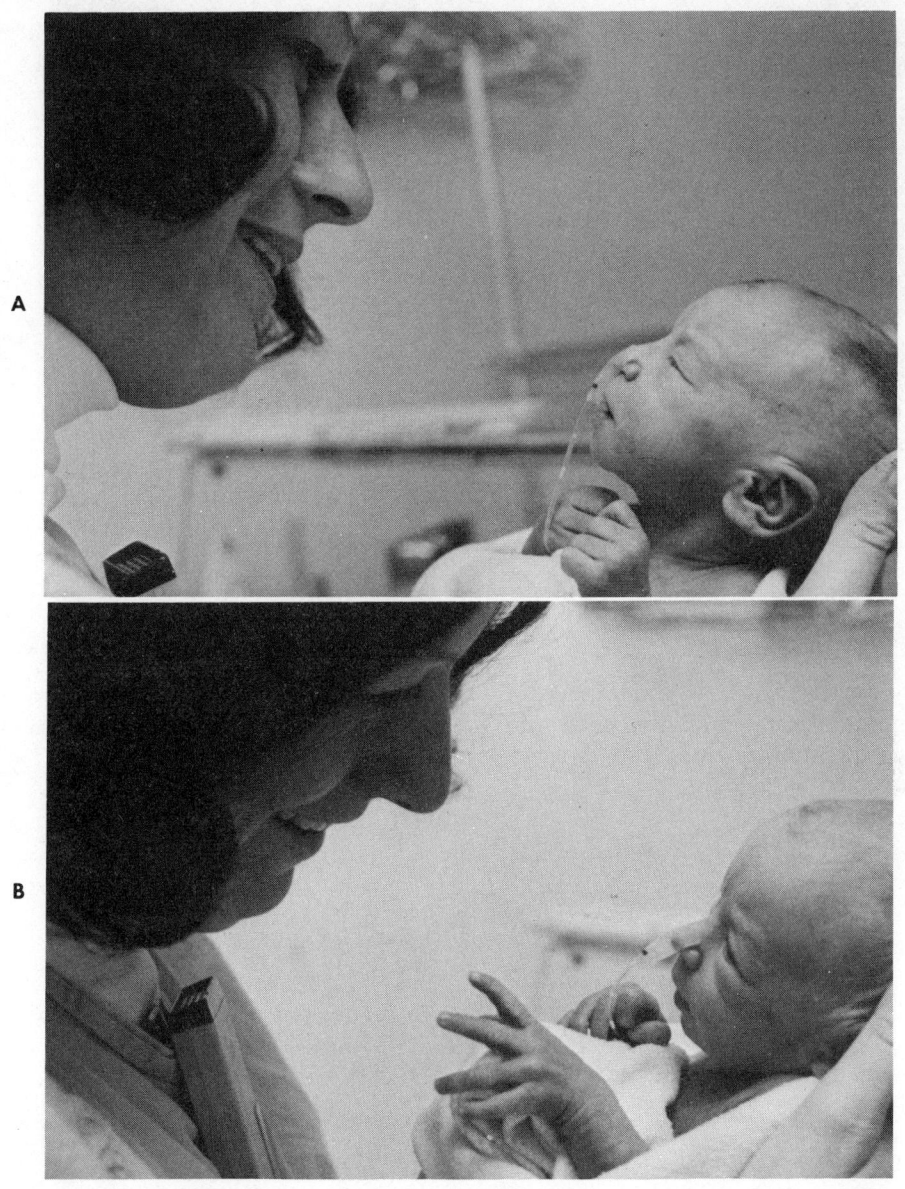

Continued.

Fig. 5-4. Alertness and responsiveness to animate and visual stimuli placed within the visual range of an infant of 32 weeks gestation at 2 days of life.

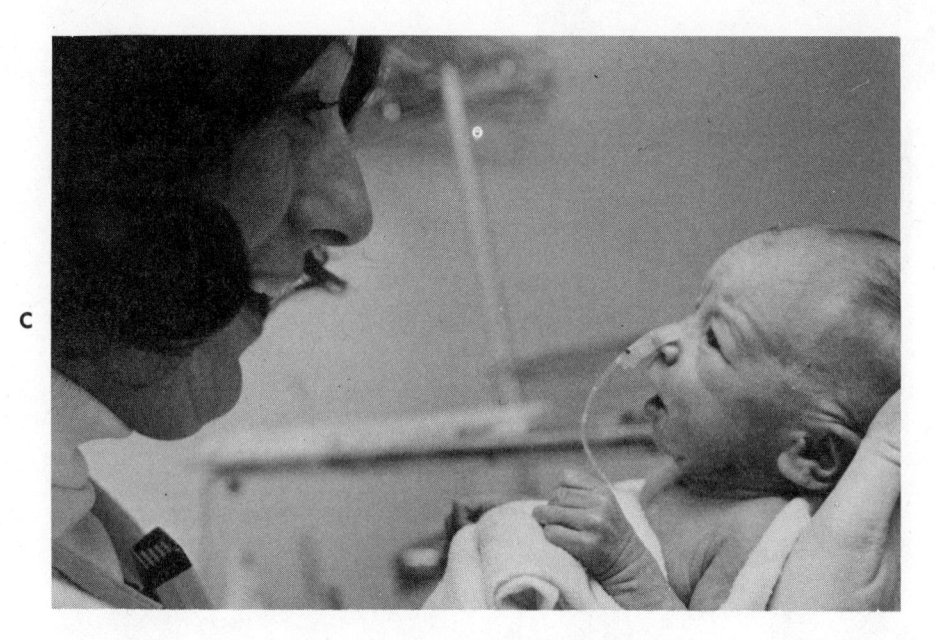

Fig. 5-4, cont'd. For legend see p. 83.

SUMMARY

Early identification of developmental behaviors enables families and infants to engage in therapeutic practices through quality of their interaction and maximal use of the health care system and its resources. Caution must be exercised by nurse-practitioners in prediction of permanent behavioral patterns and in preparing of intervention programs for premature infants. Overzealousness can lead to detrimental effects. More investigation is needed. The nursing profession can no longer afford to waste precious time and potential of its clients.

REFERENCES

1. Amiel-Tison, C.: Standardizing the physical examination during the first year. In Gluck, L., editor: Intrauterine asphyxia and the developing fetal brain, Chicago, 1977, Year Book Medical Publishers, Inc.
2. Bernard, K.: Report: the first four trimesters of life, presented at the University of Washington, Seattle, May 4-6, 1975.
3. Bobath, K.: The motor deficit in patients with cerebral palsy, Clinics in Developmental Medicine No. 23, England, 1966, Lavenham Press.
4. Bowlby, J.: Deprivation of maternal care, New York, 1966, Scholken Books.
5. Brazelton, T.: Neonatal behavioral assessment scale, Clinics in Developmental Medicine No. 50, England, 1973, Spastics Intenational Medical Publications.
6. Brazie, J. V., and Lubchenco, L. O.: Assessment of gestational age. In Kempe, C. H., Silver, H. K., and O'Brien, D., editors: Current pediatric diagnosis and treatment, ed. 3, Los Altos, Calif., 1974, Lange Medical Publications.
7. Broussard, E., and Hartner, M. S.: Further considerations regarding maternal perception of the first born. In Hellmuth, J., editor: Exceptional infant, vol. 2, New York, 1971, Brunner/Mazel, Inc.
8. Buerger, E. M.: Neuromotor development; assessment and implications. In Currie, J., and Pepper, K., editors: Mental retardation nursing approaches to care, St. Louis, 1978, The C. V. Mosby Co.
9. Buerger, E. M.: Unpublished data, 1976.

10. Carter, R. E., and Campbell, S. K.: Early neuromuscular development of the premature infant, Phys. Ther. 55(12):1333-1341, 1975.
11. Dargassies, S. S. A.: Part V: Neurological maturation of the premature infant of 28 to 41 weeks gestational age. In Falkner, F., editor: Human development, Philadelphia, 1966, W. B. Saunders Co.
12. Eastman, V.: The effects of environmentally induced influences on the neurological maturation and weight gain of premature infants, unpublished masters thesis, Loma Linda, Calif., 1978, Loma Linda University.
13. Fiorentino, M. R.: Normal and abnormal development, Springfield, Ill., 1972, Charles C Thomas, Publisher.
14. Graziani, L. J., and Korberly, B.: Limitations of neurologic and behavioral assessments in the newborn infant. In Gluck, L., editor: Intrauterine asphyxia and the developing fetal brain, Chicago, 1977, Year Book Medical Publishers, Inc.
15. Kennel, J., and Klaus, M.: Care of the mother of the high-risk infant, Clin. Obstet. Gynecol. 14:926-935, 1971.
16. Neal, M.: Relationships between vestibular stimulation and the developmental behavior of the premature infant, unpublished doctoral dissertation, 1967, New York University.
17. Netter, F.: Ciba collecton of medical illustrations, vol. 1: Nervous system, New York, 1962, CIBA.
18. Peiper, A.: Cerebral function in infancy and childhood, New York, 1963, Consultant's Bureau.
19. Prechtl, H., and Beintema, D.: The neurological examination of the full-term newborn infant, Clinics in developmental medicine, no. 12, Philadelphia, 1975, J. B. Lippincott Co.
20. Segall, M.: Cardiac responsivity of auditory stimulation in premature infants, Nurs. Res. 21:15-18, 1972.
21. Tronick, E., et al.: Clinical uses of the Brazelton Neonatal Behavior Assessment. In Friedlander, B. Z., et al., editors: The exceptional infant: assessment and intervention, vol. III, New York, 1975, Bruner Mazel, Inc.
22. Scharr, S.: Effects of early stimulation on birth weight, paper presented at American Public Health Association, Minneapolis, October 14, 1971.
23. Swyer, P. R.: The organization of perinatal care with particular reference to the newborn. In Avery, G., editor: Neonatology, physiology and management of the newborn, Philadelphia, 1977, J. B. Lippincott Co.
24. Volpe, J. J.: Neurological disorders. In Avery, G., editor: Neonatology, physiology and management of the newborn, Philadelphia, 1977, J. B. Lippincott Co.
25. Wadsworth, D.: Piaget's theory of cognitive development, New York, 1971, David McKay Co., Inc.
26. Werner, E., Bierman, J., and French, F.: The children of Kauai; a longitudinal study from the perinatal period to age ten, Honolulu, 1971, University of Hawaii Press.

CHAPTER 6

The TORCH syndrome of perinatal infection

Aarolyn M. Visintine and André J. Nahmias

Since first proposed in 1971,[13] the acronym TORCH (*T*oxoplasma, *O*ther, *R*ubella virus, *C*ytomegalovirus and *H*erpes simplex viruses) has gained wide acceptance and usage among physicians and nurses. One of the main reasons is that it has focused on a group of agents that can infect the fetus and/or newborn, comprising an important cause of mortality and of significant damage that may not be appreciated until later childhood. Furthermore, it calls attention to the need for uncovering still other agents that might be associated with similar ill effects on the quality of life.

Recognition of the clinical spectrum and identification of the known causative agents initially progressed slowly and were the result of contributions from different parts of the world. It is of some historic interest that the association of three of the agents with perinatal disease was first made by ophthalmologists, emphasizing the importance of clinical observations. Thus, in the case of toxoplasmosis,[16] a Czechoslovakian ophthalmologist, Janku, first described, in 1923, parasitic cysts in the retina of an 11-month-old infant with congenital hydrocephalus and microophthalmia. Five years later, the French microbiologist, Levaditi, suggested a possible connection between congenital hydrocephalus and toxoplasmosis. In 1937, a case of neonatal encephalitis was reported by American workers and the cause was later identified as *Toxoplasma*. Following these initial reports and aided greatly by the development of serologic tests, the wide spectrum of infection with *Toxoplasma,* from subclinical to fatal, became recognized.

Similarly, in the case of herpes simplex virus,[10] an Italian ophthalmologist, Batignani, first recorded, in 1934, the case of a newborn with keratitis from which the herpes virus, identified two decades earlier by German workers, was recovered. In 1935, the American pathologist, Hass, described the histopathologic findings in a fatal case of neonatal disseminated infection. As sporadic cases were reported from around the world during the following four decades, the wide clinical spectrum of neonatal herpetic disease was also appreciated. The differentiation of herpes simplex viruses into two types, HSV-1 and HSV-2, by the German scientist, Schneweis, provided the means for American pediatricians to demonstrate that most neonatal infections were acquired from a maternal genital herpetic infection near the time of delivery.

The association of the rubella virus[1] with cataracts and congenital heart disease was first made by an Australian ophthalmologist, Gregg, in 1941. It took another two decades, however, before American virologists isolated the rubella virus in the laboratory. In 1964, when a major rubella epidemic occurred in many parts of the world, these newly available virologic and serologic techniques permitted detailed study of that epidemic and a definition of the "expanded rubella syndrome" with its multiple organ involvement and sequelae in congenitally infected infants.

The history of cytomegalovirus (CMV)[5] has both older and newer aspects than that

Table 6-1. Summary of outcome and clinical findings that may be associated with TORCH agent infection

Condition	T	R	C	H
Abortion and stillbirth	+	+	+	+
Prematurity and/or intrauterine growth retardation	+	+	+	+
Normal-appearing; infection in first month of life	+	+	+	+
Constitutional signs				
Fever, lethargy, poor feeding	+	+	+	+
Skin				
Petechiae	+	+	+	+
Purpura	+	+	+	+
Vesicles, ulcers	0	0	+	+
Pulmonary				
Pneumonia	+	+	+	+
Reticuloendothelial system				
Hepatosplenomegaly	+	+	+	+
Liver calcification	+	0	+	+
Jaundice	+	+	+	+
Hemolytic and other anemias	+	+	+	+
Thrombocytopenia	+	+	+	+
Immunologic, humoral, and/or cell-mediated deficiencies	+	+	+	?
Cardiac				
Myocarditis	+	+	+	+
Congenital cardiac defects	0	+	+	0
Bone lesions				
Metaphysitis	+	+	+	+
CNS				
Encephalitis	+	+	+	+
Microcephaly	+	+	+	+
Hydrocephalus	+	+	+	+
Intracranial calcifications	+	+	+	+
Hearing deficits	+	+	+	+
Eyes				
Retinopathies (chorioretinitis or pigmented retina)	+	+	+	+
Microophthalmia	+	+	+	+
Keratoconjunctivitis	0	0	0	+
Cataracts	0	+	+	+
Glaucoma	0	+	0	0

Since the original compilation,[9] newer findings have expanded some of the similarities.

of the other three agents. The large inclusion-bearing cells, which give the virus its name, were first observed in the kidneys of a stillborn infant by a German pathologist, Ribbert, in 1881. Similar inclusions were later demonstrated in salivary glands of infants, so that the infection was called *salivary gland disease*. When the virus was identified by American virologists in 1956, the concept that the infection was almost always associated with overt clinical disease was proved erroneous in that the large majority of intrauterine-acquired infections was found to be subclinical in the neonatal period. It has only become appreciated recently that some of these asymptomatic cases go on to develop sequelae and that many infants can also become infected from a maternal cervical CMV infection, breast milk, or blood transfusions.

About 10 years ago, a group at Emory University and the Center for Disease Control, working on perinatal problems, realized that there was a large number of clinical and epidemiologic similarities among these agents (Tables 6-1 and 6-2). Only by specific laboratory tests, not routinely available in hospital laboratories (such as tests for syphilis or other bacteria), could these infections be most often differentiated from each other and from other infectious or noninfectious conditions. Thus, TORCH was born.

In the following sections, we discuss various aspects of each of the known TORCH agents, first in women before and during pregnancy, then in the fetus and newborn. More detailed information on these perinatal infections can be obtained in several recent publications.* We will end by briefly discussing the "O" in the complex, whose aspects particularly related to birth defects have been recently reviewed elsewhere.[11]

TORCH INFECTIONS BEFORE PREGNANCY

Of the various TORCH agents, rubella has provided the best example of what might be accomplished in managing susceptible women *before* they become pregnant to prevent infection in their offspring. There is both a good serologic test (hemagglutination-inhibition, or HI) for detecting susceptible individuals and effective rubella vaccines for prevention. Yet, even today, many women, by the time they become pregnant, are still nonimmune (10-30%). In some cases, the women have not

---

*See references 2, 5, 6, 12, and 17.

Table 6-2. Route of transmission of TORCH agents to fetus and newborn

	From mother				From other sources		
			Postnatal			Postnatal	
Agent	Transplacental	Intrapartum	Breast milk	Other contact	Blood transfusion	Other infants[a]	Other adults[a]
Toxoplasma	++	0	0	0	?	0	0
Rubella virus	++	0	?	?	0	?	?
Cytomegalovirus	++	++	+	+	?	?	?
Herpes simplex virus	?	++	?	?	0	?	?

++ = most frequent route of transmission.
+ = less frequent route of transmission.
? = Infrequent or not well-documented.
0 = Unlikely, not reported.
[a]By indirect or direct contact.

developed immunity because they were not infected earlier by the wild virus (a history of rubella is not good enough to supplant serologic testing). Such women may have escaped becoming immunized, since routine vaccination of 12- to 15-month-old boys and girls in the United States did not begin until about 10 years ago. For such cases, there has been a recommendation for vaccination of adult women and at-risk groups of females, such as nurses, teachers, and doctors, who have been shown to be serologically negative and who are not pregnant or likely to become so for at least 3 months following vaccination (the rubella vaccine virus may potentially affect the fetus). To help ensure greater immunity by the time of pregnancy, some states, such as Massachusetts and Colorado, now require a premarital serologic test for rubella.

There are even more problems related to the other TORCH agents. First, there are as yet no available vaccines, although CMV and HSV vaccines are under current investigation. A second problem is that with both of these viral infections, antibodies in the pregnant woman may not prevent infection of the conceptus,[10,18] although such transplacentally acquired antibodies may favorably affect the clinical outcome of the baby. Until further definition of these basic issues, including the possible risk of transmission of CMV to hospital personnel who might become pregnant, large-scale serologic testing for these viruses cannot be routinely recommended at present. Similarly, the benefits of premarital serologic testing for *Toxoplasma,* as done for instance in Oregon, await evaluation.

TORCH INFECTIONS DURING PREGNANCY

The most important clue to a possible risk for a perinatal infection would be diagnosing the acute or persistent infection in the pregnant woman. Unfortunately, the TORCH agents most often cause either completely asymptomatic infections or clinical manifestations that are not specific enough for a definitive diagnosis without confirming laboratory testing.

Toxoplasmosis

Toxoplasmosis is a good example of an infection in the pregnant woman that is most often asymptomatic (about 90%) and whose symptomatology in clinically manifest cases is too nonspecific — fever, malaise, sore throat, headache, enlarged lymph nodes, or a picture compatible with mononucleosis that is heterophile-antibody negative.[16] The parasite is usually acquired from eating raw or undercooked meat; contact with cat feces has also been incriminated. A recent outbreak of toxoplasmosis occurred in several individuals, associated with a horse stable, presumably because of the cats in the stable. Blood transfusion has been infrequently implicated in transmitting toxoplasmosis. Avoidance of the exposures noted above during pregnancy might therefore be helpful.

Congenital toxoplasmosis is estimated to occur in about 1 in 1000 deliveries. Overall, the risk to the fetus of acquiring transplacentally-transmitted toxoplasmosis from a mother infected during pregnancy is about 35%.[4] Both the ability of the parasite to cross the placenta and the severity of the fetal infection are related to gestational age. Thus, toxoplasmosis acquired in the first trimester is less likely (approximately 15% risk) to be transmitted to the fetus, but if this occurs, the fetal infection most often results in severe clinical manifestations. On the other hand, an infection acquired by the mother in the third trimester is more likely to be transmitted to the fetus (approximately 65% risk), but the infection is usually mild or asymptomatic in the neonatal period.

Congenital infection almost never occurs in a pregnant women with *Toxoplasma* antibodies; there is only one report of two infected infants born sequentially to the same woman. The prevalence of antibodies in pregnant women will vary both geographically and by age.[16] Thus, in one American city, only 16% of 15- to 19-year-old pregnant women were seropositive, while half of the women over 35 years of age had antibodies in their serum.

If the diagnosis of toxoplasmosis is suspected during pregnancy, serum should be obtained as early in gestation as possible with a sequential serum obtained 10 to 20 days later. Paired sera should be tested *at the same time* to attempt to demonstrate a significant rise in antibody titers. A variety of assays have been used, including the indirect immunofluorescence, Sabin-Feldman dye test, and indirect hemagglutination. Enzyme-linked immunosorbent assays (ELISA) are under investigation, as is the value of IgM *Toxoplasma* antibody testing to indicate an acute infection.

Confirmation of the diagnosis in the pregnant woman leaves one with serious dilemmas. Until these problems are resolved, it is unlikely that the widescale screening of all pregnant women by such serologic tests, although theoretically possible, will be routinized. Regarding the possibility of a therapeutic abortion if toxoplasmosis is diagnosed in early gestation, one must balance the low risk referred to above of transmission to the fetus with the great likelihood that the infection will be severe if the fetus acquires the parasite. Careful interpretation of serologic results by experts in this area is mandatory, as abortion may otherwise be performed needlessly. An alternative approach, therapy with sulfadiazine and pyrimethamine, is not advisable in early gestation because of the potential teratogenic effect of the latter drug. In addition, the effectiveness of these drugs is not fully evaluated, although they might be considered in definite cases occurring in later gestation.[16]

Transmission of toxoplasmosis from a congenitally-infected infant to others has never been proved. However, routine precautions, such as careful handwashing, are suggested when handling blood or contaminated materials from patients with an active infection.

Rubella virus

The greatest risk to the fetus occurs when primary maternal rubella occurs during the first 12 weeks of gestation.[1,5] Both the pathologic potential and evidence of infection in the fetus decline with advancing gestation. When maternal rubella is acquired during the first 8 weeks of gestation, there is about a 50% risk of fetal infection and approximately 85% of such infants will have demonstrable defects. The fetal infection attack rate declines to 35% at 9 to 12 weeks gestation (with almost half developing defects), to about 10% during 13 to 24 weeks gestation (approximately 15% showing later defects).

Only half the women who experience primary rubella will be symptomatic with a rash and adenopathy. However, these manifestations can be caused by many other agents, such as enteroviruses. Therefore, if a pregnant woman has signs and symptoms compatible with the disease, it is important to obtain a serum within 3 days and a second serum 1 to 2 weeks later. In case of suspect exposure, the first serum must be obtained within 1 week and the second serum collected 3 to 4 weeks later. Both sera should ideally be tested for hemagglutinating inhibition (HI) at the same time and in the same laboratory, since there is variability between laboratories or even when the tests are done in the same laboratory at different times.

A fourfold risk in HI antibodies occurs

rapidly after illness, usually in about 2 weeks. However, on occasion interpretation of results obtained with HI tests is difficult, and assays for IgM antibodies, which reflect a primary infection, might be needed. For more detailed information in the interpretation of serologic tests for rubella, a manual from the Center for Disease Control is most helpful.[15]

Counseling the pregnant woman regarding abortion must be done, therefore, with as good laboratory evidence of current infection as possible, with full knowledge of the relative risks of the fetal infection in relation to gestation, and with regard to the pregnant woman and her consort's convictions and desires about the pregnancy. Such counseling is even more difficult in case of inadvertent administration of the rubella vaccine to a pregnant woman in early gestation, since the risk of the fetus being affected is very small.[8]

It would be helpful to prevent contact of the pregnant woman with suspect rubella from other pregnant women in outpatient clinics or hospital wards. As emphasized earlier, it is advisable to test hospital personnel serologically and to vaccinate them if they are seronegative and not likely to become pregnant within 3 months.

Cytomegalovirus

This virus can be isolated from about 10% of women during pregnancy.[19] The most common site of isolation is the cervix; the virus can also be recovered from the urine less commonly and from oral secretions least often. Similar rates of virus isolation have been observed in nonpregnant women of comparable age and socioeconomic status. However, during the first trimester the rate of isolation is only 1% to 2%, climbing to about 5% in the second trimester, and reaching approximately 10% in the last trimester. In the large majority of such cases, the infection appears to represent reactivation of the virus in a pregnant woman with prior CMV exposure rather than an initial CMV infection. Although such women possess antibodies, it is now well documented that intrauterine, intrapartum, or postnatal infections can be acquired by the conceptus.[18] Furthermore, sequential CMV infections in the same woman have been observed. So far, CMV infections in infants born to women with past CMV exposure prior to pregnancy have largely resulted in asymptomatic infections. Whether the cases of asymptomatic infections that later develop sequelae or whether those infants symptomatic at birth are born to mothers whose CMV infection has been acquired for the first time during pregnancy still remains to be determined conclusively. Similarly, although it might be expected that the infection acquired early in pregnancy is the most harmful to the fetus, the evidence is still much more tenuous as compared with that noted above for toxoplasmosis or rubella. It should be appreciated that by childbearing age about 80% of women in lower socioeconomic groups have already experienced a CMV infection, which is approximately twice the rate found in women of higher socioeconomic groups.[5]

CMV infection in the pregnant woman is only infrequently symptomatic. Occasionally, a heterophile antibody–negative mononucleosis syndrome can be diagnosed and confirmed virologically and serologically as a primary infection. In such cases, an amniocentesis might be performed, and if the virus is isolated from the amniotic fluid, an abortion may be considered.[3] Until further data become available, routine serologic screening during pregnancy is not recommended. However, in the situation of a pregnant woman known to be exposed to an individual with an active CMV infection, for example to CMV mononucleosis or to a congenitally infected baby, serologic testing might be performed to demonstrate a primary infection. Several tests, such as indirect hemagglutination, complement fixation, immunofluorescent, or enzyme-linked antibody assays, are available; their reliability depends greatly on the experience of the laboratory performing the particular assays. It should be appreciated that there are very limited data on which to base rational decisions and that, whenever possible, experts in this area should be consulted regarding the significance of laboratory tests and possible management.

The risk of transmission of CMV to personnel working with infected patients has not been clearly established.[21] Until further information becomes available, it would seem advisable that pregnant women (nurses, physicians, and other personnel) avoid caring for known patients with symptomatic CMV infection.

Herpes simplex viruses

HSV can affect external genital sites, for example, the vulva, and internal sites, for example, the cervix, being most frequently asymptomatic in the latter site. Such genital infections are caused most often by HSV-2, although about 10% of such infections may be caused by HSV-1, the type most usually associated with oral infections. With either virus type, a genital herpetic infection in a pregnant woman near the time of delivery presents a potential hazard to the infant because the most usual mode of acquisition of HSV by the newborn (at least 80% of cases) is during passage through the infected birth canal or by means of an ascending infection through a leak or tear in the amniotic membranes.[10] Introduction of the virus has been documented to occur also following internal fetal monitoring, in which case the initial lesions are noted at the monitor site. Although there are a few cases suggestive of transplacental transmission of HSV to the fetus, on the basis of currently available data, therapeutic abortion is not recommended for a woman detected to have genital or nongenital herpes in the first half of the pregnancy. There appears to be, however, an increased risk of spontaneous abortion in case of a primary genital infection.

The pregnant woman may develop a primary infection, that is, without previous exposure to either HSV-1 or HSV-2, or may have a recurrent HSV infection. In either case, the infection may be completely asymptomatic, although when clinically apparent, primary genital infections tend to be more severe—fever, pelvic pain, lymphadenopathy, and more extensive vesicles and ulcers. A primary genital infection tends to be of higher risk to the infant because of this more extensive involvement, often with cervical infection, and longer persistence of the virus—3 to 12 weeks. The severity of the infection may cause premature labor and delivery. In addition, the woman may not have developed antibodies that would be conveyed transplacentally to her baby and provide some protection. Although such antibodies are acquired by babies of mothers with recurrent genital herpes or even prior oral herpes, the antibodies are not fully protective and the baby can still develop a severe, if not fatal, infection. Because of the risk to the infant of maternal genital herpes, either primary or recurrent, it is advisable to consider delivering the baby by cesarean section if the viral infection is present at the time of delivery. Unfortunately, the genital infection is clinically evident in only one third of such cases, and about half the time, the baby is delivered prematurely. Because of the relatively infrequent likelihood of genital herpes at the time of delivery (1:200 to 1:2000 deliveries), it is not currently practical to test every pregnant woman. Serologic testing is not helpful; the best method is to culture the virus from the cervicovaginal area and from lesions when present (results can be obtained most usually in 1 to 4 days). A more rapid and readily available method, although not as sensitive as viral culture, is the Papanicolaou smear, which can demonstrate the cellular changes associated with herpetic infections.[14]

In view of the above problems, we have focused on a group of women with greater likelihood of having genital herpes at delivery. This includes: (1) women with genital herpes before pregnancy or during earlier pregnancy, (2) women whose sexual partner(s) has (have) a past history of genital herpes, and (3) women with herpetic lesions below the waist, since these are often associated with genital herpes that may be asymptomatic. It is recommended that such women be monitored virologically and/or cytologically at the following intervals: 32, 34, and 36 weeks and weekly thereafter. This would obviate performing a cesarean section on anyone with genital herpes in the past, since the likelihood of the virus being present at the time of delivery is small; aided by negative laboratory tests, an abdominal delivery would most usually be unnecessary. If the infection is documented to be present in the mother's genital tract near the time of delivery, a cesarean section performed before the membranes have ruptured or within 4 to 6 hours of rupture is likely to prevent almost all cases of neonatal infection acquired by this route. Some failures of this practice may occur in a case of an intrauterine infection, usually because of a leak in the membranes.

Because of the possibility of postnatal transmission from mothers with genital or oral herpes, it is advisable to prevent mothers from having intimate contact with their infants until their herpetic lesions have resolved and are virus free (as confirmed by culture or Papanicolaou smear). The mother should wear a gown and gloves if she insists on holding her infant or if she desires to breast-feed. In the latter case, it is important that there be no herpetic lesions on the breasts, as virus transmission from such sites has been recorded. If the mother has oral herpes, she should be instructed not to kiss the infant and to wear a mask.

Since person-to-person transmission of herpes occurs primarily by very close contact, personnel caring for patients with active herpes should wear gloves when handling the patient or contaminated articles or if they use suction catheters if the patient has oral herpes. It would be advisable to remove hospital personnel with active herpetic infections of the hands from direct patient care in the prenatal clinic, labor and delivery areas, as well as newborn nursery, until their lesions have healed. As discussed in detail elsewhere,[20] removal of hospital personnel with cold sores appears too stringent a general recommendation, particularly because of the lack of definitive evidence for such transmission to newborns and the high frequency of cold sores among personnel (about 1 per 100 per week).

TORCH INFECTIONS IN THE FETUS AND NEWBORN

The outcome of a pregnancy complicated by some, if not all, of the TORCH infections may be fetal death resulting from abortion or stillbirth, intrauterine growth retardation, or premature delivery. The conceptus may demonstrate various types of clinical manifestations or appear normal in the neonatal period but demonstrate sequelae, sometimes only on close follow-up examination, several months or years postnatally. It is worth pointing out that in case of twin or triplet births, one or all of the babies in the set may be infected.

With the exception of herpes simplex

viruses, TORCH infections are more often asymptomatic than clinically apparent. When the infections are symptomatic in the neonate, the clinical manifestations are usually indistinguishable, so that evaluation for all of the TORCH agents, and occasionally Others (see last section), must be performed simultaneously. Moreover, the most frequent presenting symptoms are often nonspecific, such as vomiting, lethargy, irritability, and jaundice, and bacterial infections, such as septicemia, meningitis, and congenital syphilis, must be excluded. In addition, infants with certain metabolic or hematologic disorders, as well as others of still unknown etiology, such as neonatal hepatitis, may initially demonstrate similar clinical findings.

The diagnosis of TORCH infection in the neonate depends on specialized laboratory tests. Conventional serologic assays are most usually not helpful for rapid diagnosis, since it is difficult to differentiate transplacentally acquired antibodies in the infant's serum from antibodies resulting from an active infection. Only if antibody titers are found to persist several months postnatally would such serologic tests be potentially helpful. Since serum IgM does not cross the placenta, finding IgM antibodies in an infant's serum to a specific agent would be much more helpful. However, these tests are only performed in research laboratories, some state health laboratories, and the Center for Disease Control.[13] Furthermore, there are several possible reasons for obtaining false positive results, and there are occasions when IgM antibodies are not detected even in the presence of an active infection.[6] The problems with using total serum IgM levels are possibly greater because there are too many cases of nonspecific elevated levels and too many instances of normal levels in infected babies for this commonly available assay to be helpful for routine screening. Whereas diagnosis of toxoplasmosis and rubella are most often made serologically, infection with CMV and HSV is best determined by identification of the virus rather than by serologic methods.

When confronted with the problem of making a diagnosis of TORCH infection in the individual infant, all available resources and testing facilities must be used. A specific diagnosis should be sought as quickly as possible in case therapy is possible for the infection and to prevent possible transmission of the agent to other infants or personnel. Moreover, the affected infant will require close follow-up for many years. Periodic examinations, including ophthalmologic, audiometric, neurologic, and psychomotor evaluations, are necessary. Corrective surgery, hearing aids, and other rehabilitation procedures may be required for some of the infants to restore them to as normal a life as possible.

Clinical aspects and suggested diagnostic evaluation and isolation procedures of TORCH infants are discussed in the following sections.

Toxoplasmosis

The classic triad of hydrocephalus, intracranial calcifications, and chorioretinitis in the neonate had, for many years, been the syndrome most usually associated with congenital toxoplasmosis. However, as more and more cases of this entity were described, it became apparent that there may be a variety of presenting manifestations: jaundice, hepatosplenomegaly, cerebrospinal fluid pleocytosis with a rising CSF protein, and seizure disorders being among the most common. Other findings are listed in Table 6-1. It should be reemphasized that about two thirds of infants with congenital toxoplasmosis have clinically inapparent infection at birth.

In the symptomatic infant or an infant whose mother had suspect or documented toxoplasmosis during pregnancy, it is helpful to obtain sera around the same time from both mother and infant, as well as cerebrospinal fluid from the infant. These specimens are best assayed simultaneously for specific IgM and IgG antibodies to *Toxoplasma* by the indirect immunofluorescence (IF) test. In addition, these specimens are tested for indirect hemagglutinating (IHA) antibodies to toxoplasma. Serial testing of such specimens, obtained at 10- to 14-day intervals, is usually necessary to confirm the diagnosis in an infant by demonstrating a significant rise in IHA or IF IgG antibodies. The diagnosis of toxoplasmosis in the infant may be more rapidly accomplished if IF IgM antibodies are elevated. However, IgM tests for toxoplasmosis may be falsely negative as a result of either the inability of the infant to produce such IgM or its binding to the parasite.[4] Interpretation of serologic results should be done in consultation with experts knowledgeable about the specific test procedures.

Isolation of the *Toxoplasma* organism requires inoculation of clinical specimens in laboratory animals and is not performed routinely for diagnosis. Identification of the parasite is also possible histopathologically from biopsy or autopsy specimens.

Although not conclusively demonstrated to be effective, particularly since the damage induced by the parasite might be irremediable, treatment with sulfadiazine, 50 to 100 mg/kg/day, orally, in two divided doses, and pyrimethamine, 1 mg/kg/day, orally, for 3 to 4 weeks, is the standard drug regimen. Folinic acid (Leucovorin calcium), 5 mg IM, is given twice weekly to help prevent the antifolic effects of pyrimethamine, such as thrombocytopenia or leukopenia. In progressive disease, more than one course of therapy may be advisable during the first year of life. Strict isolation is usually not necessary once the diagnosis has been confirmed; careful handwashing should, however, be continued.

Rubella

Congenital rubella is a chronic viral infection that may involve one or many organ systems.[1,5] The pathologic potential of the infection continues throughout infancy and even later childhood because of this chronicity. Only about one third of neonates will show symptomatic involvement of one or more organs. The infants classically exhibit jaundice, hepatosplenomegaly, cardiac malformations with incipient or acute heart failure, purpura, neurologic involvement, such as seizures or microcephaly, and cataracts or other ocular findings. Other affected infants will only become symptomatic or have detectable abnormalities, such as hearing loss, psychomotor and language delays, or retinopathy later in infancy or childhood.

The most commonly used diagnostic assay has been the hemagglutination-inhibition test. Paired sera from mother and infant are obtained, and repeat testing is performed at 3 and 6 months of age for HI antibodies. A persistent high titer of HI antibodies in the infant's serum as compared with the mother's serum, above and beyond the level of passively received transplacental antibody, will support the diagnosis of congenital rubella. For more rapid diagnosis, the detection of specific rubella IgM antibody in the newborn period is most useful. Virus isolation from clinical specimens, such as throat or urine, is a difficult procedure that is not used for routine purposes.

Treatment at present consists only of supportive management and surgical correction of certain defects, such as cardiac anomalies. The infant should be kept in isolation while in the hospital, and pregnant women must not handle infected babies since they continue to shed the rubella virus from tears, saliva, and other secretions for many months or years.

Cytomegalovirus

It appears that, at least in lower socioeconomic populations, less than 5% of cases of intrauterine-acquired CMV are symptomatic in the neonatal period. Thrombocytopenia with petechiae, jaundice, hepatosplenomegaly, chorioretinitis, and microcephaly with intracranial calcifications were at one time considered hallmarks of the disease and may indeed be the presenting manifestations.[5] However, these and other clinical or laboratory findings may be apparent with infections by any of the TORCH agents (Table 6-1).

In asymptomatic, intrauterine-acquired CMV infection, the persistence of virus in the urine and other sites for several months or years suggests a potential for continuing damage to various organs. Hearing deficits, as well as psychomotor dysfunctions, may be a later sequelae of these silent infections.

Intrapartum-acquired cytomegalovirus infection (from an infected maternal cervix) or postpartum acquired infection (for example, from infected breast milk) is also most often asymptomatic. However, interstitial pneumonitis, occurring between 6 and 12 weeks of age has been suggestively associated with intrapartum CMV acquisition, but further studies are needed to delineate sequelae of such infections. A few cases of symptomatic disease have also been associated with blood transfusion.

When cytomegalovirus infection is suspected in the neonate, several laboratory aids may be used. A rapid presumptive diagnosis can be obtained within 30 minutes by examining urines by electron microscopy using the pseudoreplica technique.[7] In close to 90% of cases of intrauterine-acquired CMV infection, viral particles could be detected by this method. Inclusion-bearing cells may also be shed into the urine intermittently and can be detected cytologically in freshly voided specimens. It is necessary to examine at least three separate urines; but even so, in only about a third of the cases can the diagnosis be made. Although more definitive, isolation of CMV by inoculation of clinical specimens into tissue culture cells is slower, requiring several days or weeks. Serologic assays, including IgM antibody testing, are not as reliable as viral identification.

Treatment for transplacentally acquired CMV infection is supportive. Although some antiviral durgs can suppress the virus transiently, clinical benefit from any such regimen has not been convincingly demonstrated. Infected infants should be followed to determine psychomotor, ocular, or hearing defects so that possible rehabilitating measures can be established early.

Symptomatic infants with intrauterine-acquired CMV infection are best cared for in isolation. Pregnant personnel should be cautioned not to handle such infants who may shed the virus for prolonged periods.

Herpes simplex viruses

In contrast to the other TORCH agents, herpes simplex viruses are almost always responsible for symptomatic illness in the neonate, although the diagnosis is often missed clinically.[10] The disease may be manifest at any time from birth to 5 weeks of age. Although visible signs such as skin vesicles, ulcers of the mouth, or ocular involvement (conjunctivitis, keratitis, chorioretinitis) eventually occur in about two thirds of all cases, they are the presenting manifestation only about one-half of the time. Disseminated herpes, which affects visceral organs such as the liver and adrenals (with or without central nervous system involvement), most often becomes apparent between 6 and 12 days of age and is heralded by nonspecific, constitutional symptoms such as anorexia, lethargy, vomiting, and fever or hypothermia. This fulminant form of the disease results in death, usually within a few weeks, in 80% of the cases. Disseminated disease occurs more frequently in infants, especially premature infants, who have received no transplacental antibodies to HSV because their mothers had a primary genital (less frequently oral) HSV infection at the time of delivery.

Neonatal herpetic infection can also be localized to the skin, eyes, mouth, or central nervous system alone or in combination, without visceral organ involvement. Such localized infections may occur even in the presence of transplacental-acquired antibodies. Thus, recurrent maternal genital HSV can cause severe and even fatal (in the case of localized CNS infection) disease in the infant. Survivors of neonatal herpes may experience skin recurrences, which are not of serious clinical consequence, at various sites on the body.

The diagnosis of neonatal HSV infection is more readily suspected if a history of genital herpes in the mother or her sexual partner(s) is obtained. Characteristic vesicular skin eruptions, sometimes consisting only of a single vesicle, should also alert the examiner to the possibility of a herpetic infection in the neonate. Ulcerations in the mouth should be searched for carefully, and a thorough examination of the eyes should be made initially by the primary physician, and as soon as practical by an ophthalmologist. Scrapings obtained from the base of vesicular lesions or ulcers, as well as conjunctival scrapings, may reveal characteristic intranuclear inclusions when examined cytologically. Electron microscopy may detect herpesvirus particles in vesicle fluid, tears, oral secretions, and cerebrospinal fluid. The virus can be readily grown (usually in 1 to 4 days) in tissue culture cells from swabs of the conjunctiva, mouth, or vesicular fluid, or from urine, blood, and CSF.

Serologic assays are only helpful in determining whether the infant has acquired transplacental antibodies if the mother's infection was not a primary one. IgM antibodies to HSV are most often not detectable in the infant's serum until 2 to 3 weeks after birth and so are not usually helpful for diagnosing an infection early.

The most difficult diagnostic situation occurs in the neonate, without external visible lesions, who develops seizures and progressive meningoencephalitis, characterized by a relative lymphocytosis and, usually, elevated CSF protein. Besides herpes as a possible cause, such a clinical pattern may be associated with toxoplasmosis, CMV, and other viruses (for example, enterovirus), as well as bacterial or noninfectious viruses. Thus, evaluation for the several possible etiologies must be performed simultaneously and as rapidly as possible. An epidemiologic history of genital herpes in one or both parents, as well as cervical cultures from the mother, may assist in suspecting a herpetic etiology. Confirmation may be obtained by culturing the virus in the baby from such sites as the mouth, urine, or CSF. A brain biopsy may be necessary to establish a diagnosis of neonatal herpes encephalitis when visible herpetic stigmata are absent and other causes of CNS involvement have been ruled out.

Idoxuridine and adenine arabinoside are now well-documented as being helpful in the treatment of herpetic infections of the cornea and conjunctiva. Systemic therapy with idoxuridine or cytosine arabinoside has not been shown to be effective in the neonate with severe HSV infection, and both drugs are associated with toxic side effects such as bone marrow suppression, which mitigates against their use in the neonate. Clinical control trials of systemically administered adenine arabinoside are ongoing but are as yet incomplete. Several therapeutic modalities such as gamma globulin, exchange blood transfusions, transfer factor, and interferon have been used in a few cases of neonatal herpes. However, their benefit cannot be evaluated since no controlled studies were performed.

THE "O" OF TORCH

We have found over the past decade that the well-recognized TORCH agents — *Toxoplasma,* rubella, cytomegalovirus, and herpes simplex viruses — account for only about 10% of the infants born each year with clinical features of the TORCH syndrome in whom other bacterial and noninfectious causes could also not be identified. When sought in babies with congenital malformations, these agents have been found to account for a very small number of cases. Yet major birth defects occur in at least 1% of all births, of which to date only a small percentage can be explained on any basis, whether genetic, chromosomal, or environmental. Can other infectious agents be involved then with either the TORCH syndrome or birth defects?

Several infectious agents have been suspected to cause fetal and neonatal disease.* Some, such as smallpox and vaccinia, which had occasionally been noted to be deleterious to the fetus and newborn, should no longer be considered a problem since smallpox has been eradicated and vaccinia stopped. Varicella-zoster virus has been found to affect the fetus or newborn in two ways. Infants whose mothers had varicella during early pregnancy may now have a syndrome consisting of limb deformities, cicatricial skin lesions, cortical atrophy,

---

*See references 2, 5, 6, 11, 12, and 17.

and ocular abnormalities.[22] Infants may also acquire the varicella-zoster virus from a mother who experiences onset of the virus within the last 5 days of pregnancy. The infants can then develop a severe, often fatal case of disseminated chickenpox. This might be prevented by administration of zoster immune globulin to the infants soon after birth. Hepatitis B has more recently been shown to be acquired late in pregnancy or at the time of delivery from mothers infected with the virus, most usually acutely, but occasionally if she is a chronic carrier. An asymptomatic infection can usually be demonstrated in the infant several months after birth, but such infants may also develop a mild to severe liver disease. The diagnosis of both varicella and hepatitis B infection can be easily made — the former by clinical evidence of chickenpox in the mother and the latter by Australian antigen (hepatitis B surface antigen) determinations available in most hospital laboratories.

Enteroviruses, particularly some of the coxsackie B and echoviruses, can sometimes infect the newborn. Among the spectrum of such infections is a disease occasionally resembling a disseminated neonatal herpetic infection. In these cases, there is involvement of several visceral organs, including the liver and heart, coagulopathies, and meningoencephalitic signs. Coxsackie B viruses have also been associated with congenital cardiac defects in unconfirmed reports. Similarly, unconfirmed studies have associated adenoviruses, influenza viruses, and mumps viruses with birth defects, the latter also with endocardial fibroelastosis.

The list of suspects can be extended to several other microbial agents, including newly discovered viruses.[5,6,11,12] There is also the possibility that there are still undiscovered agents that require unconventional methods, such as electron microscopy, to be identified. The known TORCH agents exemplify the problems that might be expected — the usually asymptomatic or undifferentiable infection in the pregnant woman, the wide spectrum of clinical involvement of the fetus and newborn, and the difficulties in their specific diagnosis. They have also taught us the value of careful clinical and epidemiologic observations, the potential of the application of different methods for laboratory diagnosis, and the possibilities for prevention and therapy. The next decade will hopefully help resolve some of the problems still existent with the old TORCH agents and open the way to uncovering other agents that can cause deleterious effects in the fetus and newborn.

REFERENCES

1. Alford, C.: Rubella. In Remington, J., and Klein, J., editors: Infectious diseases of the fetus and newborn infant, Philadelphia, 1976, W. B. Saunders Co.
2. Charles, D., and Finland, M.: Obstetric and perinatal infections, Philadelphia, 1973, Lea & Febiger.
3. Davis, L., Tweed, G., and Stewart, J.: Cytomegalovirus mononucleosis in a first trimester pregnant female with transmission to the fetus, Pediatrics **48:**200-206, 1971.
4. Desmonts, G., and Couvreur, J.: Toxoplasmosis: epidemiologic and serologic aspects of perinatal infection. In Krugman, S., and Gershon, A., editors: Infections of the fetus and newborn infant, Progress in Clinical and Biologic Research, vol. 3, New York, 1975, Alan R. Liss, Inc.
5. Hanshaw, J., and Dudgeon, J.: Viral diseases of the fetus and newborn, Philadelphia, 1978, W. B. Saunders Co.
6. Krugman, S., and Gershon, A.: Infection of the fetus and newborn infant, Progress in Clinical and Biological Research, vol. 3, New York, 1975, Alan R. Liss, Inc.
7. Lee, F. K., Nahmias, A. J., and Stagno, S.: Rapid diagnosis of cytomegalovirus infection in infants by electron microscopy, New Engl. J. Med. **299:**1266-1270, 1978.
8. Modlin, J. F., Herrmann, K. L., Brandling-Bennett, A. D., et al.: Risk of congenital abnormality after inadvertent rubella vaccination of pregnant women, New Engl. J. Med. **294:**972-974, 1976.
9. Nahmias, A.: The TORCH complex, Hosp. Prac. **9:**65-72, 1974.
10. Nahmias, A., and Visintine, A.: Herpes simplex. In Remington, J., and Klein, J., editors: Infectious diseases of the fetus and newborn infant, Philadelphia, 1976, W. B. Saunders Co.
11. Nahmias, A., and Visintine, A.: Role of infectious agents in birth defects — an overview of still unresolved problems. In Milunsky, A., editor: Hereditary disease, New York, Plenum Publishing Corp. In press.
12. Nahmias, A., Visintine, A., and Starr, S.: Viral infections of the fetus and newborn. In Drew, W., editor: Viral infections, Philadelphia, 1976, F. A. Davis Co.
13. Nahmias, A., Walls, K., Stewart, J., et al.: The TORCH complex, Hosp. Prac. **9:**65-72, 1974.
14. Naib, Z., Nahmias, A., Josey, W., et al.: Relation of cytohistopathology of genital herpesvirus infection to cervical anaplasia, Cancer Res. **33:**1452-1463, 1973.
15. Palmer, D., Cavallaro, J., and Herman, K.: Rubella hemagglutination-inhibition tests, Atlanta, Ga., 1977, U. S. Department of Health, Education and Welfare, Center for Disease Control.
16. Remington, J., and Desmonts, G.: Toxoplasmosis. In Remington, J., and Klein, J., editors: Infectious diseases of the fetus and newborn infant. Philadelphia, 1976, W. B. Saunders Co.
17. Remington, J., and Klein, J.: Infectious diseases of the fetus and newborn infant, Philadelphia, 1976, W. B. Saunders Co.
18. Reynolds, D., Stagno, S., Reynolds, R., et al.: Perinatal cytomegalovirus infection: influence of placentally transferred maternal antibody, J. Infect. Dis. **137:**564-567, 1978.
19. Stagno, S., Reynolds, D., Tsiantos, A., et al.: Cervical cytomegalovirus excretion in pregnant and nonpregnant women: suppression in early gestation, J. Infect. Dis. **131:**522-527, 1975.
20. Visintine, A., and Nahmias, A.: Genital herpes, Perinat. Care **2:**32-41, 1978.
21. Yaeger, A.: Longitudinal, serological cytomegalovirus infections in nurses and in personnel without patient contact, J. Clin. Microbiol. **2:**448-452, 1975.
22. Young, N.: Chickenpox, measles and mumps. In Remington, J., and Klein, J., editors: Infectious diseases of the fetus and newborn infant, Philadelphia, 1976, W. B. Saunders Co.

PART THREE

Problems of assault and battery

Only recently have problems of assault and battery commanded public attention. Therefore, few health professionals have had the opportunity to become sufficiently knowledgeable to deal with such situations. Elmer focuses on infant battery—specifically infant characteristics and other factors precipitating mistreatment, effects of abuse on the growing child, characteristics of infant abusers, clues to early detection, methods of treatment, preventive possibilities, and role of the health care practitioner. An index of suspicion for identifying potentially high risk parents is included.

Star discusses similar problems as they relate to battered women. The incidence of women who are physically assaulted is underreported and underestimated and, therefore, not adequately dealt with on a local, state, or national level. Issues such as the "why" of wife beating, the natural assaults and injuries, the dynamics of abuse, fears of battered women, and guidelines for helping battered women are clearly delineated. Also included is a Battered Women's Change Potential Scale.

Awareness of the plight of the sexual assault victim is also relatively recent. Bemmann and Bundy describe the human crisis of sexual assault as it relates to pain, trauma, and disruption caused in the personal, psychologic, physical, sexual, family, and social aspects of a woman's life. Few situations demand as much sensitivity and multidisciplinary knowledge from health professionals, advocate workers, and the judicial system as does sexual assault.

CHAPTER 7

Infant battery

Elizabeth Elmer

INTRODUCTION

Less than 20 years ago. the term *battered child* was invented for a child who had been physically attacked by his or her adult caretaker.[37] Several papers concerning mistreated children had previously appeared in the literature, [8,14,66,79] but it took Kempe's phrase to arouse a "blinkered world."[65] On behalf of abused children, a stirring began that was ultimately to result in universal state laws mandating the reporting of suspected abuse, the establishment in many states of central registries to store information related to reports, and a general strengthening of child protection agencies in the United States. The National Center for Child Abuse and Neglect was established by Congress in 1974 and charged with various duties related to the study, treatment, and prevention of child abuse.

Partly as a result of these activities, which led to increased public and professional awareness of child abuse, reports of abused and/or neglected children have soared, and authorities now estimate that upwards of one million children may be abused or grossly neglected each year in the United States.[23,51] Whether the number of incidents of abuse is actually growing or whether the apparent increase is a result of more efficient reporting is moot. The important fact is that we have discovered *private* violence in the United States as contrasted with public violence, of which we have long been aware.

Despite mandated reporting in the United States, statistics concerning abuse tend to be unreliable for many reasons. Prominent among these is the lack of agreement as to definitions, lack of uniformity among the states concerning the upper age limit of childhood, differences as to who must report, and reluctance on the part of many professionals to report their suspicions. Nevertheless, we do know that abuse may strike children of all ages, including babies.

This chapter will focus on abused infants—baby characteristics that appear to touch off mistreatment, effects of abuse on the growing child, characteristics of infant abusers, precipitating factors, clues to early detection, methods of treatment, preventive possibilities, and role of the nurse. In this chapter, *infant battery* applies to babies under 24 months of age who manifest nonaccidental injuries, that is, injuries at variance with the history, or injuries that the caretaker admits inflicting. The lesions may be significant, for example, subdural hematoma, or they may appear relatively minor, for example, bruises. It should be noted that the significance of the injury bears little relationship to the degree of risk for the child.

Professionals and nonprofessionals alike deplore the willful injury of helpless babies and find it hard to deal objectively with abusing parents. Natural recoil from the abusive behavior, however, should not obscure the complexity of the issue. There is no prototype of the abused child just as there is no single model of the abusive parent. As noted by Scott,[65] child abuse is a range of syndromes, not just one, and the abuse of children describes behavior, not a clinical entity. Similarly, the precipitating causes as well as the effects on the child may show great variation. This chapter will present current thinking and also gaps in knowledge.

THE INFANTS

The true incidence of infant battery is open to question. When child abuse was first "discovered," it was thought that infants comprised the largest single group of abused children. This was probably because hospitalized infants provided the initial means of identifying the phenomenon and also because personnel in institutions other than hospitals, for example, schools, were slow to accept the possibility of abuse and slow to report suspicious cases. Nationwide figures now available indicate that age groupings of abused children are roughly the same in size.[1] Infant battery, however, continues to command attention by virtue of the extreme vulnerability of infants to rough handling.[9] During the early months of life, the normal head is disproportionately heavy for the weak neck muscles. The brain is not yet myelinated and is softer and less protected than the older brain. Also, during infancy the brain is developing more rapidly than at any other stage of extrauterine growth and is especially vulnerable to injury. The infantile bony structure, still attached only weakly to the surrounding tissues, is easily damaged. Thus infants may suffer permanent handicap, retardation, or death because of abuse.

According to current figures, victims of infant battery are about equally divided between males and females. Birth order has not been extensively investigated with respect to infants suffering abuse. However, an analysis of three surveys of abused children of all ages showed a significant predominance of large families compared with the national average.[44]

The occurrence of brutal handling so near the time of birth suggests that circumstances of the pregnancy or the perinatal period may provide important clues. Early investigators found an abnormally high rate of prematurity among abused babies and reasoned that prematurity itself might cause an infant to be especially difficult for the parents, thus leading to abuse.[15,68] The prominence of prematurity was confirmed by many later researchers.[21,39,69]

Other investigators have identified separation of mother and baby as a hindrance to the bonding necessary to ensure a healthy beginning relationship.[38] Because hospital practice usually involves placing premature infants in a special nursery and forbidding the new mother access to the infant, prematurity itself may not be a factor in the unfortunate early separation of mother and child. A prospective study of 255 premature and/or ill newborns showed that the abused children weighed less at birth, remained in the hospital longer, and were visited there less frequently.[32] All these differences were statistically significant. Further suggestive evidence comes from a survey of child abuse in New Zealand.[20] Of the 170 children living with their mothers at the time of the abusive incident, 42% had been separated for a significant period between birth and 36 months of age.

Neurologic dysfunction may accompany prematurity or be present in the newborn because of other conditions. Pasamanick[58] believes that mothers of neurologically abnormal premature infants are more tense than mothers of neurologically normal premature infants. Even though abnormal premature babies may demonstrate only slight neurologic impairment, they may be disorganized, unstable, and easily stressed, thus creating much tension for the mother and perhaps resulting in abuse.

Lynch[45] described abused infants and preschoolers as having a significantly greater number of serious illnesses during the first year of life than a nonabused sibling group. Similar findings have been reported in a study of abused compared with matched accident infants.[17] Lynch's subjects had significantly more separations from their mothers during both the neonatal period and the first six months of life. Mothers of abused infants also suffer from a high incidence of gestational illness according to ten Bensel and Paxton.[75] There can be little doubt that negative factors bearing on both baby and mother and relating to birth or the early months of life are critically important to explore in relation to infant battery. (For an excellent review, see Sameroff and Chandler.[60])

Physical handicaps, either congenital or acquired, have been designated as contributing to the possibility of later mistreatment, but findings in this area are inconsistent. Birrell and Birrell[6] found that 25% of the 42 abused children they studied had some form of handicap; on the other hand, Martin and co-workers[47] found few such conditions among the 58 abused youngsters they examined in follow-up. It is probable that a severe, visible physical handicap in a baby induces a feeling of sympathy and concern in the caretaker whereas a minor (and less visible) handicap, such as a mild neurologic abnormality, appears to the caretaker as a "mean" disposition or a deliberate attempt to thwart caretaking efforts.

Another potential source of difficulty for both mother and baby is the baby's individual temperament. Some infants like to be cuddled, while others avoid the mother's attempts to cradle or hug.[62] Such a difference is of no significance provided the mother can adapt to the infant's needs without anxiety and disappointment. Other kinds of individual differences have been identified in newborns, particularly patterns of crying and soothability.[41] Again, such innate differences do not necessarily spell trouble. The mother's ability to read the baby's cues and respond appropriately is the crucial factor. Thoman[76] notes that some babies give ambiguous cues, for example, crying or not crying under similar conditions, irregular sleep patterns, and the like. Any mother might have difficulty understanding this kind of baby, but the inexperienced mother would be especially beset and confused by such an infant.

Persistent individual differences in children have been documented by one group of investigators.[77,78] These researchers divided babies into three groups: easy, difficult, and variable, according to nine temperamental characteristics such as predominant mood, patterns of activity, and regularity. The majority of babies are thought to be "easy," thus presumably rewarding. It is when the "difficult" baby happens to have parents who themselves are difficult because of personal problems, pressures of the environment, or both, that trouble is imminent.

Aside from objective characteristics of the baby that may account for his or her abuse, some babies are endangered simply because they behave as normal infants do.[17,74] In this instance, the baby's vulnerability to abuse stems from the parent's distorted perception of infancy, which will be discussed in the next section.

In view of the marked vulnerability of infants to abuse, it is not surprising that the array of possible sequelae is also great and includes effects on physical, motor, intellectual, and social development. Note, however, that it is exceedingly difficult to link any particular outcome to abuse because so many other noxious influences associated with it might have affected the child. Examples of these influences include prematurity, early mother-baby separation, early growth failure, maternal deprivation, and distorted parent-child interaction.

The easiest results of abuse to trace are the physical effects. Among these, Caffey has designated subdural hematoma as "the most common, most injurious, and least understood lesion" resulting from what he calls the whiplash shaken syndrome.[9] He adds that this lesion is by far the most frequent cause of death in the battered baby. Very often there are no visible external signs of injury, but trauma to the brain may cause severe and permanent central nervous system damage, including visual handicap that may result in blindness.[28] Harcourt and Hopkins also note the rarity of external ocular trauma and advise, as does Caffey, that the extreme frequency of extensive intraocular hemorrhages at the time of the traumatic incident justifies detailed examination of the fundi of all battered babies as a routine measure.

Babies are prone to a special type of bone injury because of the peculiar physiology of their bone structure.[67] The causes may be grabbing the child either to hurt him or to save him from a possible fall, or twisting the limbs in anger or innocence, as when administering passive exercise. The resulting injuries may include tearing or dislodging of the periosteum, a fibrous membrane that is loosely attached to the shaft of the bone during infancy. Injuries of this kind rarely occur in accidents such as falls. Most commonly, the large bones are affected, and the lesions, usually multiple, are in various stages of healing.

Injury of the tissues over the bone causes bleeding between the periosteum and the bone of the shaft. This leads to swelling and ultimately, within a period of 2 to 3 weeks, to calcification that can be diagnosed by x-ray examination.[31] Since the formation of callus takes some time, the x-ray film may not reveal the injury immediately, and babies in whom bone damage is suspected should have repeat x-ray films several weeks following the incident. Injuries of this kind are less likely to occur as the child grows older and the periosteum attains a stronger bond with the bone.

Some parents believe that shaking a child is a safer way of punishing than spanking or beating. Many adults, often well-educated professionals, see no harm in whirling a baby about by holding to one arm and one leg. Shaking, whirling, throwing in the air—all can be exceedingly destructive for an infant.

Another physical condition that may be associated with abuse is failure-to-thrive, that is, height, weight, or both below the third percentile in the absence of organic disease. On a continuum of poor child care practices, failure-to-thrive would stand between neglect and abuse. This condition, like prematurity, often makes a child more difficult to manage because of sleeplessness, restlessness, and increased crying.[65] It may precede or be one of the causes of attack, or it may be one of the results. Koel[40] has noted an overlap between growth failure and abuse, which was also a prominent finding of mine.[15,17] The few follow-up studies available suggest that the outcome for such children is as grim as the outcome for abused children.[18,19,53]

Appelbaum[2] found a significant degree of mental and motor retardation among a group of abused preschool children when they were compared with a matched nonabused group. Sandgrund and co-workers[61] have reported significantly lower mental scores among 8½-year-old abused children compared with matched nonabused children. In my first study,[15] 55% of the abused group was judged retarded. (No comparison children were used.) In later studies, results have been more ambiguous.[17,47] Among their respective abused groups, both myself and Martin and co-workers found some brighter-than-average children, as expected in a normal distribution. At the same time, the number of children with depressed scores was also higher than expected. No ready explanation comes to mind for this array of findings beyond the possibility of differing definitions of abuse, which might have yielded quite different groups of children.

There is little doubt that the more severe forms of abuse against infants and young children are likely to result in mental retardation, and one researcher believes that child abuse may contribute a sizable proportion of cases to the hospital population of mentally subnormal patients.[55] However, Oliver's results, like those of my 1967 study, were based on subjects chosen according to unusually stringent criteria that would place them in the distinct minority of abused children, most of whom fortunately suffer much less severe injury.

The social-emotional results of abuse are thought to be manifold but unfortunately have been little studied by means of comparison groups. In a follow-up assessment of abused children, Martin and Beezley[46] found a number of problems including impaired ability for enjoyment, low self-esteem, pseudoadult behavior, and school learning problems. Whether these difficulties are significantly more frequent among mistreated youngsters cannot be answered by means of the available data. However, I found that all the study children—abused, accident, and nontraumatized alike—were beset by a host of developmental problems, and no one group of children was affected more.[16] Although some of the young subjects had been abused, physical attacks apparently were only one of many negative influences on all the children's lives. This has also been remarked by Burland and co-workers.[7]

To summarize, babies are especially vulnerable to abuse because of their immature physiology. Variables associated with mistreatment are prematurity, maternal and infant illness, and early separations. Temperamental difficulties between caretaker and baby constitute another negative influence. Possible sequelae include permanent physical handicap, retarded mental and/or motor development, and poor social and personal skills, but additional controlled studies are necessary to clarify ambiguous results.

THE FAMILIES

By far the greatest percentage of alleged perpetrators are the natural parents, although step, foster, and adoptive parents may also abuse. Note that these are designated as *alleged* perpetrators; the agent is not always known.

In most instances, establishing "who done it" should not be a goal of medical personnel. If it must be done, investigation to assign guilt is properly the job of the police. As noted by Okell,[54] facing their own violent actions may be more than battering parents can manage, especially in the early stages of identification and treatment. More important for the professional is the evidence that the child is receiving poor care and that the parent is overwhelmed; the task is to protect the child and support the parent while the problem is untangled.

An exception to the stricture against finding out the perpetrator is the possibility, in a few cases, that an older sibling hurt the baby. This is an aspect of abuse that has received little attention, but work in Pittsburgh has revealed perhaps a handful of cases in which a three- or four-year-old has been allowed to remain unsupervised with an infant, with dire results.[27]

Abusive parents may be of any religion or ethnic group. Various researchers have identified them as particularly young, but national figures from the American Humane Association analysis of reported cases show that more than half the alleged perpetrators in validated reports were over 30 years of age, and only 6% were less than 20 years of age.[1]

We know that child abuse occurs in all social classes, among rich and poor alike, but we know this only because of one or two middle- or upper-class cases in our own experience. Many investigators have remarked on the skewed reporting that causes poor people to be decidedly overrepresented among official cases.[17,24,51] Lower-class families are more often "caught" because of their visibility in clinics, welfare offices, and hospitals. Another possibility is that financial strain in the absence of necessary support systems is sufficient stress to result in child abuse, especially among single, poor mothers.[22] It should be remembered that abuse has many causes and that different stresses peculiar to the middle and upper classes may also lead to child abuse.

Ill health has been named as a prominent factor in abusing compared with nonabusing mothers.[17,45] This makes sense because an ill mother has less tolerance and is more fatigued than a mother in good health. On the other hand, this is a finding that may relate more to social class than to abuse. Lower-class families are more closely identified with child abuse and neglect than middle and upper classes, and health problems in this group are known to be greater.

Two physiologic states peculiar to women should be much more extensively studied for possible association with abuse. Premenstrual tension in otherwise loving and adequate mothers has been identified as a precipitating factor in child battery.[10] This state, easily treated by progesterone, might well be a common but overlooked influence. The postpartum mother is known to be subject to depressive moods, yet no aids have been institutionalized for this period, for example, health or lay visitors available in the home. This is a time of great physical and emotional depletion for the mother, nevertheless grandmother usually leaves, father goes back to work, and mother is left to cope on her own.

When child abuse first came into focus as an actual occurrence, it was thought that the cause must be psychosis or severe psychologic disturbance in the abuser. It is now believed that only a small percentage are psychotic but that many may have character disorders associated with deficits in nurturing during their own early childhood. A group of such characteristics that have been repeatedly identified are lack of basic trust, low self-esteem, unrealistically high expectations for the infant, and role reversal.* It can be seen that these traits fit together and may all stem from the lack of a consistent, nurturing relationship at the beginning of life. Instead, abusive parents often experienced criticism, harsh demands, perhaps even physical attack as

---

*See references 3, 29, 49, 73, and 74.

children that produced feelings of worthlessness and self-blame in them. The effect of these multiple rejections is to cause the parent to unconsciously pin all hopes for love and appreciation on the longed-for infant. Expecting impossible proofs of affection from a tiny baby, the parents are bound to be frustrated and to feel even more unloved. Worse, the parents begin to believe that the baby is deliberately frustrating them and must be punished. Distorted perception of the baby is a common research finding.[50]

Another side of faulty perception is a true lack of knowledge concerning how infants grow and develop, particularly how they develop psychologically. Anxious to have their child grow up successfully, the naive parent believes the child must be taught manners and conduct immediately or else the child will grow up as a boor and an embarrassment.

Although much the same traits as discussed above have been identified in various studies of abusive parents, very few comparison groups have been used, therefore the extent of similar characteristics in the general population is unknown. One study that did use comparisons was that of Melnick and Hurley,[48] who found several significant differences between matched groups of lower-class Black abusive and nonabusive mothers. Parke and Collmer[57] note that the lack of differences was also remarkable: no differences appeared between the two groups on 12 of the 18 variables that were tested.

Extensive therapeutic work with abusive parents in Denver showed that early abuse or deprivation was a feature common to their histories.[74] Remnants of the earlier harsh relationship could sometimes be observed when the abusive mother and her mother were seen in a joint interview.

Finding a history of early mistreatment in abusive parents does not, however, show that all abused children become abusive parents. One would need a prospective study of abused children to determine the range of child care that they provide to their offspring. Provocative findings along this line have recently been reported: the high-risk (abusive) mothers indeed had histories of early mistreatment, but their nonabusive comparisons reported an incidence of childhood abuse four times as great.[32] Clearly, this is another aspect of abuse that requires systematic study.

Perhaps the challenge of the parental role is too much for some individuals, who might function in acceptable fashion except for it,[40] and being a parent does demand resources that are not required by other roles. Solnit[72] notes the essential ambivalence associated with parenthood: children are the symbols of their parents' immortality yet also the reminder of their parents' inevitable death, therefore they stimulate conflicting and powerful feelings. The same ambivalence is expressed in soft lullabies that may hide unacceptable hostile wishes toward the baby as well as tender thoughts, for example "Rock-a-Bye Baby," which has the baby falling along with the tree and the cradle.

In summary, abusive parents have characteristics often associated with inadequate or harsh nurturing in early childhood, but the extent of similar characteristics in the general population is not known. Poor physical health appears significantly greater among abusive than among nonabusive mothers. However, the challenge of the parental role itself may be at least partly responsible for aggression against children.

THE ENVIRONMENT

The environment is implicated in child abuse in many important ways, three of which will be discussed. First is the custom of presenting violence by means of printed material, television, and radio. Scientific studies have attempted to research the effects, if any, on the aggressive behavior of young viewers. An equally important question is the effects on adults, especially parents of young children, for whom brutal behavior is repeatedly modeled. Violence *is* a way of life; it is so commonplace that hardly anyone even shudders at the evidence.

We also have a few studies indicating that physical aggression against babies is a common method of punishment. According to one early study, a fourth of the mothers in several Los Angeles clinics began to spank their babies by 6 months of age, and almost half were doing so by 12 months of age.[42] I reported similar findings on a study population that included middle- and upper-class families as well as those from the lower classes.[17]

Isolation is the second environmental force of importance for the understanding of child abuse.[15,74] Whether caused by themselves or by others, many abusive parents have no close human bonds, for example, neighbors who might drop in to chat; relatives who can be counted on in an emergency; friends to confide in, to help, and be helped by. The parents' lack of basic trust implies a suspicious view of others along with reluctance to risk themselves. This uneasiness with others and the impulse toward isolation makes abusive parents elusive and difficult to treat because they behave the same with potentially helpful professionals and paraprofessionals.

Isolation may take the form of living in remote, barely accessible areas, keeping the blinds drawn during daytime hours, having an unlisted telephone, and the like. Such living arrangements make it hard for others to help, hence abusive parents are often forced (or force themselves) into having to manage everything alone.

The third aspect of the environment that affects child abuse is stress.[25,59] Stress may be related to chronic invidious conditions such as inadequate education, poor jobs, and insufficient income, or it may be the acute blow, for example, losing a wallet. The actual events themselves are less important than how the individual perceives and responds to them. More than other parents, abusive parents perceive excessive amounts of stress impinging on them.[34] An example of this in one study was the abusive mothers' perceptions of pregnancy with the index child; although the medical records indicated fewer problems among this group than among their comparison group, abusive mothers saw more stress and more problems than did the nonabusive group.[17]

A supportive network of friends, neighbors, and relatives makes it easier to tolerate stress or perhaps reduces the perceived importance of it. A relationship may exist between stress and support such that as support increases, the perception of stress decreases in some as yet unknown fashion. As indicated by the previous discussion, the tendency toward isolation would cause support for the abusive parent to be in short supply, so the parent is left to manage everyday problems alone and to vent frustrations in the only available arena, the family.

EARLY IDENTIFICATION

Identification is important in relation to three different kinds of problems: (1) abuse that has already occurred, (2) specific subgroups who are clearly at risk for abuse, and (3) attitudes and customs in the general population that increase the probability of abuse. The third problem is outside the scope of this section, and the second will be discussed under prevention. This section will focus on signs that indicate that a child has probably suffered abuse. Only through the professional's sensitivity to such indications can the child and family receive appropriate treatment.

It hardly seems necessary to state that infants should always be examined undressed. Although this is standard practice in hospitals and clinics, public health nurses visiting in homes may find it inconvenient. In some instances the baby may not be seen at all because of naptime or some other reason. There is no way, however, to achieve early identification without a look at the patient.

Certain injuries are always suspect when they occur in infants less than 2 years of age and even more suspect in infants under 12 months of age. These injuries include bruising of the face, abdomen, or back—superficial injuries that are not normally acquired by the well-cared-for infant.[31] Any fractures in a child of less than 2 years of age should raise warning signals. Many hospitals make a practice of admitting such babies even though admission is not medically necessary. The purpose of course is to provide time for assessment of the circumstances of the injury and the childrearing abilities of the parents.

Other injuries that should alert medical personnel are burns of any kind. Unfortunately, cigarette burns on infants are not uncommon. Burns over extensive areas of the body may be caused by placing the baby in very hot water. Investigators found that the patterns of such lesions could reveal how the child was positioned in the water and whether the burns in question could be accidental.[43]

A rule of thumb is always to consider the child's injuries in the light of his or her motor development. Parents often give a history of accident to explain the child's condition. Such an explanation should be matched with the child's motor development to determine whether he or she is capable of the actions described.

Occasionally, details of the history are discrepant, for example, the parents' stories may conflict in important details such as who was with the child when the injury occurred. In such instances the examiner might conclude that no one was with the child, and the parents actually may not know what happened. Another conclusion might be that the parents do not wish to reveal the circumstances of the injuries. In either case, the next step is to learn about the family's childrearing abilities; their present health, financial, and social situation; and what supportive resources they may have. Another item of family history that may help in the assessment is information about the abused child's siblings. One investigator found that they were apt to have more injuries, accidents, and deaths than normally would be expected.[52]

Failure-to-thrive (height and/or weight below the third percentile for age and sex in the absence of organic disease) is related to child abuse in that it implies a disturbance in the parent-child relationship.[19,53] Bone-injured abused infants are frequently also diagnosed as failure-to-thrive,[15] while poor physical development may conceal the fact of skeletal lesions.[40] Parents of failure-to-thrive babies need detailed evaluation and supportive help just as do abusive parents.

The final item that may assist in early identification is the length of the interval between the occurrence of the injury and the search for medical care.[30] While abusive parents do bring their injured children for care, it may be only after a prolonged period.[17] Like the other items of history, delayed medical care in itself proves nothing but is valuable as one piece of a total picture.

TREATMENT ALTERNATIVES

The most common treatment for an abused baby and the family is to place the baby in a substitute care situation (shelter, relative's home, or foster home) while the parents receive counseling or psychiatric treatment. When the parents are thought psychologically ready to be reunited with the infant, the baby is returned to them. Criticism of this plan centers on the failure to observe parents and child interacting together; it is difficult to judge readiness for improved child care simply by means of interviews. Decisions to return the child under circumstances of this kind have resulted in death for several infants in one community.

Ideally, parents should receive appropriate help while also interacting with their infant and being assisted in learning child care skills. The infant requires protection while this process goes on, so a residential setting may be desirable. Short of that, the infant may be placed in a foster home in which the natural parent is welcomed and helped by role modeling and teaching. This type of treatment as well as residential treatment for the baby has rarely been available.[64]

According to the official evaluation of child abuse demonstration projects, more abusive parents reported being helped by means of paraprofessionals than by any other method.[5] In matters of child abuse, Kempe initiated the use of paraprofessionals, whom he called *lay therapists*. These are usually women who have successfully reared children and who work with two or three families at a time with the aim of providing a trusted confidante to act as advocate, advisor, and model of acceptable behavior.[4,36] The paraprofessional is selected, trained, and supervised by a professional in one of the areas of mental health, for example, psychiatrist, social worker, mental health nurse. She is available to the family at any hour of the day or night, either in person or by telephone, to offer support at times of crisis. She is thought of as the bridge to the community; ultimately, the family forms community ties that will take the place of the paraprofessional as a supportive resource.

Paraprofessionals also form the backbone of Parents Anonymous, a group similar to Alcoholics Anonymous, which provides an opportunity to meet with other parents struggling with the same kinds of problems in relation to children.[4] Some chapters of Parents Anonymous include professionals as consultants, others do not. A "buddy" system provides a member of the group who can be an anchor for another abusive mother at times of stress.

Other types of treatment for the abusive family include individual counseling, activity or therapy groups, and/or resources for substitute care of children. Very often, problems of the abusive family are multiple and require multiple kinds of treatment, for example, additional education, tutoring, vocational training, help in locating a job, housing, assistance in dealing with public agencies, health assessment and care, and marital counseling.

The need for substitute child care resources is very common, especially for single mothers. Without such resources, mothers may have to care for the child or children for 24 hours a day, 7 days a week. Such constant care of a minor child is wearing in the extreme and should not be necessary for anyone. Unfortunately, day care and other forms of child care are not plentiful especially in relation to the infant, for whom group care is most unusual.

According to the summary evaluation of eleven federally funded child abuse demonstration projects, only 50% of the families who were treated could be rated improved.[5] In view of these discouraging figures, it seems wise to invest greater energy and effort on prevention.

PREVENTION

It is undoubtedly impossible to completely eliminate all child abuse. Given the data on infant battery, however, reduction of its incidence is a reasonable possibility if sufficient resources, skills, and political backing are available.

Prevention efforts quickly elicit heated discussion between those who favor protecting children at all costs and those who are acutely sensitive to the possibility of intruding on parents' privacy. Philosophically, the ideal preventive program should have three attributes: (1) it should be equally available to all groups in the total population, (2) it should be noncoercive, and (3) it should have predictable benefits. Four types of possible programs will be described briefly, then discussed in terms of these criteria.

The first type of program is based on screening to identify adults who are high risk for abnormal parenting. Child abuse has been called a low base rate phenomenon, that is, an infrequent event with reference to the universe of children. Predicting who will abuse is like searching for the needle in the haystack; screening for high-risk parents might be viewed as reducing the size of the haystack. The development of suitable research instruments has focused largely on newborns and their parents. Once high-risk families are located, special supportive services are provided to help these families get off to a good start with their babies.

Although screening for high risk is still in the testing stage, considerable success has marked the effort.[26,63] The principal objection is that the process automatically labels a group of parents as potential mistreaters of children. So far the percentage of false positives is high, hence the risk of misclassification is also high.

The second possible type of program is provision of services geared to normal life crises involving parents and children. Recipients would not be identified through a screening procedure. Instead, eligibility would automatically be conferred by virtue of experiencing certain life events such as pregnancy, delivery, the neonatal period. These events (and others as well), although normal, also hold a potential for either weakening or strengthening a family depending on how well the members are able to cope with the particular event.

Kempe's idea of providing health visitors for all families with children under school age probably fits here, since rearing young children implies the need for institutionalized support.[35] Britain has found the health visitor so beneficial that the mandated number has recently been almost doubled. Many people in the United States, however, protest that the health visitor is a threat to family privacy since it would be a compulsory and universal service as it is in England.

Courses to prepare young people for parenthood are the third kind of preventive program, currently being offered in many junior high schools across the country. Developed by three governmental and educational institutions, one program offers high school students both didactic and experimental education concerning young children.[13] The program has been well received by both male and female students and appears to fill a very real need. Two possible objections are (1) that the students do not yet have full-time responsibility for children, therefore the material has less immediate relevance than desirable, and (2) that the experience with infants may encourage too early marriage and childbearing.[12]

The final possible program to be discussed is mass media education in parenting. Many organizations are currently producing audiovisual material for this purpose, but despite the power of the media, the efforts have had little apparent effect. This may be a result of the absence of an overall plan with consequent dissipation of energies, or the failure to obtain results may be more apparent than real and may stem from the absence of evaluation.

Considering the four kinds of programs in light of the criteria (available to nonselected population, noncoercive, and beneficial), only the third (high school curriculum in parenting) and the fourth (mass media parent education) appear completely satisfactory. Services for high-risk parents selected by a screening procedure are addressed to only one segment of the cohort of new mothers and babies; the health visitor concept would be compulsory. On the other hand, the educational programs, although philosophically sound, may not reach the part of the population most in need of help. It may well be true, as Kempe maintains,[35] that the health and protection of young children must be safeguarded by society and would be vastly enhanced by mandatory house calls from a trained, sympathetic health visitor prepared to support the parent.

ROLE OF THE NURSE

This chapter has discussed the characteristics of the abused baby, some of the sequelae, characteristics of abusive families, role of the environment, and methods of identification, treatment, and prevention. In conclusion, the role of the nurse will be discussed in relation to this outline. Since the professional role of the nurse varies a good deal depending on the setting, some roles will be more feasible than others.

Knowledge

To perform any role at all, it is essential that nurses understand the laws of their particular states and the regulations in their particular institutions. Although all states have laws mandating medical personnel to report all cases of suspected child abuse, variations from one state to another are great.

Within every institution whether it be a hospital, a health department, or a school, there should be a written policy governing the initiation and channeling of reports of abuse. This is important information for the nurse, who should also understand the resources available in the community and how to use them. Although the nurse may not be directly involved with these resources, the management of suspected cases is enhanced when the nurse can view the movement of the case from a wide perspective.

Sensitivity to health needs

Because the child is the victim of abuse, medical care is usually concentrated on him or her and little attention may be paid to the parents' state of health. As noted in the section on families, investigators have learned that abusive parents have significantly more health problems than nonabusive parents. The alert nurse can be instrumental in seeing that parents' health needs are specifically addressed.

Family planning

Another characteristic of abusive families is the relatively large number of children per family. This suggests the advisability of discussing with the parents some form of family planning. Many abusive parents have little interest in the idea of planned births; nevertheless, repeated discussion may eventually take hold and help change the attitudes of the parents, thus ultimately reducing the size of the family.

Observations of baby and parents

A large proportion of nurses on either obstetric or pediatric services (and also community and state nurses) are in an excellent position to observe parents and baby together. The value of such observations cannot be overstated; they form the basis for some of the screening tools currently being developed by researchers. We have seen that trouble often begins within the first few weeks or months of life and clues to such disturbances are often very clear to a sensitive observer.

Hurd[33] speaks of the opportunity on the obstetric service to observe mother-baby attachment in the formative stages. Special supportive resources can be called into play when needed; sometimes the obstetric nurse who has a good relationship with the mother becomes an outreach person to support the initial weeks away from the hospital.

The interested nurse can get help on how to develop observational skills from supervisors, colleagues, social workers, or other professionals who are studying mother-baby interaction. Videotapes and films are available from many libraries, and these can be of great help in identifying healthy and unhealthy forms of interchange.

Record keeping

Records do not need to be voluminous but should be accurate, dated, and made as soon as possible after the patient contact.[70] Occasionally the nurse may be called to testify in court, and records can be an important aid.

Referral

In many instances, the responsibility of the nurse will cease following discussion with the doctor or referral of the family to an appropriate resource. A plan for follow-up on such cases should be made at the time of referral and a file set up to act as a reminder. It is extremely frustrating to make referrals with the hope of assisting families, then to hear nothing about what happened.

Some nursing departments have established a system of screening children and families for signs of abuse. Because of the rapid flow of patients in and out of hospitals, very often the entire picture of abuse does not emerge in time for medical personnel to act appropriately unless special steps are taken. Olson describes an index of suspicion used for categorizing children and families who appear at risk.[56] The appropriate hospital response is then chosen to correspond with the degree of risk and the type of family.

In other medical facilities, the system might be an interdisciplinary team that reviews suspicious cases. Here the nurse might be the source of referral or might add valuable information in the context of the data contributed by other professional members of the team.

Community activities

Most communities are eager to include nurses in the groups that attempt to solve the problems of child abuse. Together with other professional groups, the individual nurse may help set up workshops, institutes, and training sessions.[11]

Interdisciplinary teams may include personnel from protective services, medical facilities, schools, day care facilities, law enforcement facilities, and others. The kinds of responsibility assumed by these teams differ from one community to another. Some review all new cases, some determine treatment plans, some require follow-up information to maintain accountability.

An energetic and perceptive nurse can be successful in identifying community needs and helping establish additional services. Possible kinds of services include Parents Anonymous, crisis nurseries, cooperative babysitting groups, and parent education groups, but the list is virtually endless. The most successful kinds of community services are those that have a ripple effect by

1. Attitude in dealing with staff
   ___Irrationally hostile (3)
   ___Situationally hostile (1)
   ___Verbally paranoid (project all blame on others) (3)
   ___Combative (5)
   ___Abusive (5)

2. Family structure
   ___Family together (0)
   ___Divorce (1)
   ___Separation exists (4)
   ___Child/parent role reversal (5)
   ___Foster home (3)
   ___One spouse deceased (1)
   ___Uncontrolled sibling rivalry (3)
   ___Rigid, compulsive structure (2)
   ___Loose, ill-defined structure (2)

3. Family problems (parental figures)
   ___Alcoholism (5)
   ___Drug abuse (5)
   ___Frequent visitors to emergency ward (3)
   ___Evidence of sexual promiscuity (3)
   ___History of parental figures being abused children (5)
   ___Chronic organizational problems in the home because of the child (5)
   ___Psychiatric history (3)   ___Past suicide attempt (5)
   ___Unstable job pattern (5)
   ___Documented assault and/or battery (5)
   ___Hypertension (2)   ___Ulcers (2)

4. Religious affiliation
   ___None (5)   ___Strong (0)   ___Lukewarm (2)

5. Labor and delivery
   ___High-risk pregnancy (3)
   ___Low-birth weight (5)
   ___Mental retardation in child, mother, or father figure (5)
   ___No prenatal care (5)
   ___Isolation from mother during newborn period (3)
   ___Born out of wedlock (5)

6. Cultural factors
   ___Bi-cultural home (3)
   ___Patrilineal authority (5)
      ___Jewish (0)
      ___Caucasian (3)
      ___Black (3)
   ___Interracial marriage (3)
      ___Hawaiian (1)
      ___Polynesian (1)
      ___Chicano (2)
      ___Puerto Rican (1)
      ___First generation European immigrant (1)
      ___Arab (1)

   Matrilineal authority (3)
      ___Jewish (1)
      ___Caucasian (3)
      ___Black (1)
      ___Hawaiian (0)
      ___Polynesian (0)
      ___Chicano (0)
      ___Puerto Rican (1)
      ___First generation European immigrant (3)
      ___Arab (3)

   ___Metropolitan residency (4)   ___Rural residency (2)

7. Child or siblings
   ___Frequently admitted to hospital (5)
   ___Diagnosis
      ___Long bone fractures (5)   ___Hematomas (5)
      ___Head injuries (5)   ___Failure to thrive (5)
                                      ___Malnourishment (3)
   ___Bruises (multiple) in various stages of healing (5)
   ___Multiple scratches (2)   ___Burn sites, varying healing stage (5)
   ___Described by parent figures as discipline problems (5)
   ___One child or more under 3 years of age (3)
   ___Parents contradict themselves when describing illnesses and injuries of children (5)
   ___History of not visiting children when admitted to hospital (5)

When the interview for the Index of Suspicion is completed, points assigned the parent for each item are added and the total is ranked: low risk—0 to 40 points; moderate risk—41-75 points; high risk—76 to 115; very high risk—116-149; and extreme risk—150 points or more.

Fig. 7-1. Index of suspicion. Identification of parents who are potential child abusers. (Copyright © 1976, The American Journal of Nursing Company. Reprinted from Olson, R. J.: Index of suspicion: screening for child abusers, Am. J. Nurs. **76**(l):109, 1976.)

involving more and more people. Sometimes this is accomplished by training any trainees who become interested in taking this further step. In some places, discussion groups for new parents have expanded by means of training parents after they have participated as members.

A few nurses who have had extensive experience in observing mother-baby interaction performed assessments of mothers and their infants focusing on the possibility of helping improve the relationship.[71] The evaluation of mother-baby pairs is a subtle and difficult operation, but accomplishing it may spare the baby removal from the home and may give the mother a boost at a time when she needs it most.

Professional education

Knowledge about child abuse has increased enormously in the last 10 years. This means that very few professionals had the opportunity to learn about it in the course of their professional education. This brings us to the final recommendation concerning nursing roles in relation to abuse.

Real progress with this ballooning problem requires that medical personnel as well as other professionals have a sound base of education on which to build their clinical experience. Adding material about child abuse and its ramifications increases the already heavy burden of the nursing curriculum. The same is true of other kinds of professional education with the result that young graduates are poorly prepared for dealing with the evidence of family trauma that stands out on every side.

Well-educated and experienced nurses are needed for every aspect of child abuse including sophisticated research, clinical practice, community organization, and teaching. One of the most important possible roles of the nurse is to act as a missionary for further education in the formal curriculum of undergraduates. Although similar courses could be used at every level, it is desirable to start with the earliest, then expand.

CONCLUSION

The amount of information now available about child abuse is almost unbelievable considering the scarcity of information 10 to 15 years ago. The plan of this chapter was to outline some of the main considerations, not to provide a total compendium. The interested reader will find a wealth of detail in any one of the review articles.[57,60,65]

A survey of the current situation regarding the incidence of child abuse is discouraging. There is more of it than anyone expected some years ago, and we have very little understanding of what to do about it at this time. Nevertheless, a positive aspect is the willingness to consider the problem. Until recently the ordinary way of dealing with child abuse (and especially baby abuse) was to sweep it under the rug and pretend it did not exist. Surely we have learned that no problem can be adequately dealt with unless it is first recognized and accepted as a problem.

REFERENCES

1. The American Humane Association: National analysis of official child neglect and abuse reporting: an executive summary, Englewood, Colo., 1978, The Association.
2. Appelbaum, A.: Developmental retardation in infants as a concomitant of physical child abuse, J. Abnorm. Child Psychol. 5:417-423, 1977.
3. Baher, E., Hymen, C., Jones, C., et al.: At risk: an account of the work of the Battered Child Research Department, National Society for the Prevention of Cruelty to Children, London, 1976, Routledge & Kegan Paul, Ltd.
4. Beezley, P., Martin, H., and Alexander, H.: Comprehensive family oriented therapy. In Helfer, R., and Kempe, C., editors: Child abuse and neglect: the family and the community, Cambridge, Mass., 1976, Ballinger Publishing Co.

5. Berkeley Planning Associates: Executive summary: Evaluation of the Joint OCD/SRS National Demonstration Program in Child Abuse and Neglect, 1974-1977, Berkeley, Calif., 1977, Berkeley Planning Associates.
6. Birrell, R., and Birrell, J.: Maltreatment syndrome in children: a hospital survey, Med. J. Aust. 2:1023, 1968.
7. Burland, J., Andrews, R., and Headstein, S.: Child abuse: one tree in the forest, Child Welfare 52:585-592, 1973.
8. Caffey, J.: Multiple fractures in the long bones of infants suffering from chronic subdural hematoma, Am. J. Roentgenol. Rad. Ther. Nucl. Med. 56:163-173, 1946.
9. Caffey, J.: The whiplash shaken infant syndrome: manual shaking by the extremities with whiplash induced intracranial and intraocular bleedings, linked with residual permanent brain damage and mental retardation, Pediatrics 54:396-403, 1974.
10. Dalton, K.: Premenstrual baby battering, Br. Med. J. 2(5965):279, 1975.
11. Davis, D., and Johnson, G.: A way of caring: nurses initiate community action to prevent child abuse, Assoc. Operat. Room Nurs. J. 27:631-635, 1978.
12. de Lissovoy, V.: Child care by adolescent parents, Child. Today 2:167-170, 1973.
13. Education Commission of the States: Education for parenthood: a primary prevention strategy for child abuse and neglect, Report no. 93, Denver, 1976, Education Commission of the States Child Abuse Project.
14. Elmer, E.: Abused young children seen in hospitals, Soc. Work 5:98-102, 1960.
15. Elmer, E.: Children in jeopardy. Pittsburgh, 1967, University of Pittsburgh Press.
16. Elmer, E.: Follow-up study of traumatized children, Pediatrics 59:273-279, 1977.
17. Elmer, E.: Fragile families, troubled children, Pittsburgh, 1977, University of Pittsburgh Press.
18. Elmer, E., Gregg, G., and Ellison, P.: Late results of the failure to thrive syndrome, Clin. Pediatr. 8:584-589, 1969.
19. Evans, S., Reinhart, J., and Succop, R.: Failure to thrive: a study of 45 children and their families, J. Am. Acad. Child Psychiatry 11:440-457, 1972.
20. Fergusson, D., Fleming, J., and O'Neill, D.: Child abuse in New Zealand, Wellington, 1972, Government Printer.
21. Friedrich, W., and Boriskin, B.: The role of the child in abuse, Am. J. Orthopsychiatry 46:580-590, 1976.
22. Garbarino, J.: A preliminary study of some ecological correlates of child abuse: the impact of socioeconomic stress on mothers, Child Dev. 47:178-185, 1976.
23. Gelles, R.: Violence towards children in the United States. Paper presented at the American Association for the Advancement of Science, Denver, 1977.
24. Gil, D.: Unraveling child abuse, Am. J. Orthopsychiatry 45:346-356, 1975.
25. Gil, D.: Violence against children: physical child abuse in the United States, Cambridge, Mass., 1970, Harvard University Press.
26. Gray, J., Cutler, C., Dean, J., et al.: Perinatal assessment of mother-baby interaction. In Helfer, R., and Kempe, C., editors: Child abuse and neglect: the family and community, Cambridge, Mass. 1976, Ballinger Publishing Co.
27. Gregg, G., and Elmer, E.: Infant injuries: accident or abuse? Pediatrics 44:434-439, 1969.
28. Harcourt, B., and Hopkins, D.: Ophthalmic manifestations of the battered-baby syndrome, Br. Med. J. 3:398-401, 1971.
29. Helfer, R.: The etiology of child abuse, Pediatrics 51:777-779, 1973.
30. Helfer, R., and Kempe, C.: The child's need for early recognition, immediate care and protection. In Kempe, C., and Helfer, R., editors: Helping the battered child and his family, Philadelphia, 1972, J. B. Lippincott Co.
31. Hull, D.: Medical diagnosis. In Carter, J., editor: The maltreated child, London, 1974, Priory Press Limited.
32. Hunter, R., Kilstrom, N., Kraybill, E., et al.: Antecedents of child abuse and neglect in premature infants: a prospective study in a newborn intensive care unit, Pediatrics 61:629-635, 1978.
33. Hurd, J.: Assessing maternal attachment: first step toward the prevention of child abuse, J. Obstet. Gynecol. Neonat. Nurs. 4:25-30, 1975.
34. Justice, B., and Duncan, D.: Life crisis as a precursor to child abuse, Public Health Rep. 91:110-115, 1976.
35. Kempe, C.: Predicting and preventing child abuse: establishing children's rights by assuring access to health care through the health visitors concept. Paper presented at the Ambulatory Pediatric Association Annual Meeting, Toronto, 1975.
36. Kempe, C., and Helfer, R.: Innovative therapeutic approaches. In Kempe, C., and Helfer, R., editors: Helping the battered child and his family, Philadelphia, 1972, J. B. Lippincott Co.
37. Kempe, C., Silverman, F., Steele, B., et al.: The

battered child syndrome, J.A.M.A. **181:**17-24, 1962.
38. Klaus, M., and Kennell, J.: Mothers separated from their newborn infants, Pediatr. Clin. North Am. **17:**1015-1037, 1970.
39. Klein, M., and Stern, L.: Low birth weight and the battered child syndrome, Am. J. Dis. Child. **122:**15-18, 1971.
40. Koel, B.: Failure to thrive and fatal injury as a continuum, Am. J. Dis. Child. **118:**565-567, 1969.
41. Korner, A.: Individual differences at birth: implications for early experience and later development, Am. J. Orthopsychiatry **4:**608-619, 1971.
42. Korsch, B., Christian, J., Gozzi, E., et al.: Infant care and punishment: a pilot study, Am. J. Public Health **55:**1880-1888, 1965.
43. Lenoski, E., and Hunter, K.: Specific patterns of inflicted burn injuries, J. Trauma **17:**842-846, 1977.
44. Light, R.: Abused and neglected children in America: a study of alternative policies, Harv. Educ. Rev. **43:**556-598, 1973.
45. Lynch, M.: Ill health and child abuse, Lancet **2**(7929):317-319, 1975.
46. Martin, H., and Beezley, P.: Behavioral observations of abused children, Dev. Med. Child Neurol. **19:**373-387, 1977.
47. Martin, H., Beezley, P., Conway, E., et al.: The development of abused children. In Schulman, I., editor: Advances in pediatrics, vol. 21, Chicago, 1974, Year Book Medical Publishers, Inc.
48. Melnick, B., and Hurley, J.: Distinctive personality attributes of child abusing mothers, J. Consult. Clin. Psychol. **33:**746-749, 1969.
49. Morris, M., and Gould, R.: Role reversal: a concept in dealing with the neglected/battered-child syndrome. In Child Welfare League of America: The neglected battered-child syndrome: role reversal in parents, New York, 1963, The League.
50. Morse, C., Sahler, O., and Friedman, S.: A three year follow-up study of abused and neglected children, Am. J. Dis. Child. **120:**439-446, 1970.
51. Newberger, E.: Child abuse and neglect: toward a firmer foundation for practice and policy, Am. J. Orthopsychiatry, **147:**374-376, 1977.
52. Newcombe, H.: Familial tendencies in diseases of children, Br. J. Prev. Soc. Med. **20:**49-57, 1966.
53. Oates, R., and Hufton, I.: The spectrum of failure to thrive and child abuse: a follow-up study, Child Abuse Neglect **1:**119-124, 1977.
54. Okell, C.: The battered baby syndrome: recent research and implications for treatment, Royal Soc. Health J. **92:**89-95, 1972.
55. Oliver, J.: Microcephaly following baby battering and shaking, Br. Med. J. **2:**262-264, 1975.
56. Olson, R.: Index of suspicion: screening for child abusers, Am. J. Nurs. **76:**108-110, 1976.
57. Parke, R., and Collmer, C.: Child abuse: an interdisciplinary analysis, Chicago, 1975, The University of Chicago Press.
58. Pasamanick, B.: Ill-health and child abuse, Lancet **2**(7934):550, 1975.
59. Pollock, C., and Steele, B.: A therapeutic approach to the parents. In Kempe, C., and Helfer, R., editors: Helping the battered child and his family, Philadelphia, 1972, J. B. Lippincott Co.
60. Sameroff, A., and Chandler, M.: Reproductive risk and the continuum of caretaking casualty. In Horowitz, F., and Hetherington, E., editors: Review of child development research, vol. 4, Chicago, 1975, University of Chicago Press.
61. Sandgrund, A., Gaines, R., and Green, A.: Child abuse and mental retardation: a problem of cause and effect, Am. J. Men. Defic. **79:**327-330, 1974.
62. Schaffer, H., and Emerson, P.: The development of social attachments in infancy, Monogr. Soc. Res. Child Dev. **29:**3, 1964.
63. Schneider, C., Hoffmeister, J., and Helfer, R.: A predictive screening questionnaire for potential problems in mother-child interaction. In Helfer, R., and Kempe, C., editors: Child abuse and neglect: the family and the community, Cambridge, Mass., 1976, Ballinger Publishing Co.
64. Schultz, B., Reinhart, J., and Elmer, E.: Parental stress center—two year experience. Paper presented to the American Academy of Pediatrics Annual Meeting, New York, 1977.
65. Scott, P.: Non-accidental injury in children, Br. J. Psychiatry **131:**366-380, 1977.
66. Silverman, F.: The roentgen manifestations of unrecognized skeletal trauma in infants, Am. J. Roentgenol. Rad. Ther. Nucl. Med. **69:**413-427, 1953.
67. Silverman, F.: Unrecognized trauma in infants, the battered child syndrome, and the syndrome of Ambroise Tardieu, Radiology, **104:**337-353, 1972.
68. Simons, B., Downs, E., Hurster, M., et al.: Child abuse: epidemiological study of medically reported cases, NY State J. Med. **66:**2783-2788, 1966.
69. Skinner, E., and Castle, R.: Seventy-eight bat-

tered children: a retrospective study, London, 1969; National Society for the Prevention of Cruelty to Children.
70. Slack, P.: Planning training for coping with non-accidental injury, Nurs. Times **72:**1561-1564, 1976.
71. Snyder, C., and Spietz, A.: Characteristics of abuse: a report of five families, Nurs. Pract. **2:** 23-27, 1977.
72. Solnit, A.: Changing psychological prespectives about children and their families, Child. Today **5:**5-9, 1976.
73. Steele, B.: Violence in our society, Pharos **33:** 42-48, 1970.
74. Steele, B., and Pollock, D.: A psychiatric study of parents who abuse infants and small children. In Helfer, R., and Kempe, C., editors: The battered child, Chicago, 1974, The University of Chicago Press.
75. ten Bensel, R., and Paxton, C.: Child abuse following early post partum separation, J. Pediatr. **90:**490-503, 1977.
76. Thoman, E.: The role of the infant in early transfer of information, Biol. Psychiatry **10:**161-169, 1975.
77. Thomas, A., Chess, S., and Birch, H.: Temperament and behavior disorders in children, New York, 1968, New York University Press.
78. Thomas, A., Chess, S., Birch, H., et al.: Behavioral individuality in early childhood, New York, 1963, New York University Press.
79. Woolley, P., and Evans, W., Jr.: Significance of skeletal lesions in infants resembling those of traumatic origin, J.A.M.A. **158:**539, 1955.

CHAPTER 8

Battered women

Barbara Star

Violence pervades the most intimate of interpersonal relationships. A slap across the face or a shove against the wall are common forms of marital violence. But many women also experience the thrashing, kicking, pummeling, and strangling that results in black eyes, loosened teeth, broken bones, miscarriages, ruptured eardrums, concussions, and even death.

Physical abuse within marriage occurs more frequently than most people realize. For instance, during 1975, 17,000 wife beating complaints were filed with the New York State Family Court.[32] According to the results of a recent survey, over one million women were beaten by their husbands during 1975-1977.[27] Other studies might place that figure closer to two million a year.[33] Despite the advent of hotlines and shelters for battered women, the problem remains hidden from all but a few professional groups. Usually it is the police, attorneys, and hospital personnel who are called on to deal with wife battering in most communities.

Nationwide, police respond to more family disturbance calls than to all other serious crimes combined, including murder and robbery.[20] At least 10% of aggravated assaults, those involving injury and/or a weapon, occur between husband and wife.[18] In some cities spousal assaults account for between 50% and 80% of the reported aggravated assaults.[1,2,17]

Attorneys in Legal Aid agencies find physical abuse mentioned as a major issue by approximately one third of their female clients. Of 2500 cases, a Brooklyn Legal Aid attorney discovered that 800 involved wife battering, and a California Bay area lawyer reported physical violence in 30% of his 1136 cases.[1,26] One Michigan judge estimated that 80% of the divorce cases he heard involved an allegation of physical abuse.[4]

Because wife battering is, essentially, a physical assault on a woman by the man with whom she lives that causes the victim to suffer serious or repeated physical injury, many women seek medical attention.[4,25] Boston City Hospital reported that 70% of the female assault victims treated in its emergency room had been attacked by a lover or husband.[17] Similarly, King's College Hospital in London discovered that 60% of all female assault victims over 16 years of age who needed inpatient admission were women beaten by their husbands.[7] Furthermore, an average of one battered wife each day was sent from their

Accident and Emergency department for radiologic examination. During an informal survey of physicians in the Los Angeles area, one general practitioner told me, "Any doctor who says he hasn't treated victims of wife beating cases is either lying or blind."

No social sector is immune from spousal violence. The very famous as well as the very obscure may indulge at some time or other. Various news media accounts reported that former attorney general John Mitchell, Alabama governor George Wallace, sports figure Jim Brown, and singer Fabian physically assaulted their wives.[3,4,6] Equally surprising, perhaps, was the finding from a comparison of police reports from the upper middle-class city of Norwalk, Connecticut and a Harlem, New York precinct of the same size. The comparisons showed that each received a similar number of wife abuse complaints—4 or 5 a week.[1]

Generally, information about the incidence of abuse is drawn from police and hospital records, which typically reflect a preponderance of contacts with people in the lower socioeconomic levels. A better perspective concerning the attitudes and behavior of people in middle and lower socioeconomic groups emerged from a study of conflict resolution among 2100 intact families that constituted a nationally representative sample.[33] The study discovered that:

1. Almost the same number of blue-collar and white-collar respondents approved of slapping the spouse. Twenty-six percent of blue-collar and 25% of white-collar respondents believed spouse slapping was "normal" while 11.8% of each group believed it was "good." But more blue-collar (7.9%) than white-collar (4.6%) responses indicated that slapping was "necessary."
2. When asked whether any act of violence, for example, pushing, slapping, throwing things, kicking, biting, threatening with a knife or gun, had *ever* occurred in the marriage, 29.7% of the blue-collar and 26.4% of the white-collar group indicated that it had.
3. The frequency and seriousness of spousal abuse in the blue-collar group was double that of the white-collar group (17% versus 8.9%).

The findings suggest that the attitudes toward physical abuse and the actual use of violence in marriages are very similar between middle and lower socioeconomic groups. However, when violence does erupt, it occurs more often and with greater severity in the lower socioeconomic group. This study also reaffirms that violence is *not* the norm within either socioeconomic level—75% to 80% of the respondents in each group neither condoned nor participated in spousal abuse.

WHY WIFE BEATING OCCURS

If most people do not include violence as part of their conflict resolution repertoire, why do some people occasionally or habitually resort to wife beating? Langley and Levy[14] offer several possibilities: mental illness, alcohol and drugs, public acceptance of violence, lack of communication, sex, poor self-image, frustration, change, and violence as a resource to solve problems. However, other explanations are important also. One reason revolves around the perception of people as property. Traditionally and legally, wives have been viewed as the private property of their husbands—and with ownership comes control over behavior.

In the 1800s several states granted husbands the right to "moderately" punish their wives during "emergency" situations without having to face assault and battery charges.[4] Although those laws were subsequently repealed, the belief persists that husbands have the right to determine how to treat (or mistreat) their wives without fear of reprisals. Very often battered women report that the physical violence did not begin until after the marriage, even when there was a 1- or 2-year period of living together prior to the formal ceremony. When questioned about the discrepancy in their behavior before and after the marriage rites, many husbands claimed, "It was different before. She could come and go as she pleased then. But once we were married, she was legally mine. She is *my* wife. Now she has to listen to me, and I have the right to keep her in line if she doesn't."

Another explanation is that battering constitutes an instance of displaced aggression. Displacement involves transferring the emotions felt toward a person or idea to someone or something else perceived as less likely to retaliate. Men who are unhappy at work, frustrated in their efforts to achieve success, or angry at the authority figures who rule large segments of their lives, take out their frustrations in the least threatening part of their environment—the home. Many women comment on their husband's unpredictable behavior. With no provocation from the women, the men may suddenly begin hitting their wives. It caused one woman to remark, "If things went wrong for him outside the home, *I* always got punished for it. When I greeted him at the door, I never knew whether to expect a kiss or a punch."

Not all displacements pertain to current situations, some are residuals from an unhappy childhood. The women often become aware that the anger is not really directed toward them but to a phantom from the past, usually a parent. It was common for one man, while beating his wife, to scream, "Why did you hit me so much when I was little? You shouldn't ought to have done that. I'm going to get you for it now. You're never going to hurt me like that again." Obviously the anger was not really related to his wife's behavior or to their marital relationship, but to an abusive parent who was both hated and feared.

By far the most popular explanation regards wife battering as a form of learned behavior, passed along from father to son. Several studies substantiate the linkage between witnessing or experiencing violence during childhood and exhibiting aggressive behavior during adolescence and adulthood.[11,18,28] Violent behavior between parents or from parent to child typically occurs more often in the backgrounds of battering husbands than of battered wives.

Children emulate what they see and hear. Aggressive behavior is a normal part of male socialization in this country. But, when the socialization process also includes physical aggression, children learn to view violence as a legitimate and viable reaction to stress or conflict. One battered woman decided it was time to leave the marital situation when her 4-year-old son began hitting her as he had seen his father do. "My husband watched his mother getting beaten by his father and grew up thinking it was all right to hit women," she said. "I don't want my son growing up the same way."

NATURE OF ABUSE

Although each marital relationship is unique, marital violence tends to follow certain fairly predictable patterns. Based on the literature and interviews with battered women, several general statements can be made.

The violent episodes usually result from social conflicts. Violence is an outgrowth of arguments or accusations between husband

Problems in reporting

Victims give numerous reasons for not wanting to report that they have been the victim of a sexual assault. Many just do not want anyone to find out about what happened to them, particularly their spouses, family, or friends. Others fear that publicity and reporting of the crime to the police may bring the assailant back after them. Still others are fearful of abusive treatment from law enforcement personnel, health professionals, and the criminal justice system if they prosecute. Victims may want to forget about the sexual assault as quickly as possible. They may be ashamed that they were unable to fight off their attackers. They may fear they will be blamed for the attack or fear public disclosure of their personal life in court if they prosecute.[2]

Ultimately the victim decides whether to report the sexual assault (in some cases, particularly with adolescents or children, family members may make the decision to report, or there may be witnesses to the assault), but counseling/advocacy resources encourage victims to get appropriate medical attention regardless of reporting to law enforcement authorities. Reporting of the crime to law enforcement authorities may prevent the assailant from assaulting someone else. Statistics indicate that a significant proportion of assailants suspected of sexual assault have previous arrest records, particularly in the area of violent crimes.

Recent literature has debated the probable significance of the increased rate of reporting sexual assault. It is uncertain whether the crime itself has increased or whether other factors have encouraged a higher percentage of victims to report it. Actually, there is probably a combination of causal factors. The results of a recently published study seem to indicate the rate of reporting of sexual assault crimes increases when couseling/advocacy resources are available to victims. *The Prosecutors,* volume I of the Batelle study, discusses the following factors: (1) the increased incidence of sexual assault occurs as a result of generally increased violence, (2) the change in attitudes toward victims of sexual assault may have increased the victim's willingness to report the crime to the police, (3) the criminal justice system has an increased sensitivity to the victim, (4) changes in legislation have occurred governing rape and sexual assault, and (5) there are more frequent convictions of assailants.[20]

Other statistics such as times, places, and ages

Many studies have been done in recent years on the occurrence of sexual attacks. All such studies are based on reported accounts of sexual assault, and it is assumed that assaults that are not reported are similar. For instance, the Batelle study reports that nearly half of all sexual assaults occur during the late evening and early morning hours, approximately 8 P.M. to 2 A.M. and are least likely to occur during the afternoon and early evening hours, 2 P.M. to 8 P.M. However, assaults on children are more likely to occur between noon and 8 P.M.[19] Statistics indicate that sexual assaults occur more frequently on weekends.

Women are not necessarily safe from assault in their homes. Assaults occur most frequently in the victim's residence, and the location of the crime is seen as directly related to the circumstances under which the initial contact is made between the victim and the assailant. A high frequency of motor vehicle sexual assault is associated with hitchhiking. The Batelle study[19] reports that approximately one third of the victims come into contact with the assailant voluntarily, although the assailant may use deception in making contact with the victim.

and wife. Tempers flair most often over money and jealousy, but disagreements can center around almost any theme, such as housekeeping or childrearing, with variations being replayed year after year.[3,23] As the arguments become more heated, patience snaps and physical abuse replaces verbal confrontation.

The violent episodes escalate in frequency and severity over time. What occurred once a month happens once a week; what began as a slap becomes a punch. Contrary to their hopes that violent episodes will abate over time, the longer the women remain in their marriages the more likely they are to suffer serious injuries. The most intense periods last until the participants are in their middle to late forties. After that periodic abuse is the usual pattern.

It requires less and less provocation to trigger an abusive episode. Long, haranguing arguments that promote the buildup of anger become unnecessary. The threshold to anger lowers, and it takes less verbal interaction to reach heated emotional levels. Minor incidents provoke reactions that are completely out of proportion to the situation. Once anger takes command, it is an easy next step to physical assault.

Verbal abuse accompanies physical abuse. Swearing, cursing, and verbal putdowns almost always precede and accompany physical assaults. Calling a woman "bitch" or "whore" successfully reduces her from a person to an object. It is much easier to justify hitting an object than a human being.

Alcohol use increases the likelihood of serious injuries. Even though alcohol may be involved at some time in 50% to 80% of spousal assaults, in only about a third of the cases does battering occur solely when the men have been drinking. However, women report that the men are more brutal and do more damage when they have been drinking. Whereas a sober man might slap or shove his wife, the same man, after taking several drinks, is liable to give his wife a sound beating. Drinking not only lowers inhibitions that allow social access to impulsive behavior, it offers a convenient excuse for assaultive actions. "It wasn't me, it was the alcohol talking." It is even possible that some men drink to legitimize the acting out of hostile or sexual impulses. Drug use among battering men is much rarer than alcohol use and seems to have a different effect. Most men do not batter while high on the drugs, instead they become assaultive when the drug begins to wear off.

Battering occurs in a clearly defined cycle of violence. Marital relationships that involve frequent batterings usually follow a definite three-phase violence cycle.[36] During phase one, the tension building phase, the men act edgy, irritable, and impatient. They seem to look for things to criticize in their wives' behavior. They vent their criticisms with verbal tongue lashings and occasional shoving or slapping episodes.

The second phase is the acute battering incident that results from the escalating tension. During the previous stage, the women tried to placate the husbands' anger, but in this stage violence seems inevitable. No longer able to hide their own irritations and anger, the women argue back, thus enabling the men to justify their violent actions. The battering is a way to teach their wives a lesson. This phase is the most violent and also the shortest.

The final stage is described as the calm and loving respite. The men apologize for their outbursts and make gestures of reconciliation. They promise to change their behavior in the future. The women desperately want to believe in the hope their husbands hold out to them and to forget the brutal side of their nature. Calm prevails until tensions begin to build once more and the cycle starts again.

The continuum of abuse

The term *wife battering* is an umbrella phrase that pertains to any deliberate physical asssault by a husband on his wife. But not all beatings are of the same intensity. Wife battering may progress along a four-point continuum that ranges from mild to fatal (Table 8-1).[30] Each battering incident may clearly fall into only one category or may include elements from two or more categories.

Many people exclude both ends of the continuum because they do not conform to their concept of physical abuse. They exclude the mild forms of abuse because this society possesses a high threshold of violence and usually requires bruising as the minimal medical and legal evidence that violence has occurred. At the other extreme, death is excluded because the popular concept of wife beating involves slapping or punching, neither of which is perceived as lethal. However, approximately 15% of all homicides are spouse killings; 50% of the victims in those killings are women. When women murder their spouses, knives or guns are usually involved, but weapons are less common in cases of husbands murdering their wives. Some women literally are battered to death.

NATURE OF ASSAULTS AND INJURIES

Just as assaults vary in severity, so do they vary in frequency. Many women experience physical abuse only once or twice during their marriage. But for women who are battered on a regular basis, the average seems to be monthly with some periods of greater frequency (weekly) and some periods of lesser frequency (every few months) over the years. Only a small percentage of women are battered daily.

The actual assault may last anywhere from a few minutes to over an hour. The usual pattern involves a brief, but intense, flurry of activity that ends as the anger is spent. However, some women report prolonged assaultive episodes lasting hours or even days. These incidents of serial abuse begin with an intense beating that lasts until the men tire. A short time later, when they have regained a second wind, they pick up where they left off and the beatings continue.

The majority of women do not actively fight back, instead they attempt to protect themselves by crouching or covering their head with their arms. The women who have attempted to defend themselves report their

Table 8-1. Physical abuse continuum

	Mild	Moderate	Severe	Fatal
Form of abuse	Shoving, slapping	Punching, kicking, choking	Thrashing, stomping, cutting	Pummeling, knifing, shooting, strangling
Injury	Little or no bruising	Body bruises, black eyes, contusions, cuts	Fractures, broken bones, extensive lacerations	Death
Medical treatment required	None needed	Outpatient	Hospitalization	None possible

greatest success comes early in the abuse cycle during the tension building phase. The men are still in control of their emotions and reactions and tend to back down when the women make it clear through words or actions that they will tolerate no further abuse. The time of greatest risk is a defensive action taken during the assaultive phase. Once the overt assaultive episode begins, the husbands are out of control and they use the women's self-defensive action to justify their need to punish or subdue the women.

There is a self-propelling aspect to physical abuse. Once begun, the act of punching and kicking seems to take on a life and character of its own. Unless they actively seek to stop the abusive behavior, the men become caught up in the rhythmic nature of the blows and continue over and over until they tire or until stopped by external intervention. Many men claim they felt dissociated from the arm, that it seemed to be moving by itself. So, in a sense, neither the wife nor the husband is in control during the assault, and it stops only when the man's anger is spent, when he regains contact with the reality of the situation, or when others intervene.

Fists and feet are the usual weapons, but other objects are also used in 25% to 60% of the incidents.[9,22,31] Studies mention a wide array of makeshift weapons enlisted by the men: frying pans, belts, belt buckles, knives, forks, lamps, broken glass, hot irons, brooms, lighted cigarettes, and even a piece of railroad track. Most studies show a low incidence (under 10%) of knives and guns.[3,4,6,8] By contrast, lethal weapons are apt to be present in the more serious wife battering cases. According to one study, of 40 cases reviewed, guns, knives, and other lethal weapons were present in 55% of the wife beating incidents that police were asked to investigate.[6]

Injuries may be inflicted on all parts of the body. Usually, however, the upper body (ribs, arms, and head) bears the brunt of the attack.[7] Apparently some men aim their blows to areas of the body that are more likely to be covered by clothing,[21] but for the most part, the men are not systematic in their approach. Black eyes from being punched, lumps on the head from being hit against a table or wall, and bruises on the upper arms from being grabbed and shaken represent frequent complaints. Batterings to women usually involve some combination of shoving, slapping, punching, kicking, and choking.[4,22,31]

Generally the women suffer multiple injuries with the cumulative effects producing severe, and at times, irreversible damage.[4,9,31]

injuries to the face, head, and neck—black eyes, bruised cheekbones, sprained neck, bloody, swollen, and/or broken nose, lumps and knots on the head, split and swollen lips, dislocated and fractured mandible, clumps of hair pulled out, lacerations from rings, strangle marks on the neck, inner mouth cuts, torn earlobes, and concussions

injuries to the trunk—broken collarbone, fractured tailbone, bruised spine, broken ribs, scratches and bite marks on the back, internal hemorrhage, lacerated liver, broken shoulder, bruised breast, and dislocated shoulder

injuries to the extremities—sprained wrist and ankles, torn ligaments and muscle, twisted knee, broken arm, bruised arm and leg, and burns on the feet

Contrary to theatrical portrayals of violence that depict a slap as a harmless way to calm an hysterical woman, an open-handed slap can cause serious injury. It can leave a bruise on the side of the face, dislocate a jaw, and rupture an eardrum. A punch can loosen or knock out teeth, produce a blow-out fracture of the eye, and break the bridge of the nose. There have been reported cases of retinal damage, epilepsy caused by head injuries, permanent hearing loss, headaches, dizziness, fainting spells, and back deformities. Close to 100% of the women in one sample needed some medical attention for their injuries and over 30% of the women in another study required hospitalization for their injuries.[4,31]

Pregnancy offers no guaranteed protection from assault, and sometimes triggers it. Women have been battered up to, and including, the eighth and ninth month of pregnancy. Gelles[10] suggests five factors that might account for physical assaults during pregnancy:
1. Sexual frustration — created by abstinence from sexual intercourse
2. Stress from family transition — strains produced by the transition to parenthood and the resulting changes in role relationships and family routine
3. Biochemical changes in the wife — that produce irritability, depression, and other mood changes
4. Prenatal child abuse — conscious or unconscious attempt to terminate the pregnancy
5. Defenselessness of the wife — her inability or unwillingness to retaliate because of her condition

Studies indicate that 25% to 50% of the women who had children suffered at least one assault while pregnant.[4,10] For some (4 out of 20 in one study), the assaults resulted in a miscarriage.[4]

DYNAMICS OF ABUSE

According to the profile yielded by personality tests, as a group battered women are reserved, withdrawn, depressed, and anxious people with low self-esteem, poorly integrated self-images, and low coping abilities who are easily upset and overwhelmed by life's problems.[28,29,31] Although some of these traits might be anticipated among people who live in constant fear of impending danger, the personality tests measure fairly stable, long-term characteristics. Therefore, these traits are not necessarily created by the marital situation but are definitely reinforced by it. Reserved people maintain an emotional distance from others and are not given to demonstrative behavior.[29] Most of the women described themselves as nonovertly affectionate people. It is not that they disliked being hugged or kissed, they just felt uncomfortable giving that type of affection, especially to other adults. A look at the family of origin revealed parents who were also generally undemonstrative in their display of love toward their children.

Their emotional reserve created difficulty for the women when they left their family of origin and entered the marital relationship. Their husbands interpreted the women's reserved attitude as a sign of rejection. They accused the women of being frigid and demanded more proof of their love. As one woman explained, "My husband wanted me to be more flirtatious and seductive toward him, to set a different environment. But I couldn't be that way without acting." As a result, the woman felt rejected. "To me that was like saying, 'You don't turn me on as you are,' that I wasn't acceptable to him as myself." So the woman pulled back from the relationship even further.

Battered women have a tendency to reproduce the conditions of their early family situation in their marriage.[12] Most battered women are not raised in families in which they witness or experience physical abuse. Interviews with the women do reveal, however, that they are raised in families that severely restrict emotional expression.[30] They learned to suppress their strong emotions, especially anger, and not to expect physical demonstrations of affection from their parents. Even though many are the oldest children in the family and carried a large share of the housekeeping and child-rearing responsibilities, they were denied opportunities to make decisions about their own activities. Instead, their parents encourage compliance. The usual widening of social contacts that normally takes place during childhood and adolescence doesn't materialize for many battered women. "I was pretty much of a loner as a kid and never had many friends," is the frequent response.

The same pattern prevails in their premarital dating behavior. One study reported that the women in their sample had dated fewer than five men prior to marrying the person who subsequently battered them.[31] In some cases social contacts are limited by the women's lack of comfort in social situations, in other cases the limits come from parents who insist that their daughters wait until late adolescence before allowing them to date. Frequently the women marry to escape their confining families.[31]

So, while physical abuse within the family of origin is not the norm, restrictions on individuality and personal freedom are very much evident in the backgrounds of battered women. They approach the marital situation with feelings of low self-worth that are the result of a diffuse self-identity and a devalued sense of their own potentials and abilities.

The women commence what for most is a first marriage, with men who appear strong and purposeful, men who offer secure boundaries. "It was his strength and gentleness that most attracted me to him," the women recall. "He really seemed concerned about me."

One study discovered that several of the women in their sample (49%) had seen at least one violent outburst directed toward themselves or others by their husbands prior to marriage.[31] But these were considered significant only in retrospect. At the time the women did not treat the premarital violence as an omen of later marital assaults.

The men tend to come from families in which they witnessed or experienced violence.[28] The women describe their husbands as possessive, strict disciplinarians, with their children as well as their wives, highly dependent on the women, uncommunicative, unable to talk about their feelings, exhibiting unpredictable mood swings, and blaming the women for everything that goes wrong. The men perceive the women as nagging, pushing, never satisfied. "She never let up, always telling me I should ask for a raise or get a better job. She just kept backing me into a corner."

Although they enter marriage with the hope of finding greater personal freedom, in reality the women exchange a restrictive family life for an equally restrictive marital life. The women report that the men are very jealous. They accuse the women of being unfaithful, they check up on the women during the day, and some even accompany their wives on shopping trips to select the type of clothes they think appropriate for them to wear.

The mechanisms that trigger abuse are usually trivial: leaving a carton of cream in the refrigerator too long, knitting an article of clothing the wrong size, losing a handbag, or talking to another man at a party.[5] During an interview one woman described a bloody battle that resulted from an argument about whether to open the Christmas presents on Christmas Eve or Christmas day. Sometimes there is no triggering mechanism and no warning. The men simply start hitting the women. Most often the battering begins in response to the women when they argue or assert themselves. Eventually the women measure every word and monitor every action lest they inadvertently trigger an assault.

All women who are physically battered are emotionally battered as well. In addition to being the object of the swearing or cursing that accompanies the abuse, they bear the brunt of daily verbal put-downs: "You are stupid. You are ugly. You can't cook. You are a terrible housekeeper. Nothing you say is important. If it weren't for me, nobody would want you." Day after day, the most important person in their lives tells them how incompetent, insignificant, and inconsequential they are. Heard often enough, the women begin to believe it. It reinforces their already low self-esteem and, over time, may create more damage to their functioning than the physical abuse.

Once the women accept their own incompetence as fact, it becomes easy for them to believe they are responsible for the batterings they receive. One of the most noticeable psychologic effects of wife battering is the degree to which battered women internalize the blame for the problems in the marriage. The women incorporate the blame the men project. "You know it's your own damn fault," accuse the men. "If you would clean the house better (or discipline the children, or not spend so much money, or keep your mouth shut), I wouldn't get angry. And, if I didn't get angry, I wouldn't hit you." Their accusations provoke guilt in the women and make them believe that they are failing to perform their roles of wife and mother adequately.

Both the men and women hold rigid sex-role stereotypes about the behavior appropriate for men, women, spouses, and parents. Overtly, the women hold the belief that marriage is a 50-50 partnership. Yet, covertly, many of the same women cling to the traditional ideas about marriage, such as that men should be the heads of the household and that a woman's greatest joy should be that of wife and mother.[31]

The men share those same beliefs and, as one newspaper account revealed, feel betrayed if the women act differently.[35] "When I married my wife she was a pretty, sweet girl who wanted what I wanted out of life. Or so I thought. Then she gets her consciousness raised and all of a sudden all that I'm giving her is not enough. She turns into a whining bitch. I think that's ungrateful. Damn ungrateful. If I had known that she had wanted a different style of life from the one I wanted I never would have married her. . . . My wife always told me that I didn't own her. Like hell I didn't! I did own her, that was part of the deal and she knew it. She knew just what kind of woman I wanted and she agreed to be it." Raised consciousness or not, it is the nature of relationships to change with time. But among battering couples, relationships are less flexible and change is perceived as a threat, a loss.

The fear of loss is a motivating force underlying much of wife battering. In his study of assaultive men, Schultz[24] discovered that the assaults were preceded by a perceived threat that the women would break off the marriage. Depending on the emotional needs of the assaulter, loss resulting from the threat of separation or divorce can trigger a variety of fears in the men. Elbow[5] identified four basic fears. For men whose basic need is autonomy, women signify objects needing control. The underlying message is, "I cannot be in control unless I control you." Men whose basic need is to protect, perceive loss of their mate as loss of acceptance. It is as if they are saying, "I cannot be an assertive person without you." Men who need confirmation of approval equate the loss of their spouse with the loss of self-esteem. They believe, "I cannot be as I see myself unless you see me as I want to be seen." Finally, to men who need affirmation or validation of being (existing), the loss of their mate symbolizes the loss of self. They seem to be saying, "I cannot exist without you."

The factor of control dominates the relationship. The men decide where the women can go, whom they can see, whether they can work, and whether they can return to school. The men determine the couple's social life. Some men become extremely jealous of any activities their wives engage in outside the home and force the women to give up many of their interests. "It got so I had no friends because he refused to let me go visit them," complained one woman. "Can you imagine, I had to ask his permission to leave the house!"

The women feel like prisoners in their own homes, and the isolation that results severely impairs their reality testing abilities. With no outside contacts, the women do not receive needed feedback about their behavior. They are without the input that could counteract negative self-conceptions or modify inaccurate perceptions of their capabilities. Neither can they evaluate how far their own marriages deviate from the general population.

Fortunately, one of the personality characteristics battered women possess is self-sufficiency.[29] Theirs is a self-reliance born of the realization that no one else is available on whom they can depend. They become accustomed to making decisions alone. It is mainly their resourcefulness that gives them the strength to survive in the marital relationship.

WHY WOMEN STAY

Some of the same factors that lead the women into the relationship also keep them there. The stereotype of the perfect marriage as a union that lasts a lifetime prompted one woman to say, "I thought it was my duty to stick by him, no matter what. I didn't want my marriage to be a failure."

Women who possessed few friends and very little social sophistication when they entered the relationship do not have the opportunity to change that situation during the marriage. The restrictive quality of the relationship keeps them isolated, unable to form a broad support network or to know what resources exist, or even to know that there is a different way to live. "It wasn't until I started working and heard some of the other women talking that I realized not all marriages were like mine," recalled a woman who finally left her abusive husband. "And not just about the beatings either. They seemed to do more things with their husbands and go more places. They enjoyed each other and they enjoyed life."

The passivity and compliance shown by so many battered women is one of the most difficult characteristics for them to overcome. Because they have been used to letting others take the initiative, the women are not equipped to act on their own behalf. "You can't imagine how hard it was," said a woman who broke away from a 10-year marriage. "I was used to letting him make all the decisions and I believed him every time he'd say I didn't have a brain in my head. I kept hoping someone would just come and take him, or me, away. I probably would still be there if he hadn't started beating up our little boy. That gave me the strength to leave."

The severity and frequency of abuse the women receive also influences their decision to stay or leave. Gelles[11] discovered that women who received mild physical abuse, such as a push or a shove, tended to seek no outside intervention either from friends, relatives, counselors, or police. The more frequently a woman was beaten, the more likely she was to dissolve the marriage.

One popular belief contends that some women are trained to remain in abusive relationships because they witnessed violence between their parents.[4] The assumption is that these women learn to expect and accept physical violence in their own marriages. Findings from a recent study tend to contradict that belief.[29] Among a sample of 70 women, those who came from nonviolent families remained in the marriage twice as long as those who came from families in which they witnessed or experienced abuse. It may be that women who have seen abuse realize that the violence will get worse, not better, whereas those who have not witnessed violent behavior do not know what to expect and, when violence does occur, are less well equipped to deal with it.

Wife beating, like rape, is one of those criminal acts in which the victim stands to lose more than the assailant. Very few men actually are prosecuted for assaulting their wives. In part this occurs because police are reluctant to intervene in family problems and, in part, because battered women are reluctant to press charges. Consequently, the women who flee from the violent situation risk losing their home, their possessions, and, sometimes, their children. Women arrive at shelters with little more than the clothes on their backs. Occasionally it is possible to gain entry into the home with a court injunction that offers police protection to enable the women to remove their belongings. "A lot of good that was," a woman remarked bitterly. "He had already sold, thrown out, or ripped up most of my things, including the stereo and the television. I was the one who was uprooted and left with nothing. It just isn't fair."

Nonetheless, usually it is incumbent on the women to leave, and the fewer their educational and economic resources, the less likely they are to go. Most women do not possess the job skills that would allow them to earn a large enough salary to support themselves and their children.

One of the many considerations involved in leaving is the impact such a move would have on the children. If the husband assaults the wife but not the children, the woman is hesitant to deprive her children of a two-parent family life. If the woman decides to go but leaves the children behind, she can be charged with desertion in some states and risk losing the children permanently. If she believes the home environment is destructive for the children and wants to take them with her, she must have a place to go and the means to support them. "I was ready to leave months ago," the women say, "but until I heard about the shelter I had no place to go." The fact is that resources for battered women are scarce, so their usual options include staying with friends and relatives or applying for welfare. Neither alternative offers sufficient incentive to leave anything but the most intolerably abusive situation.

External factors alone cannot fully account for their reluctance to leave, internal constraints play a large part also. The internal constraints consist of those thoughts, perceptions, and psychologic needs that affect behavior. Hope, fear, and depression top the list.

Most women cling to the hope that their husbands will change. Their hope blinds them to the seriousness of the assaults and encourages a denial system that misperceives the reality of the danger they face. They consistently underplay the damage done and seek rationalizations to explain their husband's behavior. Reinforcing their false hope further is the fact that battering men do not batter all the time. There are periods of calm, of pleasure, even of love.

The women receive sustenance during these times that counteracts the pain.

However, at some level of awareness the women realize that their husbands are capable of causing severe, perhaps irreversible, injuries. They fear not only for their own lives, but also for the welfare of their children and the possible reprisals to relatives and neighbors who attempt to intervene. They react to the constant potential threat to their existence with what Symonds[34] calls *frozen fright*. Their fear is so overwhelming and they feel so hopeless about escaping that they bury or freeze their fear. From their viewpoint, survival depends solely on appeasing the assaulter. The women use passive avoidance rather than active resistance to cope with the situation. Their attempts to cajole and comply lead others to the false conclusion that the women condoned, produced, or participated in the battering act.

People who perceive themselves as victims and who believe none of their actions will influence the outcome of a situation eventually become depressed. Depression is a major characteristic of battered women. It underlies their actions and colors their perceptions. Struggle seems useless; they give up fighting and concentrate on day-to-day survival.

Among battered women, fear knows many hiding places. When asked why they remain despite the pain, the women mention fear of the unknown and fear of loneliness. Ours is a society that stresses togetherness. Women are not encouraged or taught how to live alone or how to be on their own. The women imagine themselves in a strange apartment, penniless, no one to talk with, nothing to do, and not even the sound of a radio to comfort them. They prefer a familiar world with its occasional pain to a strange world filled with untold dangers. At least marriage offers the illusion of being cared for and cared about.

Relationships are complex and, once formed, not easily dissolved. People often remain in relationships long after they cease being satisfying, beneficial, or productive. The same tendency holds for battered women. What we sometimes label masochism may be nothing more than passivity coupled with the fear of leaving.

GUIDELINES FOR HELPING BATTERED WOMEN

All battered women should be told of the available options and resources even though not all are prepared to act on the information they receive. However, interventions work best when they correspond to the person's motivation for change; so it is always best to attempt some assessment of the women's readiness to seek and use help. A Change Potential Scale, based on my research and experience, was devised to aid in the assessment process by identifying those women who would be most amenable to change efforts (Fig. 8-1).

The Scale was developed specifically for inclusion in this book and has not been subjected to extensive prior testing. It should be used only as a guide until determinations have been made about its reliability and validity.

The Scale contains 10 items that focus on gathering information within three broad categories — family and work responsibilities, support network, and physical abuse patterns — that have been found to influence the women's willingness and ability to promote change. Each item contains a list of possible responses. The responses are assigned a numerical value of 1, 2, or 3. The total score, the sum of all the responses checked, ranges from a low of 10 to a high of 30. A low score indicates a low change potential, that is, the woman will be less likely to take the steps necessary to change or leave the relationship. A high score indicates a high change potential, that is, the

BATTERED WOMEN'S CHANGE POTENTIAL SCALE

Directions: Mark the response that seems most accurate for each item. Compute a total score by adding the numbers in parenthesis next to the answer that was checked. Also analyze the scoring patterns by counting the number of 3's, 2's, and 1's checked. High scores indicate a high change potential while low scores indicate a low change potential.

1. Length of relationship
    ____ Less than a year   (+3)
    ____ 1 to 3 years   (+2)
    ____ 3 to 5 years   (+2)
    ____ Over 5 years   (+1)

2. Number of children
    ____ None   (+3)
    ____ 1   (+3)
    ____ 2 - 4   (+2)
    ____ 5 or more   (+1)

3. Who else lives in the home
    ____ A boarder or stranger   (+3)
    ____ Her relative or friend   (+3)
    ____ His relative or friend   (+2)
    ____ No one   (+1)

4. The number of her relatives who live within a few miles
    ____ Several   (+3)
    ____ A few   (+2)
    ____ None   (+1)

5. The number of friends she has
    ____ Several   (+3)
    ____ A few   (+2)
    ____ None   (+1)

6. The woman holds employment
    ____ Full-time   (+3)
    ____ Part-time   (+2)
    ____ Not at all   (+1)

7. Whom has she told about the abuse
    ____ Several people   (+3)
    ____ A few people   (+2)
    ____ No one   (+1)

8. How often does the abuse occur
    ____ Daily   (+3)
    ____ Weekly   (+3)
    ____ Every few weeks   (+2)
    ____ Every month   (+2)
    ____ Every few months   (+1)
    ____ Once or twice a year   (+1)

9. How severe is the abuse
    ____ One or more hospi-   (+3)
         talizations
    ____ Frequent medical treat-   (+2)
         ment
    ____ Occasional medical   (+1)
         treatment
    ____ Never needed medical   (+1)
         treatment

10. Frequency of abuse during past year
    ____ Increased   (+3)
    ____ About the same   (+2)
    ____ Decreased   (+1)

Fig. 8-1. Battered Women's Change Potential Scale.

woman is more likely to consider and implement long-term change because of discomfort, exasperation, and/or fear.

Once a total numerical score is obtained, go back over the scale and count the number of responses checked for each of the numerical values 1, 2, or 3. If most of the responses bear a value of 1, the change potential is low. If most of the responses are assigned a value of 3, the change potential is high. If most responses checked have a value of 2, the change potential is not conclusive and can go either way. If responses are mixed and no clear-cut pattern emerges, the woman may feel too ambivalent about the situation to initiate change at that time.

Nursing personnel are in an excellent position to offer assistance to battered women. Not only do nurses have the opportunity to witness the physical injuries, but battered women often perceive nurses as supportive and sympathetic and may feel more comfortable confiding in them than they do with doctors. Regardless of the women's change potential, all battered women can profit from the following.

Encourage the women to talk about the battering and the injuries. Most women have not had the opportunity to talk about the physical assaults to an objective person. Some have felt too embarrassed to confide in anyone, including their parents. Even if no further action results, talking itself provides therapeutic benefits. Talking allows a release of pent-up feelings and, equally important, establishes a dialogue through which fresh input can be gained.

Encourage a realistic appraisal of the situation. Many battered women would like reassurances for their fantasy that the beatings will not happen again. Rather than try to comfort them with words that convey the message, "Everything will be just fine," or frighten them with predictions that, "He's going to kill you," the nurse should provide an answer that is more in keeping with reality. One such response might be, "I certainly hope it won't happen again, but the usual pattern is that not only will it occur again, but it will become increasingly worse."

Know community resources. Remember that battered women are isolated from the general community. They probably do not know about hotlines, legal services, shelters, or counseling agencies available to them. Make a list of those services for the women to take with them and keep for future reference.

Involve the social service department in the hospital. Usually battered women only make contact with the medical social worker if they require inpatient care. Some social service divisions would be willing to offer short-term outpatient counseling if they were aware of the problem. The women need this type of outreach service because the resolve to change so often fades within a few days after the assault.

Remain patient with battered women. Change is not easy for the women because they feel ambivalent about their situation. Their lack of follow through or their unwillingness to leave the battering relationship is frustrating and infuriating to those people trying to help. Attempting to force the decision-making process or to gain early closure adds more weight to the women's already heavy burden and undermines the change effort. Be available to serve as a sounding board for ideas and to help clarify options but allow the women to make their own decisions at their own pace.

Keep records to document the extent of the problem. On a larger scale, programs designed to eliminate wife battering will develop only if there is proof that a problem exists. Since no mandatory reporting systems similar to those for abused children have yet been instituted for battered women, agencies must keep their own records. Because hospital personnel change shifts and wards so frequently, there is a tendency to underrate the number of wife battering cases needing treatment. A concerted record keeping effort can go a long way to present an accurate picture of the problem.

REFERENCES

1. Barden, J.: Wife beaters: few of them ever appear before a court of law, New York Times, 10-21, 1978.
2. Boudouris, J.: Homicide and the family, J. Marriage Fam. 33:667-682, 1971.
3. Carlson, B.: Battered women and their assailants, Soc. Work 22:455-460, 1977.
4. Eisenberg, S., and Micklow, P.: The assaulted wife: Catch 22 revisited, thesis, University of Michigan Law School, Ann Arbor, 1974.
5. Elbow, M.: Theoretical considerations of violent marriages, Soc. Casework 58:515-526, 1977.
6. Flynn, J., Anderson, P., Coleman, B., et al.: Spouse assault: its dimensions and characteristics in Kalamazoo County, Michigan, master's thesis, School of Social Work, Western Michigan University, 1973.
7. Fonseka, S.: A study of wife beating in the Camberwell area, Br. J. Clin. Pract. 28:400-402, 1974.
8. Gayford, J.: Battered wives, Med. Sci. Law 15: 234-236, 1975.
9. Gayford, J.: Wife battering: a preliminary survey of 100 cases, Br. Med. J. 1:194-197, 1975.
10. Gelles, R.: Violence and pregnancy: a note on the extent of the problem and needed services, Fam. Coordinator 24:81-86, 1975.
11. Gelles, R.: The violent home, Beverly Hills, 1972, Sage Publications, Inc.
12. Hanks, S., and Rosenbaum, C. P.: Battered women: a study of women who live with violent alcohol-abusing men, Am. J. Orthopsychiatry 47: 291-300, 1977.
13. Holt, D., and Cumming, J.: The messy Wallace divorce, Newsweek 91:23, 1978.
14. Langley, R., and Levy, R.: Wifebeating: the silent crisis, New York, 1977, E. P. Dutton & Co., Inc.
15. Marsdén, D., and Owens, D.: The Jekyll and Hyde marriages, New Soc. 8:333-335, 1975.
16. Martha loses temper, Detroit Free Press, December 13, 1974.
17. Martin, D.: Battered wives, San Francisco, 1976, Glide Publications.
18. McCord, W., McCord, J., and Howard, A.: Familial correlates of aggression in nondelinquent male children, J. Abnorm. Soc. Psychol. 62:79-93, 1961.
19. Mulvihill, D., and Tumin, M., editors: Crimes of violence, vol. 11, Washington, D.C., 1969, Government Printing Office.
20. Parnas, R.: The police response to domestic disturbance, Wis. Law Rev. 914:914-960, 1967.
21. Pizzey, E.: Scream quietly or the neighbors will hear, London, 1974, Penguin Books Ltd.
22. Prescott, S., and Letko, C.: Battered women: a social psychological perspective. In Roy, M., editor: Battered women, New York, 1977, Van Nostrand Reinhold Co.
23. Roy, M: A current survey of 150 cases. In Roy, M., editor: Battered women, New York, 1977, Van Nostrand Reinhold Co.
24. Schultz, L.: The wife assaulter, J. Soc. Ther. 6: 103-112, 1960.
25. Scott, P.: Battered wives, Br. J. Psychiatry 125: 433-441, 1974.
26. Senate Subcommittee on Nutrition and Human Needs: Family violence, Sacramento, Calif. 1975.
27. Spouse abuse cases top one million, Public Administration Times, 1:6, 1978.
28. Star, B.: Comparing battered and nonbattered women, Victimology 3: in press.
29. Star, B.: The psychological dynamics of battered women. Paper presented at the California Attorney General's Conference on Domestic Violence, Los Angeles, April, 1978.
30. Star, B.: Treating the battered women. In Hanks, J., editor: Toward human dignity: social work in practice, Washington, D.C., 1978, National Association of Social Workers.
31. Star, B., Clark, C., Goetz, K., et al.: Psychosocial aspects of wife battering. Paper presented at the American Orthopsychiatric Association Annual Meeting, San Francisco, 1977.
32. Steinmetz, S.: Violence between family members, Marriage Fam. Rev. 1:1-16, 1978.
33. Straus, M.: Normative and behavioral aspects of violence between spouses: preliminary data on a nationally representative U.S.A. sample, Durham, 1977, University of New Hampshire.
34. Symonds, M.: Victims of violence: psychological effects and aftereffects, Am. J. Psychoanal. 35:19-26, 1975.
35. Thomas, I.: A wife-beater tells his story, The Village Voice, August 1, 1977.
36. Walker, L.: Treatment alternatives for battered women. In Chapman, J., and Gates, M., editors: The victimization of women, Beverly Hills, 1978, Sage Publications, Inc.

CHAPTER 9

Sexual assault: social, legal, medical, and psychologic aspects

Kathryn C. Bemmann and Susan C. Bundy

INTRODUCTION

Few human crises are greater than an experience with sexual assault for the pain, trauma, and disruption caused the victim in personal, psychologic, physical, sexual, family, and social aspects of her life. Few situations demand as much sensitivity and widely disparate multidisciplinary knowledge from health care workers—initially under time pressure, subsequently over a long time—sensitivity and knowledge not only of health care professionals, but also of the law enforcement and legal systems. Interdisciplinary understanding and cooperation are essential for the best short-term and long-term resolution of the crisis for the victim, the victim's family, and society.[15]

For these reasons, sexual assault counseling and advocacy groups have been formed in many areas, involving specialists in this complex situation serving not only victims' needs but also often acting as advisers to the community. Where such a group does not exist, the responsibility for good evaluation and care and evidence collection is even greater for the health care professional.

Awareness of the plight of the sexual assault victim is relatively recent, having gained momentum in the mid-1970s with the women's liberation movement. New concepts about it are now accepted by feminists and nonfeminists alike and are applicable to both sexes and to adults and children. Two researchers who have contributed the most widely known and comprehensive studies on victims of sexual assault and of the institutions that deal with them are Burgess and Holmstrom.[7-10,14,15] Their publications are very highly recommended for more detailed information.

The language in this chapter will reflect the assailant's gender as male and the victim's as female (known as male-on-female sexual assault). Male-on-male sexual assault occurs and is equally traumatic for the victim: reports of it and more information about it are just emerging as the taboo against reporting it lifts. The overwhelming majority of victims are female, however, and especially because of the gynecologic nature of this text, discussion will be limited here to the female sexual assault victim. Female-on-female and female-on-male sexual assaults have been known to occur, but appear to be relatively rare with the possible exception of child sexual abuse.[6] Information here is still being gathered. Sexual assault seems to be almost entirely a crime peculiar to the male. Hence, although there are exceptions, the assailant will be referred to in the male gender.

Our choice of the term *sexual assault* rather than *rape* deserves some explanation. *Sexual assault* is perhaps preferable, since *rape* often is thought of in stereotypic, ill-defined ways, steeped in myth rather than reality. The use of a new and different term sometimes enables a rethinking of a subject.

DEFINITIONS

Legal terms and definitions of sexual assault or rape vary from state to state. Many states have rewritten or are rewriting laws to reflect changes in thinking on sexual assault including sex-neutral language and degrees of assault and penalities; other states have a long way to go to update their laws.[5] It is especially important for health professionals dealing with the problem to familiarize themselves with the sexual assault or rape laws of their state.

Sexual assault is generally defined legally as sexual intercourse with a person, by force, and against that person's will. The slightest penetration fulfills the requirement for "sexual intercourse"; neither full penetration nor emission is required. "Force" can be actual physical force or verbal threats of death or bodily harm to stymie resistance.[13]

Sexual assault, then, is a crime, an act of violence and force, initiated by the assailant, using sex as a weapon, and without and against the victim's will and consent. This definition spells out the realities and counters some of the myths. These myths are myriad, but the general underlying themes are that the victim is a responsible and not an innocent party to the incident, while the assailant is an innocent, sick, or duped party to it.

The range of actual sexual assault experiences is wide, from surprise "blitz" attacks with threats of bodily harm or death, to an insistence on sexual intercourse in a social or family situation in which sexual contact was either unexpected or not agreed on. The latter type of event is often misinterpreted or overlooked as nonconsent by many dealing with the sexual assault victim because of erroneous, widespread assumptions that certain social situations, such as dates, imply consent for sexual contact.[10,22]

INCIDENCE OF SEXUAL ASSAULT
General statistics

Sexual assault is considered the most underreported violent crime in this country. Because this crime is less likely to be reported by its victims, statistics vary considerably and the actual incidence is still unknown. The most recent sexual assault statistics have been published by the Batelle Law and Justice Study Center in Seattle, Washington, and most information in this section is taken from the published results of that study.[19]

It is estimated that although 250,000 sexual assaults are committed each year, only about 56,000 are reported to law enforcement authorities. These statistics can be further broken down to show that approximately one in four sexual assault complaints results in an arrest and only one in sixty results in a conviction. Previous reports from the Batelle Center indicate that in 1974 the rate of sexual assaults was 26.1 per 100,000 inhabitants. The statistics show a 115.7% increase in the rate of reporting of sexually assaultive crimes from 1965 to 1974. Approximately every 9 minutes an American woman is sexually assaulted or sexually abused.[2]

A large proportion of reported sexual assaults involve stranger-to-stranger attacks, but authorities assume that sexual assaults involving nonstrangers (acquaintances, family, friends) may be very underreported.

Alcohol or other drugs are often involved in assaults—usually on the part of the assailant, often by both the assailant and the victim, and sometimes by the victim alone. Sexual assaults, contrary to myth, tend to be intraracial, rather than interracial, and members of minorities appear overrepresented as both victims and offenders. Minors are either assailants or the victims, each in approximately 10% to 20% of all offenses. Female infants under 1 year of age are raped as are women in their 80s and 90s.

Physical force is used against victims in at least half the reported sexual assaults, and guns and knives are the most common weapons used. The victim's resistance is most commonly verbal. Approximately one fourth of the victims of sexual assaults suffer physical injuries that are serious enough to require medical attention or hospitalization, and it is likely that a large proportion of assaults that are unreported involve no injuries. Medea and Thompson[17] report that over 70% of assailants use some form of force and may use more than one form, including threats, blows, weapons, beatings, and attempted choking. Nearly half the victims report awareness of being led into a dangerous situation, what might be referred to as a hunch or "gut reaction." Most victims resist physically (over 80%), nearly a fourth resist by trying somehow to dissuade their attackers verbally, and a sixth of victims scream. Victims who resist the attack are more likely to be injured than those who do not resist. However, the effect of resistance in a sexual assault depends more on the motives of the assailant than on the resistance or show of strength by the victim. From one fourth to half of assaults involved more than one assailant,[1] a factor that significantly reduces the victim's hope or opportunity for resistance against an assault. The presence of two or more assailants is in itself overwhelming and overpowering.

Approximately one fourth of sexual assaults involve oral sex acts, which has important implications for medical procurement of evidence for prosecution. Initial reports of the assaults are generally made to law enforcement authorities, and more than half the assaults are reported within 1 hour of the assault. Eyewitnesses who are not co-conspirators appear to be very rare. Most sexual assaults are premeditated—an assailant plans to assault someone and finds an opportunity to do so. Of course, the plan is to not be discovered.

THE "WHYS" OF SEXUAL ASSAULT
General profiles

Increasingly, sociocultural views hold that sexual assault is a battleground for power and control, an interface of violence, between the sexes. Human beings have been traditionally reared to expect certain behaviors from each sex. Anatomy and physiology have contributed to these expectations because of differences between the sexes in size, muscle mass, and reproductive tasks. Males were encouraged to be the doers, the movers, the takers, in short, the aggressors, rewarded for being physically active, achieving, accomplishing, dominating, winning—the "actors." Females, conversely, had to be, or were supposed to be, the "reactors," the passive recipients, submissive, physically inactive, the childbearers and caretakers of the human race, first and foremost. This contrast tended to result in a significantly lower evaluation of women in a society that depended on physical prowess for survival.

A strong tendency toward physical violence is prevalent in American society.[6,13] The phenomenon is difficult to study in the population as a whole, but it has been studied in prison populations by sociologist Curtis and reported by Brownmiller.[6] Curtis formed profiles of felons convicted for three types of violent crime—aggravated assault, rape, and robbery—and found that the profile of the rapist was midway between the other two in several ways: age, use of force and alcohol, and locale and victim focus of the crime. The man convicted of aggravated assault was in the oldest age group of the three, used the most force and alcohol, stayed in his own neighborhood, indeed, usually in his own home, to commit the crime, and mostly assaulted people in his own race and those known to him. The robber was in the youngest age group, used the least force and alcohol, went out of his neighborhood, and robbed strangers. Taking some characteristics from both was the rapist.

No separate psychopathology has been identified for the rapist aside from the individual quirks and personality disturbances that might characterize any other offender.[1] There is often disordered sexual behavior with distortions and admixtures of sexuality, anger, and power issues, not yet recognized as unique pathology.[8]

Brownmiller calls the rapist "an unextraordinary, violence-prone fellow."[6]

Forcible sexual assault and the assailant

Nevertheless, several patterns of sexual assault and assailants have been identified in the assailants' aims: the power aim, the anger aim, and the sadistic aim.[8,11]

In the *power aim,* the most common, the object is to gain control over the victim, and only necessary force is used to accomplish that goal. Verbal threats, weapons, and some physical force may be used. This type had earlier been called the *sexual aim* by researchers. The attempt to compensate for feelings of inadequacy finds expression in sexual conquest, but the basic issue is power and control. Other personality defects include low self-esteem, feelings of vulnerability and helplessness, and immaturity. Both fantasies and behavior tend to be highly repetitive, and the rapist does not get the satisfaction for which he is looking; he is anxious and desperate, but not really angry. Assaults are likely to be planned. The assailant characteristically fantasizes that his prowess and charms will make the victim hopelessly enamored of him and sexually turned on to him, and he may keep the victim captive for prolonged periods. He often distorts and misperceives some verbal or physical behavior on the part of the victim as consent for sex. A common theme involves his feeling of being controlled by others, including women, and the sexual assault is an attempt to reverse the order of power. His first conviction probably is not for his first offense. Often the victim is younger, thereby easier to overpower because of age, size, and naivete. The same victim may be chosen again.

Called the aggressive aim by researchers at one time, the object of the *anger aim* is degradation, humiliation, and brutalization of the victim. Far more force and aggression are used than are needed to merely gain control of the victim. About 20% of sexual assaults fit this category. The assailant characteristically experiences some precipitating stress in a significant relationship, releasing sudden anger and rage that are misdirected toward the victim in an attempt at retaliation. More sporadic and more impulsive than in the power aim, the time span of the assault is short. Sex is seen by the assailant as dirty and degrading, and he uses it to humiliate; other acts considered "dirty" by the offender may also be performed. Language used toward the victim is hostile and obscene. There may be no sexual arousal, and the assailant may be impotent unless the victim performs the requested act or acts. The victim may be much older than the assailant. The same victim is highly unlikely to be chosen for an assault again by the same rapist. Psychologically, the brutality of the assault ensures a higher conviction rate.

Fortunately fewer than 2% of offenders fit the pattern of the *sadistic aim,* referred to as sex-aggression diffusion at one time by researchers. This has the deadliest potential of all sexual assaults. Aggression has become eroticized in the assailant; the more violent he becomes, the more sexually excited he becomes and vice versa. Homicide is most likely to occur in this type. These assaults are ritualistic, repetitive, premeditated, and carefully calculated. The same type of victim is chosen, and the same situation is reenacted. The rape may not involve sexual areas of the assailant at all; that is, vaginal penetration may be accomplished with various instruments and weapons. Definitely intentional, the violence is interspersed with other types of assaultive and nonassaultive behavior. The assailant is more apt to be diagnosed as psychotic.

The victim's part in the forcible sexual assault

It is obvious from the discussion of the types of sexual assault that a victim's behavior may be significant in the outcome of the assault. We do not intend to blame but only to emphasize that no specific behavior is "right" all of the time. Sometimes only passive compliance will save a victim's life; at other times, it is not the better defense, and active, effective resistance might save a victim's life.

Symonds[24,25] describes two responses that immediately follow the shock and disbelief of sudden, unexpected violence—frozen-fright or anger. Even though the latter is rooted in fright, the victim recalls only the anger and the fighting behavior. A human being usually experiences the same type of response in different assaults or crises. These behaviors are regressions to adaptive and innate patterns of early childhood. Although actually self-preservation, this behavior may seem to be friendly, even cooperative, causing confusion for all, including the rapist, the victim's family and friends, the police, and even the victim herself. Symonds also describes resistance patterns that may be passive or active. Passive patterns of response are generally seen in those persons raised in middle and upper socioeconomic families and who were not exposed to violence in early life. They include verbal or physical efforts to stop the rapist by pleading and attempting to induce guilt or appealing to his conscience. Generally failing, the responses may make the rapist angry rather than guilty. Active (or aggressive) resistance includes verbal threats or physical fighting and is directed toward producing fear in the rapist,—fear of either being hurt, caught, or exposed if he persists. While there is growing evidence to indicate that in the majority of cases of attempted rape an actively resisting woman is only slightly injured, this knowledge is not much help to the woman exposed to a violent rapist. She has only a short time, if any, to evaluate her crisis and react to it.

Researchers are attempting to find ways to enable women to learn to tell rapidly and with assurance which response in a given assault is preferable and why. This topic will be further expanded in the heading under Prevention. Until more is known, victims should be supported for doing what they can and what they know how to do for survival.

Nonforcible sexual assault

Although the most widely recognized form of sexual assault is "forcible rape," Burgess and Holmstrom's study has defined two other types—accessory-to-sex and sex-stress assaults.[10]

The *accessory-to-sex assault* is defined as a sexual situation in which the victim assists or aids the offender in a secondary way but is unable to or incapable of consent to the sexual situation because of the stage of her personality or cognitive development, as in the case of children or extremely disturbed, deprived, drugged, psychotic, or mentally retarded adults. The assailant may have a power relationship to the victim because of age or authority, for example, and uses that power to manipulate her. The assailant may pressure the victim into accepting money, candy, or other material goods, lure her to accept human contact through sex, or talk her into believing the sexual activity is appropriate and enjoyable, even "good" for her. The sexual activity may well be enjoyable for the victim. The trauma may be expressed through a withdrawal, both social and psychologic, from the victim's usual activities, particularly evident if the victim has been pledged or threatened to secrecy by the assailant.[14]

The *sex-stress assault* is probably the least understood by everyone. Medical, law enforcement, and legal authorities are the least sympathetic or understanding with this type of assault, which Burgess and Holmstrom define as an anxiety reaction resulting from the circumstances around sexual activity to which both partners initially consent, but something goes wrong later, for example, demands for acts of sexual perversion or the expression of violence.[14] Often the victims of the sex-stress assault are sexually inexperienced adolescents and nonassertive or submissive adult women inexperienced in dealing with sexual demands, but prostitutes who discover themselves in situations for which they did not bargain also fit into this category. Also included by Burgess and Holmstrom are several sex-stress reactions that are confusing when classified in "assault" categories, for example, an adolescent or adult women has consented to sex, but later denies consent and claims assault when confronted by authority figures, such as police, parents, or other adults. Thus, because an accusation of sexual assault is made, medical attention may be requested or demanded for the "victim." It is important to point out that Burgess and Holmstrom have included these types of assault to encourage a nonjudgmental approach to all cases of alleged sexual assault. Spurious complaints comprise only 4% or 5% of the total reported, and it is not to the credit of the health care system to be judgmental of those seeking services for any reason, especially in the complex area of human sexuality.

The crime of opportunity

Just as normal sexuality activity is response to opportunity, so is sexual assault, and rapists are indeed opportunists. Men's upbringing, and perhaps their hormones, have made some of them susceptible to thinking they can gain power and self-esteem or satisfy sexual urges through the use of violence. Women's upbringing and low social, psychologic, and economic status have made them vulnerable to men's violence by means of sexual expression. When this is combined with racial inequities, as in the case of minorities, the combined impact of all forces makes for an even greater sexual assault problem.

FEELINGS OF THE SEXUAL ASSAULT VICTIM
Rape trauma syndrome

The type of sexual assault, the victim's reaction to it, and the prevailing attitudes of the institutions or systems that deal with sexual assault victims all have an enormous impact on the level of distress experienced by victims in the rape trauma syndrome. Holmstrom and Burgess[15] have defined the rape trauma syndrome as the physical, emotional, and behavioral stress reactions that result from a person's being placed in a life-threatening situation through a sexual attack. Rape trauma syndrome involves the acute or immediate phase, most frequently seen by medical, legal, and counseling personnel immediately following the assault, and a long-term reorganization phase.

Acute phase. A complete disruption of the victim's lifestyle occurs. The style of the victim in the immediate or impact phase of the reaction to sexual assault can be described as expressed, in which feelings of anger, fear, or anxiety are overt, or controlled, in which feelings are masked or hidden, the victim's affect appearing calm or composed. In the past, medical, law enforcement, and criminal justice personnel lacked sensitivity in dealing with the victim who appeared subdued and calm after reporting a sexual attack. Professionals who work with victims of sexual assault are now more aware of the variety of emotions expressed by the victim — from crying, hysteria, and fear, to anger, to appearing calm or withdrawn.

Physically, because of the force used in the assault, victims may complain of soreness all over their bodies or in specific areas that were the focus of the assailant. They may complain of disturbances in sleep patterns, an inability to fall asleep, frequent and early wakening, and so on. Disturbances in normal eating patterns are also common and may include a decreased appetite, stomach pains, or nausea. Nausea could also be a reaction to antipregnancy medication. Victims may have symptoms that are specific to the focus of the assault. For example, victims forced into the act of oral sex may have feelings of irritation and pain in their mouths and throats; those who have had a vaginal assault may complain of vaginal discharge, itching, and burning on urination; others forced to have anal sex may feel rectal pain or complain of bleeding.

Victims often feel ashamed or guilty; this is the feeling most often expected of her by those with whom she comes in contact. Various kinds of fears of physical injury, mutilation, or death are commonly expressed; such feelings are acute stress reactions to the actual or implied threat of being killed and result in the development of a rape trauma syndrome. Attempts are made to block all memories of the assault, but such memories may continue to haunt the victim, and flashbacks or vivid memories of the attack may recur. Victims may have a strong need to go over details of the assault repeatedly, trying to think of ways to change or undo what happened, but this frustrates and additionally distresses them. The reaction of fear is added to by other emotions: humiliation, degradation, shame, embarrassment, self-blame, anger, and revenge. As mentioned earlier, some victims may be willing, even eager, to talk about their emotional reactions, and a supportive person who can allow them to express these emotions is an asset to their recovery.

Long-term phase. In the long-term process of reorganization that follows the acute crisis phase, a variety of factors affects the victim's coping strengths — personality style of the victim, supportive people to respond to her distress, and treatment she receives from those with whom she comes in contact following the assault. Disruption or changes in the victim's lifestyle are common. Victims may resume no more than minimal functioning, such as agreeing to go out but only with a companion. They may turn for support to family members with whom they normally do not have daily contact, although they may keep the occurrence of the sexual assault from their friends and family. Some victims react with a strong need to get away and may take a trip or change residences and phone numbers.

Victims often complain of dreams and nightmares of two main types: in the first, dreams consist of an event similar to that of the attack with vain attempts to escape. The second type of dream may be disturbing to the victim; she may dream that she commits an act of violence, such as killing or stabbing someone. The victim may report a feeling of control in the dream itself, but she then must adjust to this new, violent image of herself.

Phobias that are specific to the circumstances of the assault are another reaction. Victims in Burgess and Holmstrom's study sample expressed a fear of being in crowds, fear of being alone, or fears related to some characteristic of the assailant, such as a similar moustache or beard, the smell of alcohol, and so on. Because victims may think that everyone knows about the assault, they may express feelings of suspicion or paranoia or a fear of everyone. A fear of sex and disruption in their normal sexual style, as well as a suspicious reaction to men in general, is not uncommon. If, later, a second upsetting situation occurs, such as a purse-snatching, or if there is a prior psychiatric or physical condition, a compounded reaction may result for which more than crisis counseling is indicated to deal with additional symptoms.

Children and adolescents

The expression of rape trauma syndrome in children and adolescents is essentially similar to that seen in adults, with the major differences being in the personality of the young person as compared with the adult, the developmental crises facing the child, the young person's degree of ability to report the distress being experienced, and the manner in which the distress is expressed. The immediate or impact reaction of the child or adolescent may be either expressed (crying, talking about other concerns, complaints of physical symptoms) or controlled (fear of retaliation or parental reaction, fear of telling what happened because of verbal or physical threats, and shy, subdued demeanor). Somatic or physical reactions are similar to those expressed by adult victims, and fear and embarrassment are common emotional reactions. In the long-term or reorganization process, child or adolescent victims may want to change schools, be truant, argue with classmates, or have difficulty keeping up with their assignments. Nightmares involving violence are common. Phobias often develop such as fears of being alone, going to school, and sex. Characteristics of an assailant such as color of hair or type of beard may become the focus for phobic reactions.

ATTITUDES OF SOCIETY AND ITS INSTITUTIONS

Societal attitudes toward rape and sexual assault are becoming more sympathetic to the trauma suffered by the victim. This change in attitude is a result of the interest aroused by the women's movement in the needs of women as well as of the increased interest and research into the psychology of victims.

Law enforcement

Law enforcement authorities are most often the first professional group that the victim of a sexual assault encounters, and the attitude of officers may have serious impact on the reaction of the victim to the assault and on her recovery from the assault. Burgess and Holmstrom's research reported a minority of negative responses to victims of sexual assault by law enforcement authorities.[10] It is unfortunate that this minority has received a majority of media coverage and has contributed to the reluctance of victims of sexual assault to report the crime.

Most law enforcement officers are well aware of the violent nature of the crime of sexual assault and may hold punitive attitudes toward the rapist. In dealing with a charge of any kind, however, the officers make a judgment as to the validity of the charge and put their professional competence on the line.[10] This fear of being wrong and the concern for erroneously convicting someone contribute to the officers' careful checking of all complaints. Too often, after carefully checking out a complaint, arresting a suspect on the charge of sexual assault, and making an enormous investment of time and effort, officers find that the victim refuses to follow through the criminal justice process and the suspect must be released. These factors contribute to the skepticism of officers in dealing with sexual assault complaints.

The opening statement by a police officer can set the tone for the entire interview. A statement that puts the victim at ease and gives consideration for the crisis state can provide for a more profitable interview. Officers develop a professional detachment from those they serve, as do those in other professions, and victims may misinterpret the professional demeanor of officers as noncaring, nonsympathetic, or judgmental. Victims, on the other hand, must remember that the focus of law enforcement is to determine the validity of the complaint and gather evidence that will make an arrest possible. Questioning by officers immediately following the assault may lead authorities to a quicker arrest, preventing further assaults by the same assailant on other women. Such questioning may be perceived as distressing by victims, however.

Medical system

The medical or health care system is usually the second "institution" that the sexual assault victim encounters, brought there as a rule by law enforcement officers.[15] By far, most health professionals maintain professional politeness toward victims, concentrating on technical competence accomplished with smiling faces and reassuring comments. Neither a great deal of sympathy nor overtly negative feelings are shown. This polite, nonjudgmental approach is good.

Especially positive reactions are expressed toward young victims, and in the case of adults, toward pretty and articulate victims of forcible rape.[22] Expressed negative reactions are relatively few, consisting of comments about "lack of cooperation" or openly moralistic and degrading remarks to patients' faces. A handful of other reactions are hard to classify as either positive or negative; they have been called "conscientious harassment." Wanting to give good care to patients and meeting with resistance at times for varying reasons, the health care staff may talk, persuade, bargain, and push, and depending on how hard they push, their behavior may begin to be more harassing in nature, infringing on patients' freedom of choice.

"First do no harm" is learned by all professionals in the health care system; "first do no more harm" should be the dictum for dealing with sexual assault victims. Most frequent attitudinal or behavioral problems on the part of health workers result either from continued beliefs in the myths of rape, rather than a knowledge of its realities, or from unthinking and uninformed violations of patients' rights to privacy, confidentiality, and knowledge and feedback about their condition.[10,15] The right to have their own bodies treated with human respect and dignity is important to sexual assault victims who have just experienced a most severe violation of their bodies. Probably the best professional attitudes toward patients or clients are summed up by Symonds[25] in the following three simple statements: (1) I'm sorry it happened, (2) I'm glad you're all right (alive), and (3) You did nothing wrong.

Family and friends

Persons in the assault victim's immediate emotional environment, of course, are as subject to misconceptions and myths about sexual assault as are other members of society. Reactions to the crisis by family and friends, therefore, are often a very painful mixture of caring and blaming attitudes, and empathy and support are again needed. Burgess and Holmstrom have also described acute and long-term phases of these reactions.[10] In the acute phase, close family members and friends may experience a severe shock or impact stage. Somatic distress, such as nausea, occurs. Insomnia may be a factor as well as various obsessive ruminations about the assault. Fear of their own violent potential may be significant, as is a fear of the reappearance of and retaliation by the assailant.

Friends and relatives feel anger much sooner than the victim does. Raging against the assailant may provide some relief from the anger, but it provides little comfort to the victim. Another target of blame is the victim, for example, Did she provoke the attack somehow? Didn't she fight enough to prevent the assault? Finally, friends and relatives may blame themselves, feeling the assault could have been prevented if they had been with the victim or had not had that confrontation with her before she left for the movies, and so on.

Some long-term aspects of recovery for the victim's "significant others" deal with the issue of sexuality. Examples of responses are aversion to the victim or overprotectiveness and overconcern in making sexual overtures to her. Another problem may be an impatience with and intolerance of the victim's need for time to resolve the rape trauma syndrome. Families and friends recover from their crises faster than the victim.

Initially, many victims suffer some added trauma because of their families' and friends' inappropriate ideas and resultant behaviors relative to the assault. As family and friends understand and accept the facts of the assault, they begin to recognize the damage that the victim has suffered. The resultant guilt feelings may trigger an overprotectiveness toward the victim that can further retard her recovery, and this problem needs resolution.

Legal system

Legal authorities suffer from attitudes similar to those of law enforcement officers: a demeanor of professional detachment and a skepticism about victims following through the criminal justice process may be misinterpreted by sexual assault victims as a negative response. Like law enforcement officers, prosecutors put their professional competence on the line when evaluating charges of sexual assault and taking the case into the courtroom. Even though legal authorities may believe a sexual assault case is appropriate for prosecution, victims, as primary witnesses in the case, may be unable to identify defendants, may be unwilling to press charges, or may drop the charges once filed.[10] Legal authorities must rely on law enforcement officers to make arrests and may need to plea bargain or consider lesser charges to get guilty pleas from or convictions of defendants. Victims may interpret plea bargaining as disbelief on the part of legal authorities.

In prosecuting cases of sexual assault, legal authorities are reported by Burgess and Holmstrom as being most interested in victims considered "good witnesses."[10] Courtroom dispositions of cases depend on impressions created by victims on the witness stand. A victim/witness whose appearance and demeanor are appropriate and whose testimony is consistent, is considered a "good witness." Holmstrom and Burgess have identified a "good district attorney" as one who takes the claim of sexual assault seriously, shows concern for the victim's privacy, pays attention to social niceties, refrains from moralistic comments, and provides explanations and advice to the victim.[15]

It should be noted that the attitudes of legal and law enforcement authorities also depend on the structure of state statutes regarding the crime of rape or sexual assault. Legislation is currently changing, and there are several states (Minnesota and Wisconsin, for instance) whose sexual assault legislation is considered progressive in that convictions can be more easily obtained by providing for a range of degrees or specific charges. Marked restriction of questioning into a victim's past sex life removes from her some of the burden of testifying. Legislation in some states has not changed in hundreds of years, and therefore a complete understanding of sexual assault as a crime of violence is lacking. Outdated legislation adversely influences professional attitudes of people in the criminal justice system.

Counseling

The attitude of counseling resources to victims of sexual assault varies. Many communities, particularly those in urban areas, now have rape, sexual assault, or victim counselors who may be trained volunteers or professionals. Our experience has shown that not all counseling professionals are sensitized to the trauma and to the victim's needs. Recent interest in victimology has led to research and concern for dealing with people who have been victimized by sexual assault and other crimes.

The primary focus of the sexual assault counselor who is called in to deal with a victim immediately following the assault is to be supportive to the victim. In providing this supportive function, the counselor is primarily concerned with the victim's needs and requests and secondarily concerned with dealing with other institutional (medical, law enforcement, and legal) authorities' responses to the victim.

Counselors are accepting of the victim, her response to the assault situation itself, and her trauma reactions afterward. Counselors are nonjudgmental, noncritical, and nonblaming of the victim. Although some counselors have experienced a sexual assault themselves, a similar experience is not a prerequisite for becoming a sexual assault counselor. More important than having been assaulted oneself is an understanding of the victim's situation and the ability to empathize with the victim's response to the assault. Nor is it necessary to be a woman to empathize with sexual assault victims; for one thing, not all victims are female. Male counselors with an understanding of the victim's situation can be valuable in two areas: in working with males, both adolescents and adults, who have been victims of homosexual assaults, and in helping the spouses and families of female victims deal with their responses. A sensitive experience with a male following the crisis of a sexual assault can be a very positive experience for the female victim,[23] whether the male is a police officer, physician, nurse, counselor, family member, or friend.

THE ENTIRE MANAGEMENT PROCESS
Law enforcement

Law enforcement authorities are responsible for interviewing the victim of a sexual assault and collecting evidence for prosecution. Evidence is collected to prove that an assault occurred, that it was committed by force, and that it was committed against the victim's will, or rather, without her consent.[10] Statutes governing the crime of rape or sexual assault vary from state to state, and legal definitions of these criteria may differ. Much of the physical evidence of sexual assault is collected by medical authorities in cooperation with law enforcement and legal authorities.

Law enforcement authorities interview the victim to obtain information such as a detailed description of the assailant and details of the assault itself.[17] The police are concerned with several elements of the sexual assault: sexual penetration (legal requirements vary in different states), identification of the perpetrator, and the lack of consent on the part of the victim.[18] Law enforcement officers may make statements meant to impress on the victim the seriousness of the charges she is making.[15]

Medical system

Space does not permit a careful step-by-step discussion of evaluation and care of sexual assault victims. Highlights only will be discussed here. Reference is made again to the comprehensive works of Burgess and Holmstrom[15] for the best aids in establishing procedures and protocol; every community has its own peculiar mix of resources, of positives and negatives, and thus each protocol will have at least slight variations.

The health care system has dual roles in sexual assault areas: healer and detective. The patient who is a victim of sexual assault has a right to expect good, nonjudgmental physical and psychologic evaluation and treatment, and she and society have a right to expect good evidence collection. Evidence collection is often considered a bothersome task, extraneous to health care.

Professional politeness combined with an accepting, nonjudgmental attitude is the best overall approach to the patient. It is not the role of the health care worker to decide whether or to what extent an assault occurred; that is a complex issue decided carefully and over a prolonged period by a number of people and systems, particularly the legal system. The patient/client should best be treated as a consumer, and her requests and needs dealt with carefully and with dignity.

Attention should be given to the patient's medical risks: pregnancy, venereal disease, and trauma, both physical and emotional. Too often there is concentration only on the physical condition. Learning to recognize emotional trauma and learning to describe it are vital for good health care and for good legal records.

The time it takes most victims to recognize the possibility of pregnancy varies from victim to victim; then preoccupation with that possibility is intense. Anxiety diminishes greatly with attention and reassurance.

The importance of treating the victim with dignity and respecting her right to control her own body, regardless of her age or condition, is dealt with in other areas of this chapter, but is stressed again.

Information about procedures should be continually given to victims in appropriate language, keeping in mind the severe stress they are experiencing, and they should similarly be told results of examinations and tests and significant details of treatment. Written instructions and appointment times for follow-up are very helpful.

The health care worker should be aware that timetables and rules of the complex systems in which the victim is enmeshed may leave her enormously pressured at times, and at other times, neglected and depersonalized by all concerned. Lack of continuity of care, for example, is a real and acute problem for most victims. It should be remembered that it is not therapeutic to abandon the patient.

The patient's right to privacy is also discussed elsewhere. Care must be taken to remember that busy corridors, busy nights in the emergency room, and bulletin boards are not conducive to confidentiality. Further care must be observed in what is told to the victim's social network and to the criminal justice system.

In keeping records, helpful information such as a careful, nonjudgmental description of the victim's emotional condition should be included. "Damning" information such as prior sexual experience or activity, although often necessary to know medically, is a potential criminal justice problem; certainly, very great consideration and thought at least should be given to its inclusion in any way in the record. The medical record is, of course, a potential legal document in all health care, but especially in sexual assault cases. A carefully kept record will not only help the prosecution of a case, but will drastically cut down the number of times a health professional is subpoenaed to testify in court.

Finally, attention is drawn to the incredible problems of professional intercommunication. Often, great knowledge and expertise have developed, but in marked isolation from other systems. The professions, all of society, and the sexual assault victim would benefit from professionals' educating and communicating with one another.

Family and friends

When first seen by health professionals, the victim's family is also likely to need support, understanding, and attention. It is also important for health care workers to be aware that there are two complex areas in which difficulties can develop between the victim's social network, the victim, and the health care system following an assault. These areas are invasion of the victim's rights in terms of confidentiality or privacy and "territorial" rights to ownership of one's body. Both issues are particularly sensitive in the case of adolescent victims.

Holmstrom and Burgess state that family members or friends were often given requested information by health professionals with explicit or implied consent by victims, but at other times, victims were not asked at all.[15] It is perhaps assumed too readily that parents, for example, have a right to any and all information about an adolescent victim because they had to give written consent for the examination.

The issue of who has the right to give permission for an examination of a victim is somewhat related and also complex. There are instances when medical personnel must wait for parents to arrive to give permission for examination and treatment, the delay making a perilous situation for a victim. At other times, parents have demanded that an adolescent be examined when the adolescent strongly opposed it. Such an examination would constitute a second "violation of the body" in the opinion of experts.

These are ethical, sensitive, problem-filled areas; the medical system would do a service to itself and to patients to discuss and attempt to clarify them, rather than to settle each case on a confused and confusing ad hoc basis.

Legal system

Legal authorities have the responsibility of evaluating and preparing a sexual assault case for court. The prosecuting attorney may ask the victim to repeat details of the assault that she has already told police and perhaps medical authorities in determining the potential legal soundness of the case and types of charges to be pressed. Questions asked are similar to those asked by law enforcement authorities, and by the time they arrive at the district attorney's office, victims may tire of repeating their story, although such repetition may be encouraged by the prosecutor to prepare the victim for her appearance in court. Test questions, such as those likely to be asked by the defense attorney, may be used to determine how the victim will respond in court. Legal authorities, unfortunately, may give limited information on the workings of the criminal justice system to victims.

Counseling

Counseling personnel may provide a variety of specific services to sexual assault victims to increase the victim's personal functioning in her lifestyle following the crisis. These may include supportive services and advocacy and liaison between the victim and medical, legal, and law enforcement authorities. This involves staying with the victim during the medical examination, during the police and district attorney's questioning and throughout the criminal justice process. Burgess and Holmstrom state that counseling victims of sexual assault is designed to deal with the problems experienced by victims as a result of the assault and to provide educational information on sexual assault to the community at large, that is, how to avoid becoming a victim, and what to do if assaulted.[10]

Overworked law enforcement and legal authorities and harried medical personnel do not always have the time nor the expertise to provide counseling services to victims of sexual assault. Counselors provide emotional support to the victim, are people to whom the victim can talk about the assault, and from whom she can receive specific information about the medical, legal, or court process.[10] They are generally more available to the victim than are other professionals and can be reached by phone or seen in person. The counselor's availability as well as support can be valuable to the victim over the short-term crisis or over the long-term reorganization process following the trauma. Counselors, can provide a variety of follow-up services to assault victims. They encourage victims to receive immediate medical, as well as follow-up, testing or treatment for pregnancy and venereal disease, prepare victims for court appearances by familiarizing the victim with the court setting and procedure, are available when the victim needs someone with whom to talk, and may provide transportation or referral to other community resources. They can also be instrumental in dealing with the family or friends of sexual assault victims at the time of the assault and/or during the victim's long-term recovery process. Although counselors are available to victims and may have been called into the case by medical or law enforcement authorities, they generally follow up on the cases they have accepted. Of course, victims are free to refuse counseling services.

THE UNIQUE ROLE OF THE NURSE
Support and communication

Sexual assault victims are generally treated in hospital emergency rooms or treatment centers designed to meet the needs of such victims, but some victims may prefer to see their private physicians or receive treatment at local clinics. In any of these settings, the nurse is often the health professional who has the most contact with the victim and, even with counseling services available, is in an important position to provide a positive response to the victim's needs.

The current trend in some sexual assault treatment centers is to have gynecologic nurses fully responsible for the examination of and evidence collection from the victim. In cases of severe injury to the victim, physicians or hospital services may be required. During most examinations, the nurse remains as a support person to the victim and to the physician and acts as an important intermediary between the victim and the health care system. In the emergency room, clinic, or physician's office, the nurse possesses ". . . the skills and attitudes necessary to provide comprehensive, supportive, and sympathetic care for rape victims."[4] The nurse can use her skills to decrease the victim's fear and anxiety by providing explanations about the medical protocol and treatment, by listening to the victim's account and requests with understanding, and by giving her information on the availability of counseling services and medical follow-up treatment.[16]

Prevention of further victimization

In recent research on treatment of victims, one major area of concern has been the further institutional victimization of sexual assault (and other) victims by inappropriate or inconsiderate interactions with them. Burgess and Holmstrom have provided much of the comprehensive research in the area of sexual assault victimology and have written about nursing implications in the medical setting.[7,9] The nurse can be influential in encouraging other medical staff to work through their personal feelings and attitudes toward sexual assault, since personal biases, ambivalent feelings, and moralistic, judgmental comments can be detrimental to the victim. Local counseling services may be available to provide staff in-service training and sensitivity training, and the staff should be aware of community resources that have been established to aid victims of sexual assault.

Specific guidelines

Although most hospitals have established protocol for the medical treatment and gathering of evidence from sexual assault victims, priorities should be instituted that provide for the immediate care of all sexual assault victims. This care is an important consideration for anyone who has already suffered serious emotional and often physical trauma, but law enforcement authorities are in need of the results of the examination and laboratory testing and may be waiting to interview the victim. Sometimes prompt apprehension of an assailant may be frustrated by delays in the medical examination.

Before the examination, the victim should not be left alone and calm, sympathetic support can be provided by the nurse. Victims should be placed in a private examining room, out of the mainstream of hospital, clinic, or office activity. The nurse can encourage but should avoid forcing the victim to talk and can listen carefully to her thoughts and feelings, evaluating her distress and unique problems. Prior to and during the medical examination, the nurse can give the victim a full explanation of the procedures of the examination and the reasons for each part of the examination, with the victim able to ask questions while having them answered in a reassuring way. Since this may be the victim's first gynecologic examination, this explanation can be an important preparation for the victim's cooperation during the examination. The nurse can provide physical comforts to the victim as needed: tissues; coffee; warm water, soap, and towels for washing (only after the examination); and something to wear home if the victim's clothing has been taken as evidence. The nurse can see that adequate records are maintained because the records of the medical examination are often used as evidence in court proceedings. Subjective observations could be erroneous and detrimental to the assault case and should be avoided, or staff who have provided inadequate medical records could be subpoenaed to testify in court.

The nurse can provide information on the medical care of concerns related to the sexual assault, such as pregnancy and venereal disease. Although the probability of pregnancy is small (about 1% in a 1973 study),[12] a discussion of pregnancy with the victim is very appropriate. For those victims at a high risk for pregnancy, an antipregnancy medication may be prescribed; the victim should be made fully aware of any potential side effects or adverse reactions. The nurse can reiterate any of the physician's instructions for follow-up care or testing for venereal disease, and, if possible, schedule an appointment for that follow-up appointment before the victim leaves. The victim's discharge should be handled caringly, including a provision for transportation and someone to accompany the victim home. With the victim's consent, the nurse can refer her to local resources for continued contact and counseling. In summary, the nurse has an opportunity to provide support and comfort to the victim of sexual assault and to see that her medical treatment is a positive rather than a further traumatizing experience.

PREVENTION
Education

Prevention of the crime of sexual assault begins by educating the public, as well as state legislators, that sexual assault is not an attack motivated by desire for sexual gratification, but is a violent assault on another individual, as are the crimes of assault and battery and homicide. In a sexual assault, however, the weapon is sex, used to humiliate and dominate another person, and other weapons may also be used to force the submission of the victim to the assailant. Changes in state legislation provide for degrees of assault, sexual intercourse, or sexual contact, and the use or threat of force. Such legislative changes make convictions easier to obtain because charges more specifically fit the circumstances of the sexual assault. The public needs to be aware of the laws for the prosecution of crimes committed against them and the manner in which complaints can be made. In states with more progressive sexual assault laws, much of the burden of testifying is removed from the victim. For example, information on the victim's past sexual history is inadmissible in open court, except when it relates to her sexual relationship with the defendant prior to the assault. Sexual assault victims who are aware of legislative changes that more actively protect their interests may be more willing to report the crime. It is to be hoped that the higher the rate of reporting, the higher the rate of apprehension and conviction of assailants.

Public education involves the important task of dispelling myths that place responsibility on the victim rather than on the assailant. Such myths only serve to keep victims from reporting the assaults and provide excuses for state legislatures to avoid changing their outdated laws.

Precautions

Most old solutions for the prevention of sexual assault attacks involved restrictions on women (staying at home after dark and so on) that are no longer realistic in modern society. Society's expectations of women's and men's behaviors are changing, but until the time when conditions have become safe, there are precautions that women can take to reduce their chances for a sexual assault.

Medea and Thompson give a fairly complete listing of precautions women can take to avoid a sexual assault.[17] Women can take self-defense courses to become strong, healthy, and skillful at defense techniques and to gain confidence and the ability to think clearly in any situation. Several demonstrations and some limited practice, however, are not adequate to develop these skills; such measures may, in fact, produce a false sense of confidence that may put a woman even more at the mercy of an aggressive, violent assailant. The following can be learned, however, by all women: an understanding of sexual assault and how and when it is likely to happen; an understanding that a woman's manner of relating to men may lead her into the kind of situation in which sexual assault occurs; the knowledge and practice of taking common sense precautions (in the home, in the car, on walks, on public transportation, and so on); learning some elementary self-defense such as how to use commonly carried items (purse and keys) as weapons to protect oneself; and being aware of what to do if one or one's friend is sexually assaulted and what community resources are available to provide support in this situation. It is a good idea to try to think out and plan a response to an assault ahead of time. Women need to try to estimate the amount of anger and cool-headed practicality of which they are capable and the possible methods of avoiding an aggressive confrontation with an assailant.[17]

When an attack is unavoidable

If an attack is imminent, screaming can clear one's head, start the flow of adrenalin, scare off the attacker, or summon help. Concentration on the assailant's weak points and the vulnerable parts of the human body may give the victim the opportunity to get away from the situation. Research has shown, as mentioned earlier, that the less involved the victim is in the fight, the less likely she is to be physically injured. The victim's objective is to end the sexually assaultive encounter, however, and even if the assault itself cannot be avoided, one should remember anything that may be helpful to law enforcement authorities in apprehending and identifying the assailant. During the assault, the victim can, for example, try to focus her attention on the car, its model and year, color, license plate; the location of the assault; the assailant—his physical characteristics, unusual marks or attributes, clothing, or anything he may say.

No specific passive or aggressive behavior can be recommended as a response to all sexual assaults. Such behaviors depend on the ages and physical strengths of the victim and the assailant, on the location of the attack, and on other variables. In any case, the point is not to win the fight, but to gain the opportunity to escape from the assailant. Some suggestions have been made.[3] Fighting or verbal abuse increases the chance of the victim's being injured or killed, although statistics state that only 2% of sexual assault victims lost their lives in the assault. It is easier to escape violence than to disarm the assailant. Thus if passivity or stalling fails, the victim can attempt aggressive resistance; it is not likely that resorting to passive resistance, following an aggressive initial reaction, would be successful. Forceful resistance initiated prior to the actual physical assault is relatively less dangerous for the victim. Aggressive resistance is safer if the victim and assailant know each other than if they are total strangers or may have met in a social situation that involved alcohol and drug consumption. Fear demonstrated by the victim may escalate the assailant's anger, and screaming, running, crying, and pleading may incite violence on the part of the assailant. Any action that may increase the assailant's fear of apprehension or identification may lead to a panic reaction on his part and cause him to inflict unwarranted violence on the victim. It is important to note, however, that a woman's prior acquaintance with the assailant, use of passive resistance to the assault, and lack of physical injuries may jeopardize the court case, and women should be aware of this issue in determining whether or not to resist their attackers by fighting.

Ultimately, however, the victim of a sexual assault must make her own decision on how to prevent, or whether to resist, the assailant's attack. Her decision may depend on a variety of factors—her preparation for the occurrence of such a situation, her emotional control in dealing with the assailant, prior self-defense training, and/or the opportunity to resist. There are simply no reliable guidelines as yet applicable to all potential victim-assailant combinations. It cannot be emphasized enough that the woman should depend on her initial "gut" reactions to a sense of danger and try to avoid the sexual attack before the assailant has the opportunity to gain some control over her. It is much easier to deal with feelings of foolishness, if one has misjudged the nature of the situation and it was not going to be an assault, than it is to deal with the long-term effects of victimization by sexual assault.

SUMMARY

Sexual assault involves complex psychologic and physical reactions of the victim. Health care professionals as well as family and friends, law enforcement and legal authorities, and sexual assault counseling/advocacy groups have enormous potential impact on the resolution of this crisis and the victim's return to normal functioning. The presence of an empathetic, nonjudgmental, and supportive health care professional has the advantage in particular of encouraging the victim's cooperation during the medical examination and throughout subsequent follow-up treatment, rather than leaving her with the impression of further violation or victimization.

REFERENCES

1. Amir, M.: Patterns of forcible rape, Chicago, 1971, University of Chicago Press.
2. Barkas, J. L.: Victims, New York, 1978, Charles Scribner's Sons.
3. Behavioral Medicine: Newsletter, 15(11):3, November, 1978.
4. Bellack, J. P., and Woodard, P.: Improving emergency care for rape victims, J. Emer. Nurs. 3:32-35, 1977.
5. Bode, J.: Fighting back, New York, 1978, The MacMillan Co.
6. Brownmiller, S.: Against our will: men, women and rape, New York, 1975, Simon & Schuster, Inc.
7. Burgess, A. W.: The rape victim: nursing implications, J. Pract. Nurs. 28(11):14-15, 1978.
8. Burgess, A. W., and Groth, N.: Sexual assault: victim and offender, Abuse of Women—Midwest Conference, May 19-20, 1978, St. Louis, Mo.
9. Burgess, A. W., and Holmstrom, L. L.: The rape victim in the emergency ward, Am. J. Nurs. 73:1740-1745, 1973.
10. Burgess, A. W., and Holmstrom, L. L.: Rape: victims of crisis, Bowie, Md., 1974, R. J. Brady Co.
11. Cohen, M. L., Garofalo, R., Boucher, R., et al.: The psychology of rapists, Sem. Psychiatry 3(3):311, 1971.
12. Hayman, C. R., Lanza, C., and Noel, E. C.: What to do for victims of rape, Med. Times 101:44-51, 1973.
13. Hilberman, E.: The rape victim, Baltimore, 1976, Garramond/Pridemark Press, Inc.
14. Holmstrom, L. L., and Burgess, A. W.: Assessing trauma in the rape victim, Am. J. Nurs. 75(8):1288-1291, 1975.
15. Holmstrom, L. L., and Burgess, A. W.: The victim of rape: institutional reactions, New York, 1978, John Wiley & Sons, Inc.
16. LeFort, S.: Care for the rape victim in emergency, Can. Nurs. 73(2):43-45, 1977.
17. Medea, A., and Thompson, K.: Against rape, New York, 1974, Farrar, Strauss & Giroux, Inc.
18. National Institute of Law Enforcement and Criminal Justice: Forcible rape: a manual for

sex crime investigators, Police, vol. III. Washington, D.C., 1978, U.S. Government Printing Office.
19. National Institute of Law Enforcement and Criminal Justice: Forcible rape: a national survey of the response by police, Police, vol. I, Washington, D.C., 1977, U.S. Government Printing Office.
20. National Institute of Law Enforcement and Criminal Justice: Forcible rape: a national survey of the response by prosecutors, Prosecutors, vol. I, Washington, D.C., 1977, U.S. Government Printing Office.
21. National Institute of Mental Health: Victims of rape, U.S. Department of Health, Education and Welfare, 1976. U.S. Government Printing Office.
22. Notman, M. T., and Nadelson, C. C.: The rape victim: psychodynamic considerations, Am. J. Psychiatry **133**:408-412, 1976.
23. Silverman, D.: First do no more harm: female rape victims and the male counselor, J. Orthopsychiatry **47**:91-96, 1977.
24. Symonds, M.: The rape victim: psychological patterns of response, Am. J. Psychoanal. **36**:27-34, 1976.
25. Symonds, M.: Victims of senseless violence, Psychiatric Worldview **1**(1):1-3, 1977.

PART FOUR

Selected Ob/Gyn problems and issues

The problem of sexual dysfunction, as discussed by Doran, is of long-standing nature and often not readily acknowledged. Doran's intent is to assist practitioners working primarily in women's health care to become aware of their client's sexual problems and to intervene appropriately.

Premenstrual tension syndrome (PMT) is another health problem often inadequately managed. In chapter 11, Abraham discusses various etiologic theories and presents his current research findings that have led to a proposed plan for the classification, evaluation, and management of PMT. The illustrations clearly delineate his classification according to type and date of ocurrence of symptomatology, which, in turn, provides the necessary data for appropriate management of PMT on an individual basis.

Chapter 12 focuses on the source, causes, cure, and sequelae of vulvovaginitis, a gynecologic problem managed by nurse-practitioners and midwives. For each type of problem, Ivory discusses the chief complaint, clinical course, microscopic examination, and management. The illustrations are extremely helpful in identifying and differentiating microscopic findings.

Rocereto's discussion of the differential diagnosis of cervical pathology appropriately follows Chapter 12. The focus is primarily on the work-up and management of a Pap smear with abnormal results.

In Chapter 14, Berman and Berman review the problems associated with pelvic muscle relaxation and degeneration, a condition contributing to much distress in many women. They also describe the historical research leading to simple, physiologic methods for restoring or maintaining muscle function, including the four phases of restoration and Kegel exercises.

The use of real-time ultrasound, as described by Sipos, Platt, and Manning, has increased greatly. Its application in obstetrics and gynecology has enabled health professionals to confirm diagnoses and intervene accordingly.

CHAPTER 10

Sexual dysfunction

Maureen O. Doran

INTRODUCTION

The purpose of this chapter is to acquaint obstetric and gynecologic nurses with the etiology and treatment of human sexual dysfunction and to assist nurses working primarily in women's health care to be aware of their patient's possible sexual problems, to be able to conduct a preliminary investigation into the cause of their concerns, and to refer patients and couples for treatment when indicated. Many of the females for whom nurses care are involved with a single sexual partner in an ongoing relationship. Because of the interrelatedness of the couple's sexual functioning, one partner's sexual difficulty will most definitely affect the other's sexuality. Therefore, in addition to reviewing female sexual function and dysfunction, male sexual aspects will also be discussed. Finally, possible physiologic causes will be discussed to familiarize nurses with the possible sexual implications involved in patients with established physical problems. The basic premise remains, however, that sexual functioning is a natural phenomenon and, with the exception of possible physiologic factors that inhibit such functioning, all other disruptions must be considered psychopathologic in nature.

HISTORICAL PERSPECTIVES

The current revolution in public awareness of sexuality and sexual function began with the revealing Kinsey publications in 1949 and 1954.[3] These research studies were the first collected data on sexual practices in the United States. Masters and Johnson brought sexuality out of the realm of statistics and into that of medical science.[6] Their greatest achievement was research based on actual case studies of sexual physiology. As a result of this extensive research, they defined specific concepts for treating sexual dysfunction. The general public first became aware of these treatment principles with the publication of *Human Sexual Inadequacy* in 1970.[7] In this work, Masters and Johnson demonstrated a new approach to treating sexual dysfunction involving brief, directive counseling of the couple aimed specifically at symptom removal. This type of therapy was significantly different from the more traditional psychotherapeutic approaches that focused on the attainment of insight into unconscious conflicts often associated with sexual dysfunction. Further research regarding sexual dysfunctions and treatments has resulted in an expansion of the theoretical base and treatment techniques.

PHYSIOLOGY OF THE SEXUAL RESPONSE

A brief review of normal sexual response is important in understanding the mechanisms of the various sexual dysfunctions. Figs. 10-1 and 10-2 demonstrate the four basic phases of the human sexual response as noted by Masters and Johnson.[6] During the first two stages of both female and male sexual response—excitement and plateau—the vasocongestive phase of normal sexual physiology occurs. In the female, the vasocongestive phase results in specific vaginal changes, including lubrication, color variation, and expansion. Along with these genital changes, other physiologic changes oc-

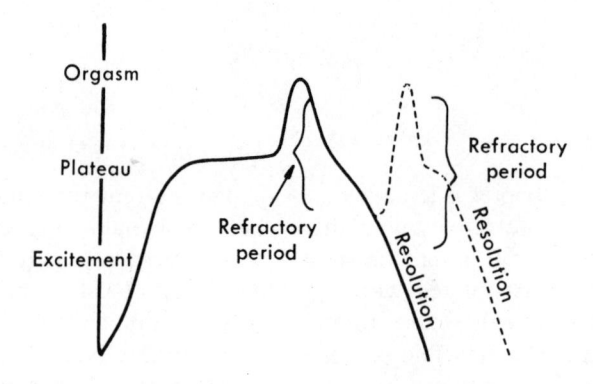

Fig. 10-1. Male sexual response cycle. (From Masters, W., and Johnson, V.: Human sexual response, Boston, 1966, Little, Brown & Co.)

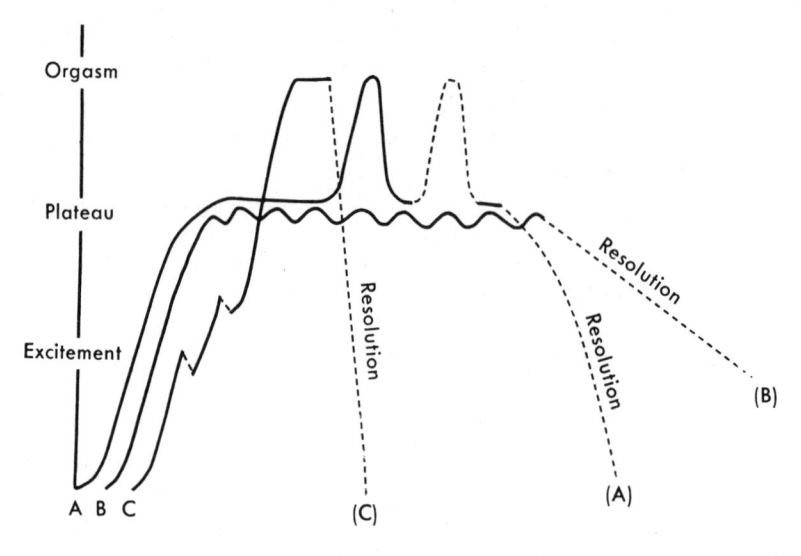

Fig. 10-2. Female sexual response cycle. (From Masters, W., and Johnson, V.: Human sexual response, Boston, 1966, Little, Brown & Co.)

cur including flushing, breast enlargement, and nipple erection. In the male, this same phase results in a pumping of blood into the penile cavernous sinus causing a firm erection. Psychologically, in both females and males, there is a heightened tension and excited anticipation during the vasocongestive phase.

The latter two stages—orgasm and resolution—make up the orgastic component of sexual response. In the female, the orgastic response results in rhythmic contractions of the vaginal walls as well as the raising of the uterus from the pelvic floor. During the resolution phase of the orgastic component, the female sexual organs return rapidly to prevasocongestive stages. In the male, the orgastic component results in ejaculation, which is actually divided into two closely occurring stages. The first stage, emission, is the initial movement of seminal fluid into the urethral bulb, at which time the male feels the point of inevitable ejaculation. In the second stage, ejaculation proper, the semen is expelled. At the resolution phase of orgasm, the male passes through a phase known as the refractory period. During this time-limited phase, regardless of the amount of stimulation he may receive, the male is incapable of achieving a second, immediate, full erection or repeating his orgasm. In contrast, however, the female does not experience this refractory period and is capable of rapid restimulation to orgasm.

ETIOLOGY OF SEXUAL DYSFUNCTION

Masters and Johnson,[7] Kaplan,[2] and other noted theorists view sexual dysfunctions primarily as psychosomatic disorders that prevent the individual from performing and/or enjoying coitus. Regarding the sexual response cycle, the vasocongestive and orgastic phases may occur together or separately.

Female sexual dysfunctions can be divided into two general categories: (1) frigidity and (2) orgastic dysfunction. Females with the first dysfunction have absolutely no response to sexual stimulation, while the orgastically dysfunctional female reaches the vasocongestive phase of sexual response but has difficulty in achieving orgasm. A third female sexual difficulty, not considered a true psychosomatic disorder, is vaginismus. In this condition, an involuntary muscle spasm of the vaginal opening prevents penile penetration.

Male dysfunctional syndromes include: (1) erectile failure, commonly known as impotence; (2) inadequate ejaculatory control, otherwise known as premature ejaculation; and (3) ejaculatory overcontrol, sometimes called retarded ejaculation. The latter two problems pertain to the control of orgasm.

FEMALE SEXUAL DYSFUNCTION

For a number of years and for a variety of reasons, female sexuality has not been as well understood as male sexuality. Obviously, female genitalia are somewhat more mysterious and only recently has female sexuality, apart from childbearing, achieved significance comparable to that of the male. Most female sexual difficulties were routinely called *frigidity*, which was used to describe conditions ranging from total sexual inhibition to minor orgastic difficulties. It has also implied that any woman with such difficulties is necessarily hostile toward men. Nothing could be further from the truth. Most women seeking help for their sexual difficulties are warm, arousable individuals very much interested in male individuals. Female sexual problems involve either the vasocongestive or the orgastic phase of sexual response. Kaplan[2] categorizes the former phase as general female sexual dysfunction and the latter as orgastic dysfunction.

Frigidity

This condition is characterized by an inhibition of the arousal aspect in the vasocongestive phase of sexual response. Physiologically, a woman with this dysfunction experiences no lubrication or expansion of the vagina and never reaches the orgastic platform. Psychologically, this woman lacks erotic feelings. Essentially, she does not become excited. Such women demonstrate a universal sexual inhibition varying in severity from true aversion toward sexuality to simple disinterest.

Orgastic dysfunction

Orgastic sexual dysfunction, the most common female sexual complaint, involves a specific inhibition of the orgastic component of sexual response. Thus, in contrast to the female with general sexual dysfunction, the woman with orgastic dysfunction experiences erotic feelings and excitement, as well as vaginal lubrication and expansion. However, despite sufficient stimulation, she is unable to reach orgasm. This clinical condition can be divided into primary and secondary orgastic dysfunction. The woman suffering from the primary condition has never achieved orgasm through any means. In the secondary condition, the woman has achieved orgasm successfully, perhaps for many years, and develops the problem subsequently. It is important to note however, that as a secondary consequence to orgastic dysfunction, the initial or vasocongestive phase of such a woman's sexual response may also become inhibited. Thus, it is essential that a thorough history be obtained to distinguish between this consequential condition and frigidity.

Physiologic and psychologic etiology

As opposed to male sexual responses, especially the male erectile response, female sexual response is remarkably free from dysfunction resulting from physical factors, such as genital malignancies, endocrine disease, and neurologic disorders that, although rare, must be ruled out by physical examination and appropriate laboratory analysis.

Psychologic etiology of female sexual dysfunction stems primarily from cultural influences, especially those that espouse the "good girl" Puritan ethic, religious conditioning, and moralistic training, all of which have exerted enormous influence in repressing full expression of female sexuality.[7] Deeper intrapsychic factors, such as unresolved childhood conflicts involving sexuality or early traumatic sexual experiences, may also result in sexual inhibition.[2] In addition, situational factors leading to sexual dysfunction need to be assessed. Inadequate sexual stimulation, inability to relax and abandon oneself to erotic pleasure, and poor communication with one's sexual partner often impede pleasurable female sexual functioning.

Vaginismus

Vaginismus, which is a relatively rare condition, is technically not a true dysfunction because it does not involve either of the two phases of sexual response. Vaginismus is a condition in which the muscles located at the entrance of the vagina involuntarily contract when penile penetration is attempted. This is a conditioned response that occurs gradually and generally secondary to painful penile penetration. Women suffering from this condition are often otherwise quite responsive sexually. While anxiety from anticipation of penetration alone can trigger such a response, this clinical entity is often seen in women suffering from chronic vaginal infections. Typically, these women continue to attempt intercourse, even though very painful, to please their sexual partners. As a result, this involuntary, protective condition precludes intercourse. For this reason, it is important that women receive prompt treatment for vaginal infections and be counselled against attempting intercourse when it is painful. A series of vaginal dilatation procedures may be necessary. The dilatation technique can be done by the woman at home and consists of gradually increasing the diameter of dilators inserted into the vagina until the woman is comfortable with a dilator approximately the size of an erect penis. When vaginismus is secondary to anxiety, education alone may relieve the stress and, thus the problem. Psychotherapy may be initiated when the condition is secondary to more deeply rooted psychologic conflicts or trauma as can occur, for example, in a victim of rape.

MALE SEXUAL DYSFUNCTION
Erectile failure (impotence)

Erectile failure involves a dysfunction in the vasocongestive aspect of the sexual response. Specifically, there is a failure of the reflex mechanism to supply sufficient blood to the penile cavernous sinus to render a firm erection. Regardless of the amount of stimulation he may receive or that he may feel aroused and desires to engage in coitus, the male is unable to achieve an erection. Of particular importance is that the vasocongestive and orgastic components of the sexual response are separable and a man may, with sufficient stimulation, ejaculate despite a flaccid penis.

Erectile failure has been divided into two clinical categories. Primary impotence refers to the condition in which a man may be able to achieve spontaneous erections in sexually stimulating situations or through masturbation but has been unable to do so with a woman.[5] This condition is, by far, less frequent than secondary impotence in which the male has had satisfactory sexual relations prior to erectile failure.

While the majority of erectile failures have a psychologic basis, it is essential to rule out possible physiologic causes. Because of the particular sensitivity of the erectile response to physical disease, a thorough physical history and examination should be conducted prior to diagnosing the illness as psychosomatic. Some key physiologic conditions to consider include surgical procedures affecting the nerve pathways to the penis, diabetes, general debilitating illness, hepatic problems, neurologic diseases such as multiple sclerosis, and tumors affecting the lower spinal cord. Special note should be made of drug abuse and chronic alcohol ingestion, both of which can result in erectile failure. All medications that the patient is taking must be reviewed. A direct correlation can often be made between the time the patient began a certain medication, such as many of the antihypertensive drugs, and the onset of his sexual difficulties. Medications affecting the parasympathetic system are of special concern.

As mentioned before, it is necessary to determine through laboratory tests any possible hormone deficiency before prescribing a course of hormonal treatment. This is true for both males and females when a hormone insufficiency is suspected. Unfortunately, this has not always been standard procedure, and many patients who do have a sexual problem, especially impotence, have already been given a hormone by a well-meaning but uninformed physician. Such a practice is totally contraindicated.

For the male suffering from physiologically related, irreversible impotence, the possibility of a penile prosthesis should be considered and discussed with the patient and his sexual partner. One relatively simple surgical procedure involves the implantation of an acrylic or teflon device into the penis that results in a permanent, partial erection. A newer, more surgically complicated device, allows the male to pump fluid into the prosthesis for a firm erection when desired.[8] These prostheses do not inhibit urination and do allow the male to achieve penetration during intercourse. For many men, although unable to regain predysfunctional pleasure, this procedure does allow them to satisfy their sexual partner during intercourse. The ability to achieve this function again can significantly increase the self-esteem of the male who believes strongly about the need to sexually satisfy his partner through penetration.

Psychologic factors that cause erectile failure range from marital incompatibility, power struggles, and lack of trust to deeper, unconscious phenomena including unresolved Oedipal conflicts, anxieties involving intimacy, and cultural inhibitions. Masters and Johnson were the forerunners in identifying even more immediate causes of this type of dysfunction. Particularly prominent for the male suffering from erectile failure is the fear of failure and subsequent performance anxiety. Most therapists agree that such anxiety alone can initiate and potentiate the problem of erectile failure.

Inadequate ejaculatory control (premature ejaculation)

Kaplan[2] states that premature ejaculation is usually cited as the most common form of male sexual dysfunction. All theorists have had difficulty, however, in specifically defining this condition because of individual variability. Masters and Johnson define premature ejaculation as the inability of a man to control his ejaculation for a sufficient length of time to satisfy his partner in at least 50% of coital situations.[7] Essentially, prematurity is a condition in which a man is unable to exert voluntary control over his ejaculation. Thus, once sexually aroused, he may wish to postpone the ejaculatory process but cannot and oftentimes will ejaculate even prior to penetration, or at best, shortly thereafter. Extensive study has shown this condition to exist primarily in younger men with no history of erectile dysfunction. These men tend to have never experienced good ejaculatory control and date their first awareness of the problem to their first coital experience. Another essential element in the male with premature ejaculation is his inability to recognize the point of ejaculatory inevitability. Kaplan has described this condition as a type of genital anesthesia, in the sense that the male cannot feel this crucial point.[2] An essential element of the treatment of premature ejaculation is helping the patient to recognize this point to control his orgasm.

As opposed to erectile failure, which can have a variety of physiologic causes, inadequate ejaculatory control is seldom physiologically based. However, a thorough physical examination is indicated for the male who functioned well for a period prior to developing premature ejaculation. This development is highly suspicious and may indicate serious neurologic or urethral disease.

A variety of psychologic factors contribute to premature ejaculation, including unsatisfactory sexual experiences that require rapid completion, such as situations involving prostitutes or lack of complete privacy when fear of observation is acute. These situationally conditioned factors are in contrast to more analytically oriented considerations. Some theorists believe that the condition is prompted by a deep-rooted dislike of women (for the problem does result in frustration and dissatisfaction for the female partner) or by conflict-ridden anxiety that peaks as the male reaches orgastic levels.

Ejaculatory overcontrol (ejaculatory incompetence)

Ejaculatory overcontrol is defined as a specific inhibition of the ejaculatory reflex of the sexual response. The initial vasocongestive phase of the sexual response, for the most part, remains intact. Thus, a male with ejaculatory incompetence responds to sexual stimulation with a firm erection. However, even with sufficient stimulation and an urgent desire, he is incapable of ejaculating. This is a relatively rare form of sexual dysfunction and is in direct contrast to the condition of the male with erectile failure. The male with impotence can, if sufficiently stimulated, ejaculate regardless of his nonerect penis, while the male with ejaculatory overcontrol has a firm erection but cannot ejaculate.

Masters and Johnson preferred not to further categorize this clinical condition, believing that its relative rarity did not warrant it.[7] Kaplan, however, did divide males suffering with this condition into two clinical categories: primary and secondary retarded ejaculators.[2] Primary retarded ejaculators have never experienced a time without this condition. Many of these patients are able to achieve extravaginal orgasm either through female stimulation or masturbation yet are unable to ejaculate once penetration has occurred. This category also includes the absolute primary retarded ejaculators who have never experienced an orgasm through any means.

In contrast, secondary retarded ejaculators functioned well prior to the onset of the condition. In many of these cases, the medical history reveals that the condition had an acute onset following a specific traumatic event such as being found engaging in undesirable sexual activity.

Physiologically, as with premature ejaculation, there are few organic components implicated in the etiology of this condition. However, as with all of these conditions, a thorough examination is indicated to rule out possible organic components.

PRINCIPLES OF TREATMENT

For over 20 years, Masters and Johnson have researched the physiology of the human sexual response and developed treatment techniques for the disruptions of these responses.[6,7] These major treatment techniques are discussed in three inclusive categories: patient, therapist, and procedural considerations. While these principles have been based on couple-oriented therapy, which is the primary approach to treating sexual dysfunction, they can also apply to the individual seeking treatment.

Patient considerations

A basic yet overlooked fact is that a certain percentage of sexual dysfunction is based on the physiologic or metabolic conditions discussed earlier. These conditions must first be ruled out by appropriate medical history and examination before beginning treatment for a psychopathologic condition.

A significant principle of all sexual therapy with couples is that there is no such thing as an uninvolved partner. This concept was not recognized in earlier treatments of sexual dysfunction in which one partner was the identified and treated patient. The relationship between the couple was not even considered. It is now understood that all sexual dysfunctions are shared disorders. Regardless of the initial cause of the dysfunction, both partners are responsible for future change and the solution of their problem.

Sexually dysfunctional individuals need educational orientation. Most patients suffering from a dysfunction are woefully ignorant of both basic biology and sexual techniques. Sometimes this ignorance alone can directly lead to the development of anxiety, which in turn produces a sexual problem. Masters and Johnson believe that a substantial number, about 20%, of dysfunctions could be reversed with education alone.[7]

The major focus of this form of therapy is not specifically the actual dysfunction, but the relationship between the couple. Along with the educational aspect provided in the treatment, techniques are offered to help the couple improve their communication. It is only through this focus that lasting results can be obtained.

Sexual dysfunction is not merely a symptom of a deep emotional problem, it can also be a conditioned response. Two of the greatest roadblocks to pleasurable sexual experiences are fears of performance and the subsequent observer role assumed by the anxious, nonfunctioning partner. In this vicious, cyclical situation, the sexually dysfunctional partner, for example, a female with a minor orgastic dysfunction, begins to fear that she will fail; that she will not "make it" or will be ridiculed by her sexual partner. (Indeed, many patients have described that they begin to worry about their performance days in advance of an anticipated sexual encounter.) As her fear increases, she becomes someone outside herself, watching herself and her performance. As a result, anxiety triggers an interruption in the normal physiology of the sexual response and she does fail. This cycle continues and worsens as failure repeats failure, and often she will begin to avoid any type of sexual situation, much to the perplexity and concern of her partner. Interestingly, this type of situation had initially been found most frequently with men. However, with the current rise in awareness of female sexuality along with changes in female assertiveness, performance anxiety and subsequent spectatoring are becoming more frequent problems among women.

One of the major principles in all of Masters and Johnson's work is that sex is the ultimate level of communication between a couple and not just a mechanism for reproduction or tension release.[6] Thus, the concept of "sensate focusing" came into being and is now an initial element in all therapy techniques with couples, regardless of the primary complaint. Sensate focusing is a nonverbal means of communication accomplished through pleasuring touch. Considering that dysfunctional patients must be freed from anxiety about their sexual performance, the couple is told to stop keeping a score card, to stop being goal centered on erection or orgasm, and to focus on the process of lovemaking. For example, in virtually all cases, the couple is initially forbidden to have intercourse or even to touch especially erogenous zones such as breasts or genitals. They are directed instead to enjoy mutual kissing, hugging, and body massage. If all goes well and the couple begins to relax, they are then allowed to include previously forbidden activities, up to and finally including intercourse. This plan of treatment reduces performance anxiety markedly since the activities producing fear are forbidden while the joy of communicating with each other and the pleasure of bodily contact are enhanced.

Therapist considerations

A broad-based educational background is essential for qualified sexual dysfunction therapists. Knowledge of anatomy, physiology, and metabolic systems, as well as skill in psychotherapy, are basic requirements.

To treat sexual dysfunctions, the therapist must be aware that sex is a natural function. This concept is not a readily accepted one in our society, which imposes many restrictions and taboos on sexual practice. To demonstrate that sexual response is a natural function, research has shown that a majority of female babies lubricate their vaginas 4 to 6 hours after birth and that male babies are born with erections. In adults, during sleep, this natural function is continued. In the majority of cases, at about 90-minute intervals, women will lubricate their vaginas and men will have an erect penis. These facts demonstrate that sexual function cannot be taught. Therapy involves removing the psychologic roadblocks that inhibit this natural function.

Masters and Johnson strongly believe that sexual dysfunction therapy teams composed of a female and a male therapist are important to have optimal communication within the therapeutic setting involving couples.[7] They believe that neither sex can really understand the opposite sex in terms of life experiences or sexual sensations. Therefore, it is helpful to each member of the couple to have the support and understanding of a therapist of the same sex.

In any type of psychotherapy, including sexual dysfunction therapy, there is the question of transference. Transference is the unwarranted feeling toward the therapist that is carried over by the patient from previous relationships. A certain amount of transference should be encouraged by the therapists because it allows the therapy team to be viewed as authorities, which in turn facilitates therapy and increases compliance with the therapists' directives and home assignments. The advantage in the dual-therapy team is that such an approach neutralizes and dilutes the flow of transference and encourages the emotional flow between the partners in treatment.

Countertransference, or the unwarranted feelings of the therapist toward the patient, must also be considered, especially when dealing with seductive patients. Under no circumstances, should a therapist act out fantasies toward a patient. Unfortunately, there is a lack of peer review or a regulatory agency to certify those conducting sex therapy. This is a true concern for all qualified and ethical therapists and one being actively considered on both state and national levels.

Lastly, in considering treatment principles involving the therapists, there is the issue of sexual values. The therapist must always be aware of the possibility of imposing his or her own sexual values on the couple receiving treatment. The basic goal of treatment, it must be remembered, is to help the couple define and feel comfortable with their own treatment and sexual goals.[1]

Procedural considerations – couples

To receive maximum nonverbal communication, outside distractions must be kept to a minimum. It is essential for the couple to schedule time for home assignments away from time pressures, distracting children, and job concerns. Sex cannot be the last priority if treatment is to be effective. While the Masters and Johnson treatment program espouses social isolation for the couple, this method is very costly and not very practical for many couples. (Their St. Louis program is 2 weeks in length with the couple undergoing intensive daily therapy sessions followed by assignments in the privacy of their hotel room.) Many therapy programs now offer more traditional sessions of two to three times a week, while the couple continues regular schedules. Clinical follow-up of treated couples is essential for the continued development of sexual dysfunction theory. Research results from such follow-up provide continuous data on patients and demonstrate the effectiveness of this newer type of treatment for sexual dysfunction.

Procedural considerations — individuals

For those females and males who are not involved in a steady sexual partnership and who do not believe that they have someone with whom they can approach treatment as a couple, other treatment plans have been developed. For females with sexual dysfunction, the vast majority of which center on orgastic complaints, a group approach is ideal. Such a group, composed of all females, including the therapist, offers a unique supportive and educational setting in which the woman can share concerns, experiences, and ultimately achievements. The group treatment is time limited and structured toward reducing anxiety about orgasm through homework assignments aimed at developing methods for successful masturbation. As with the couple approach, education and communication techniques are also included in the group sessions. It is through this approach that the woman can learn about her own sexuality and can practice relaxing and experiencing orgasm. Hopefully, then, she will be able to enter sexual relationships in a more confident and knowledgeable fashion.

Males who also must necessarily approach treatment individually have been successfully helped in a group setting. While treatment groups generally are composed of males with a similar dysfunction, groups have been conducted in which the participants have a variety of sexual dysfunctions. As opposed to females, however, clear treatment steps are difficult to define for such groups. The very nature of male sexual function, especially in the erectile response, requires that something occur, that is, erection, to even initiate sexual intercourse. The male who is receiving treatment as an individual can profit from the support and education offered in a group but will need eventual practice with a female to reduce the anxiety triggering his dysfunction.

Individual therapy for females and males having a sexual complaint is another mode of treatment for sexual dysfunction. Generally, this approach is far more time consuming and associated with less than adequate treatment results as compared with couples or group treatment. Such an approach could be the therapy of choice, however, when the sexual complaint is couched in more predominantly psychologic concerns such as depression. Regardless of the approach to be considered, a thorough evaluation is indicated for each patient to determine the optimum treatment plan.

TREATMENT RESULTS

Statistical data resulting from various studies give an indication of the success rates of the various treatment methods. Kaplan has reported in detail the findings of these studies, having divided the results according to the specific dysfunctions.[2] While the results of these studies should be carefully considered, for example, what constitutes a "cure," the overall findings for the newer forms of treatment are impressive. Masters and Johnson report that 83% of totally inorgastic women were cured through the couples approach in their program, while 77% of situationally inorgastic women were reported as cured.[7] Data on same-sex groups is as yet scarce in the literature. Reports on individual therapy for sexually dysfunctional individuals remain unimpressive. Kaplan reports that individual therapy, in this case psychoanalysis, had only a 25% cure rate after 3 to 5 years of treatment.[2] The entire area of sexual dysfunction treatment is relatively new, and further research data will be necessary to describe therapy approaches and their results.

CONCLUSION

Professional nurses have an obligation to be concerned about every health aspect of patients under their care. Obstetric-gynecologic nurse-practitioners have a special opportunity to explore possible sexual concerns with their patients. We cannot all be sex therapists, but we can all be open, aware, and concerned about this important part of our patients' health. By conducting a thorough investigation into the history of the dysfunction, the knowledgeable nurse-practitioner can assess for possible physiologic or psychologic etiologies. Educational orientation can be provided and misconceptions, some of which are lifelong, can be eliminated. Perhaps, most importantly, patients need a competent, understanding, and honest professional with whom they can discuss a sometimes frightening health problem. There have been numerous instances in which a single, complete interview alone has reversed a sexual dysfunction. It is gratifying, also, to note the increase of self-esteem at the conclusion of such an interview when the patient is assured that she is very much a woman, despite some sexual problem.

Should the presenting condition appear complicated or in need of specialist treatment, the patient or couple should be referred to a competent sexual therapy clinic or private practitioner. To ensure the reliability of such a referral, several measures can be taken. In a city with a university medical center, contact the department of psychiatry to learn if a sexual dysfunction clinic exists. If such a medical center is unavailable, call the local nursing and medical associations, requesting names of competent professionals in the area. Be certain that the referral is an established and specially trained person. Our patients' welfare depends on our reliable referral.

A final reminder—do not be afraid to approach the subject of sexual functioning with your patients. Remember that you are viewed as a helping authority figure, interested in all aspects of your patients' health. The patient or couple will not be embarrassed if you are direct and open. It will be through this type of accepting attitude that nursing can help a patient suffering from a sexual dysfunction to take that first, very important step toward a fuller, more satisfying life.

REFERENCES

1. Green, R., editor: Human sexuality: a health practitioner's text, Baltimore, 1975, The Williams & Wilkins Co.
2. Kaplan, H. S.: The new sex therapy, New York, 1974, Brunner/Mazel, Inc.
3. Katchadourian, H. A., and Lunde, D. T.: Fundamentals of human sexuality, New York, 1972, Holt, Rinehart and Winston, Inc.
4. Lobitz, W. C., and LoPiccolo, J.: New methods in the behavioral treatment of sexual dysfunction, J. Behav. Ther. Exper. Psychiatry 3(4):265-271, 1972.
5. LoPiccolo, J., and Lobitz, W. C.: The role of masturbation in the treatment of primary orgasmic dysfunction, Arch. Sex. Behav. 2:163-171, 1972.
6. Masters, W. H., and Johnson, V. E.: Human sexual response, Boston, 1966, Little, Brown and Co.
7. Masters, W. H., and Johnson, V. E.: Human sexual inadequacy, Boston, 1970, Little, Brown and Co.
8. Wood, R. Y., and Rose, K.: Penile implants for impotence, Am. J. Nurs. 78(2):234-238, 1978.

CHAPTER 11

The premenstrual tension syndromes

Guy E. Abraham

INTRODUCTION

The term *premenstrual tension* (PMT) was used for the first time in 1931 by Frank[18] to describe a condition characterized by premenstrual nervous tension, usually associated with weight gain, edema of the face, lower abdomen, and extremities, and headaches. Using a bioassay technique, he found increased estrogenic activity in blood and decreased estrogenic activity in urine. He then postulated that PMT was caused by an excess of peripheral estrogens caused by decreased renal clearance. His treatment consisted of calcium lactate for sedation, theobromine and caffeine as diuretics, and magnesium citrate as a saline laxative. In severe cases, he used irradiation of the ovaries.

Since Frank's publications, many symptoms have been added and many theories postulated for the cause of PMT. Treatment by physicians depended on their individual theories. Moos[35] identified seven major clusters of symptoms related to behavior, autonomic system, dysphoria, arousal, pain, concentration, and water retention. He proposed the term *premenstrual syndromes* to emphasize the proteiform aspect of PMT.

Unfortunately, well-controlled studies of PMT are scarce and most of the conclusions drawn from PMT studies may not be valid. Unless otherwise stated, studies reported here were not performed in a controlled double-blind fashion. Since there are many excellent and extensive reviews on PMT,* this chapter will discuss only three postulated causes of PMT, namely hormonal imbalance, malnutrition, and stress, showing how these three postulates are not mutually exclusive but are in fact closely interrelated. Areas needing more research will be emphasized, and a proposed plan will be detailed for the classification, evaluation, and management of PMT.

SOME POSTULATED PATHOPHYSIOLOGIES
Hormonal imbalance

This theory pioneered by Frank[18] states that PMT is caused by hyperestrogenemia, which results in the psychologic and somatic changes observed. Morton[37] was able to elicit some symptoms of PMT by administering large doses of estrogen to castrated women. His studies made him reason that there was also a progesterone deficiency, and he recommended human chorionic

---

*See references 17, 28, 37, 40, 42, 45, 48, and 52.

gonadotropin (HCG) injection to stimulate progesterone secretion by the corpus luteum. Dalton[15] postulated that progesterone deficiency was the cause of PMT and reported excellent results with exogenous progesterone. Backstrom and Carstensen[8] recently confirmed the hyperestrogenemia and low progesterone in a group of PMT patients whose main complaint was premenstrual anxiety.

As to what causes the hyperestrogenemia, there are three proposed postulates. To understand how these postulates interrelate, let us review what happens to estrogens in the normal woman. Estrogens are secreted mainly by the ovaries. A small amount of peripheral estrogens come from conversion of adrenal and ovarian androgens. Estrogens are bound to plasma proteins very tightly, except for a small fraction (1% to 2%), which is believed to be the active fraction available for tissue utilization. The liver conjugates estrogens, making them more water soluble and inactive. The conjugated estrogens are then cleared by the kidney and excreted in the urine.

Backstrom's postulate. Backstrom and co-workers observed premenstrual elevated FSH levels in some PMT patients with elevated estrogen levels.[9] Since FSH is known to stimulate ovarian estrogens, he postulated that hyperestrogenemia was caused by ovarian hypersecretion resulting from elevated FSH. He would then have to explain what caused the elevated FSH. This postulate would imply an increased urinary excretion of estrogen, assuming normal hepatic and renal functions.

Biskin's postulate. Biskin concluded from a series of experiments that the excess peripheral estrogen observed in PMT was caused by decreased liver metabolism of estrogens resulting from vitamin B complex deficiencies. He reported excellent results using vitamin B complex therapy.[11] These studies remain to be confirmed using individual B vitamins and accurately measuring hepatic and metabolic clearance rates of individual estrogens.

Frank's postulate. This postulate states that a decreased renal clearance of estrogens is the cause of hyperestrogenemia. With present knowledge of estrogen metabolism, renal malfunction in the presence of normal liver function would result in peripheral elevation of conjugated biologically inactive estrogens, not unconjugated biologically active estrogens. More studies are needed to confirm the elevated estrogen levels and to explain the factors involved.

Nutritional deficiencies

This theory was pioneered by Biskin in 1943[11] following his observations that patients with overt vitamin B deficiency had PMT symptoms that responded favorably to vitamin B therapy. He experimented with rats and found that the liver could not metabolize estrogens when the rats were made deficient in vitamin B. Estrogen metabolism returned to normal following vitamin B complex therapy.

In 1950, Morton[36] observed that in a subgroup of PMT, characterized by premenstrual increased appetite, craving for sweets, fatigue, and fainting spells, there was an increased glucose tolerance level with a flat GTT curve premenstrually, but not postmenstrually. These patients responded favorably to a regimen of high protein–low carbohydrate diet and vitamin B.

In 1971, Nicholas[39] postulated a nutritional deficiency in magnesium as the cause of PMT and treated 192 PMT patients with magnesium nitrate, 4.5 to 6 gm per day for 1 week premenstrually and 2 days menstrually. The best response was observed for mastalgia, nervous tension, and weight gain. However, less than half the patients

Table 11-1. Effect of magnesium nitrate* on premenstrual tension in 192 patients†

Symptoms	Patients with symptoms		Favorable response	
	Number	Percent of total	Number	Percent of total
Nervous tension	179	93	159	89
Mastalgia	162	84	155	96
Weight gain	62	32	59	95
Headache	37	19	16	43

*4.5 to 6 gm per day orally for 1 week premenstrually and 2 days menstrual.
†Adapted from Nicholas, A.: Traitement du syndrome pre-menstruel et de la dysmenorrhee par l'ion magnesium. In Durlach, J., editor: First international symposium on magnesium deficiency in human pathology, Paris, 1973, Springer-Verlag.

Table 11-2. Effect of pyridoxine* on premenstrual tension in 70 patients†

Symptoms	Patient with symptoms		Favorable response	
	Number	Percent of total	Number	Percent of total
Irritability	57	81	32	56
Depression	50	71	30	60
Edema	32	46	19	59
Mastalgia	23	33	12	52
Lethargy	19	27	10	53
Headache	16	23	13	81
Lack of coordination	15	21	4	27

*40 to 100 mg per day starting 3 days before expected symptoms and continuing until menses.
†Adapted from Kerr, G. D.: The management of the premenstrual syndrome, Curr. Med. Res. Opin. **4**:29-34, 1977.

with headache responded to magnesium therapy (Table 11-1).

Pyridoxine at a dose of 50 mg per day was reported as successful in treating premenstrual depression,[54,55] but this could not be confirmed in a better controlled study.[50] Recently, Kerr[30] reported the results obtained in 70 PMT patients treated with pyridoxine, 40 to 100 mg per day. Significant relief of symptoms was observed in over half the patients, with headache showing the highest response rate (81%) and lack of coordination showing the poorest (27%) (Table 11-2).

Stress

It is generally agrees that mental or physical stress aggravates PMT. In 1953, Rees[42] did an extensive review of the literature and concluded that PMT is a complex psychophysical state determined by a multiplicity of factors with stress being an important factor and that treatment could be applied at varous etiologic levels. A recent study by Englander and coworkers[16] suggests that women with high premenstrual symptomatology have a higher perception of tension (stress) in interactions with others than women with low premenstrual symptomatology. In other words, PMT patients have an increased susceptibility to stress, a decreased threshold in their perception of stress.

CLASSIFICATION OF PMT

Since PMT is an abnormality of the menstrual cycle, the logical approach in defining it both qualitatively and quantitatively is to

Table 11-3. Results of Multiple Affect Adjective Check List (MAACL) test during the follicular and luteal phases of fourteen normal menstrual cycles

	Anxiety*	Hostility*	Depression*
Follicular phase	7.7 ± 1.3	10.9 ± 1.1	17.4 ± 2.2
	(36.7 ± 6.2)	(39 ± 4)	(43.5 ± 5.5)
Luteal phase	8.2 ± 1.1	11.1 ± 1.0	17.7 ± 2.1
	(39 ± 5.2)	(40 ± 3.6)	(44 ± 5.3)

*Mean ″ S.D. of mean values obtained for each menstrual cycle.
( ) = expressed as percent of maximum score.

start by defining the normal menstrual cycle in terms of the same parameters evaluated. The term *normal* is based on the goal of optimal or near optimal function and of perfect health.[34] In the studies performed on the *normal* cycle, researchers usually state that subjects evaluated were menstruating regularly and in apparent good health. This implies that they were *normal* and that the values obtained may be used to compute the normal range. The assumption is made that optimal health has been defined and that the subjects studied were in optimal health. However, most researchers use the word *normal* to describe *average*. The fact is that, even today, we do not have a good understanding of optimal health. For this reason, our *normal* values are *average* values for the population studied. The study of the optimal menstrual cycle is an unexplored area. In this chapter, the normal menstrual cycle is defined as the average cycle observed in a population of apparently normal women, not the optimal menstrual cycle expected in optimally healthy women.

Comparison between the normal and PMT menstrual cycles

From menarche to menopause, women undergo cyclic changes. These changes originate in the neuroendocrine system and result in periodic vaginal bleeding of uterine origin called *menses*. The interval between the first day of menses and the first day of the next menses represents one menstrual cycle. Ovulation, which usually occurs at midcycle, divides the menstrual cycle into two phases: the follicular phase and the luteal phase. Some behavioral, endocrine, and somatic parameters studied during the normal and PMT menstrual cycles will now be reviewed.

Behavioral parameters

Moods. It is assumed that mood state is positively correlated to the corresponding behavior and that behavior would be expressed if appropriate environmental stimuli were present. Recent studies by Moos[35] and Golub[23] have indicated that variations in sex hormones during the normal menstrual cycle may be associated with changes in affect (mood, feelings, emotion). They reported increased anxiety, hostility, and depression premenstrually. However, during 29 normal menstrual cycles, Persky[41] found no significant changes in these negative moods. Our data in 14 normal menstrual cycles concur with the findings of Persky (Table 11-3). Although Golub[23] reported a significant increase in state anxiety and depression premenstrually in normal women, the scores were much lower than in patients with psychiatric disorders. State anxiety is a transitory phenomenon, in contrast to trait anxiety, which is a relatively stable personality characteristic. The magnitude of the premenstrual mood change was not great enough to affect intellectual function.[22] Persky also reported that serum androgens were positively related to depression scores in menstruating women.[41]

Demonstration of an association between sex steroid profiles and behavior during the menstrual cycle is no proof of a cause-and-effect relationship. Further studies have indeed shown that exogenous sex steroids do have an effect on mood. A review and controlled study by Culberg[14] on the effect of various hormonal contraceptives suggests that progestins may have a tendency to produce depression, whereas estrogens tend to stimulate anxiety and nervous tension. Bardwick,[10] using a verbal anxiety scale to score interviews with subjects taking contraceptive pills of various estrogenic and progestogenic potencies, concluded that subjects on estrogen-dominant pills described themselves as higher in assertiveness, aggression, and hostility when compared with those on progestin-dominant pills. The latter described themselves higher in deference, nurturance, and affiliation. Grant and Pryse-Davies[24] studied the responses of 794 women taking a wide variety of oral contraceptives. They concluded that when the level of estrogen in the pill was low, there was a high probability of depression. Depression and a low sexual interest was most common when the pill was strongly progestogenic and had low levels of estrogen. They found the lowest depression levels among women who were taking pills high in estrogen.

Arousal. Arousal refers to a state of alertness that is accompanied by a number of physiologic changes. The sensory organs become more sensitive to incoming stimuli, and the capacity to filter out irrelevant stimuli at the precortical level is enhanced. Asso and Beech[6] tested the postulate that a significant fluctuation in levels of arousal occurs during the menstrual cycle. Using the galvanic skin response, they observed a greater susceptibility to acquire a conditioned galvanic skin response premenstrually than intermenstrually, suggesting a higher level of arousal premenstrually. Lunde and Hamburg[33] used four different tests to evaluate cyclic changes in arousal during the menstrual cycle: reaction time, galvanic skin potential, two-flash threshold,* and time estimation. Reaction time and skin response did not show significant variation, but time estimation and two-flash threshold showed significant changes during the menstrual cycle: a distinct tendency to estimate the given time interval as longer and a rise in two-flash threshold during the premenstrual phase. Depending on the methods used to assess arousal, cyclic variations were either absent throughout the cycle or present as an increased arousal premenstrually. No such studies have been published on PMT cycles.

Food consumption. Very little work has been done on changes in either appetite or food consumption during the human menstrual cycle. Moos' Menstrual Distress Questionnaire (MDQ)[35] originally contained an item asking about "change in eating habits," but it was dropped because it did not consistently locate with any of the other factors.

Data collected from baboon females (*Papio ursinus*) by Gilbert and Gillman[19] showed very convincingly the effects of phase of menstrual cycle on eating behavior. Calorie (or protein) intake was relatively low prior to ovulation, increased during the luteal phase, peaked 0 to 5 days prior to menstruation, and dropped precipitously

---

*The "flicker fusion threshold," which consists of a light flickering at increasing frequency until the subject does not detect the flickering but sees the light as continuous. Adrenergic stimulation gives the ability to detect flickers at higher frequencies. A rise in two-flash threshold suggests a decreased ability to detect flicker at higher frequencies.

after onset of menstruation. Krohn and Zuckerman[31] showed that in Macaca mulatta females, the dry weight of food consumed was greater during the second half compared with the first half of the cycle. The disadvantage of the primate studies is that they were conducted in captivity and therefore may not reflect what occurs in the wild. However, the presence of a significant effect shows that at least in one specific environment this relationship holds. More work of a precise nature is needed in this area in normal women and PMT patients.

Cognitive performance. A recent review by Sommer[46] on the effects of menstruation on cognitive behavior revealed that studies utilizing objective performance measures generally fail to demonstrate menstrual cycle-related changes. Socially mediated expectations are suggested as a possible basis for observed changes in some studies. Well-performed studies on cognitive performances in PMT patients are greatly needed.

Endocrine parameters

Hormones, Among the peptide hormones studied, increased luteal phase levels of prolactin[25] and FSH[9] have been reported in PMT patients compared with normal women. Increased luteal phase serum estrogen and decreased serum progesterone levels were found in PMT anxiety,[8] but Smith reported normal estrogen and progesterone levels during the luteal phase in PMT depression.[45] Some PMT patients with premenstrual edema and weight gain were found to have elevated serum levels of the mineralocorticoids aldosterone and corticosterone.[44] However, this is not a consistent finding.

Glucose tolerance. Spellacy and co-workers[47] performed a 2-hour glucose tolerance test (GTT) in 19 normal premenopausal women during the follicular and luteal phases of the menstrual cycle. A normal response was observed during both phases of the cycle. Morton performed a 4-hour GTT in 17 PMT patients complaining of premenstrual increased appetite, craving for sweets, fatigue, and sometimes the "shakes."[36] He observed a normal GTT curve during the follicular phase but an increased carbohydrate tolerance with a flat GTT curve during the luteal phase. This paradoxic effect of increased carbohydrate intake on carbohydrate tolerance may be explained by the recent finding that a glucose load increased the affinity of target cells to insulin by as much as eleven-fold[38] therefore increasing the biologic activity of insulin. A high carbohydrate–low protein diet would be expected to produce the same effect.

Somatic parameters

Body weight. In 1934, Sweeney[51] studied body weight fluctuations during the menstrual cycle in 42 women. She observed premenstrual weight gain of less than 3 lbs in 70% of the subjects and weight gain greater than 3 lbs in the remaining 30%. In 1957, Golub and co-workers[21] studied 65 female college students 18 to 22 years of age and observed that weight gain during the menstrual cycle was always less than 3 lbs above the cycle mean value. During that same year, Chesley and Hellman[13] could not substantiate premenstrual weight gain as a consistent phenomenon in 23 normal subjects. More studies are needed to define clearly the upper normal limit of premenstrual weight gain. Since Chesley and Hellman[13] have shown that by chance alone random weight fluctuations would show the maximum rise during the 7 to 10 days premenstrual one third of the time and since it is generally accepted that random fluctuations of body weight during the menstrual cycle show a range of less than 3 lbs, one criterion for PMT would require a premenstrual weight gain of greater than 3 lbs during three consecutive cycles.

Pain threshold. In 1933, Herren[27] studied pain and touch threshold during the follicular and luteal phases of 11 normal menstrual cycles. He found a lower threshold for pain and two-point touch discrimination during the luteal phase. In 1960, Archangeli[5] compared pain and touch threshold during the normal and PMT cycles. He observed a decreased pain and touch threshold during the luteal phase in normal and PMT cycles, but the degree of change was greater in the PMT patients. In 1968, Buzzelli[12] studied pain threshold serially during 118 normal menstrual cycles. He reported an increased threshold at midcycle and a decreased threshold premenstrually. There is great need to standardize the methods of measuring pain thresholds and to quantitatively define upper normal limits during the normal menstrual cycle. Until then, we will have to rely on subjective reports related to pain threshold in response to various stimuli to which PMT patients are exposed during their daily activities.

Extensive studies have been performed on the role of anxiety on pain threshold.[49] It is generally agreed that anxiety is positively correlated with sensitivity to acute pain and lowers the threshold to painful stimuli. If this also applies to PMT patients, treatment aimed at lowering anxiety level should also improve symptoms related to pain.

Subgroups of PMT

The lack of an internationally accepted scheme for classifying and grading the severity of PMT has been a prime source of confusion and controversy concerning the incidence, etiology, and pathophysiology of PMT. In 1976, Kashiwagi and co-workers[29] set some criteria, both qualitatively and quantitatively, for the diagnosis of PMT but did not attempt to form subgroups of PMT. In 1977, Kerr[30] subdivided PMT into 3 subgroups: Group I: progesterone deficiency during the luteal phase, Group II: excess prolactin during the luteal phase and Group III: normal progesterone and prolactin during the luteal phase. However, this classification is not symptomatic, but retrospective and endocrine.

In my experience, patients with PMT may belong to one or more of the following five symptomatic subgroups:

1. PMT-A: chief complaints of anxiety, irritability, and nervous tension, occurring as early as midcycle, becoming progressively worse during the luteal phase, sometimes followed by mild depression, and improving with menses.
2. PMT-C: characterized by premenstrual increased appetite craving for sweets, (mainly chocolate), headache, palpitation, fainting spells, and fatigue.
3. PMT-D: characterized by premenstrual depression, lethargy, confusion, withdrawal, and thoughts of suicide sometimes followed by attempts at suicide.
4. PMT-H: the hyperhydration syndrome, characterized by premenstrual weight gain (3 to 20 lbs), edema of the face and extremities, abdominal bloating, and mastalgia. With increasing age, the PMT weight gain is not completely lost with onset of menses and overweight problems occur.
5. PMT-P: characterized by general aches and pains (the hyperesthesia syndrome) with lower threshold for pain premenstrually. This syndrome is usually associated with dysmenorrhea, and in the French literature, magnesium deficiency has been implicated as its cause.[39]

The postulated pathophysiology of PMT that best fits the available data is outlined in Fig. 11-1. I believe that the primary causes

The premenstrual tension syndromes 177

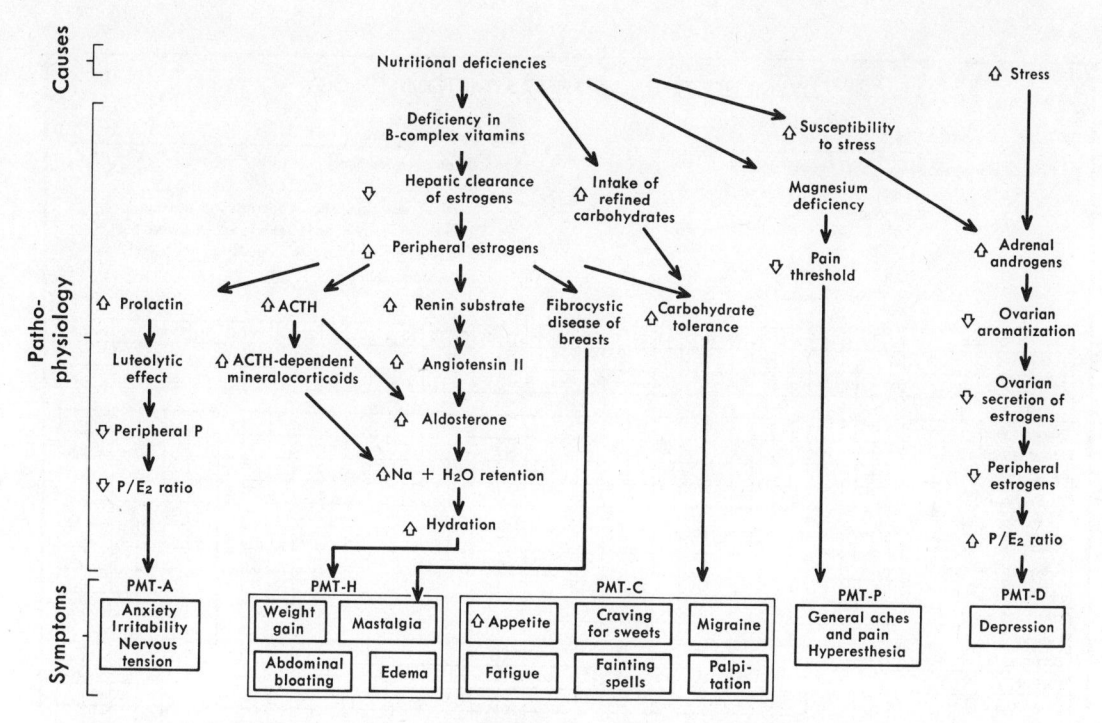

Fig. 11-1. Postulated pathophysiology of PMT. In this postulate, nutrition and stress play the more significant roles.

of PMT are: (1) nutritional deficiencies from inadequate diet, inadequate intestinal absorption, or increased demands for certain nutrients and (2) increased stress and/or susceptibility to stress with a decreased ability to cope with stress.

EVALUATION OF PMT

Premenstrual discomfort, also called premenstrual molimina, occurs in the majority of women. The symptoms are mild and often used as an index of normal ovulatory cycles. In contrast, PMT symptoms are moderate to severe, interfering with normal activity, often being incapacitating.

The evaluation of PMT patients should include a complete history with special emphasis on nutritional status. Extensive nutritional surveys by computer analysis are commercially available. The patient records her food and liquid intake. By programming the computer with the average content of nutritional factors in each of these foods, a printout furnishes the average daily intake of proteins, fats, carbohydrates, vitamins, and minerals. A 6-hour glucose tolerance test is recommended in PMT-C patients during the midcycle phase to confirm the increased carbohydrate tolerance. In the evaluation of stress factors, remember that in some PMT patients, the anticipation of menses may represent a significant stress.

Since there are so many symptoms, it is helpful to have a form with a listing of the most common symptoms (MDQ)[35] and a grading from none to severe (Fig 11-2). The patient is asked to complete these forms

DYSMENORRHEA AND PMT SYMPTOMATOLOGY

NAME: _____

Grading of menses: 0-none   3-heavy
                          1-slight   4-heavy and clots
                          2-moderate

CYCLE 1 2 3 4 5 6 7

Grading of symptoms:
0 - none
1 - mild-present but does not interfere with activities.
2 - moderate- present and interferes with activities but not disabling.
3 - severe-disabling.

DAY OF CYCLE	1	2	3	4	5	6	7	8	9	10	11	12	13	14	15	16	17	18	19	20	21	22	23	24	25	26	27	28	29	30	31	32	33	34	35	36
DATE																																				
MENSES																																				
I. PMT-A																																				
Nervous tension																																				
Mood swings																																				
Irritability																																				
Anxiety																																				
II. PMT-C																																				
Headache																																				
Craving for sweets																																				
Increased appetite																																				
Heart pounding																																				
Fatigue																																				
Dizziness or faintness																																				
III. PMT-D																																				
Depression																																				
Forgetfulness																																				
Crying																																				
Confusion																																				
Insomnia																																				
IV. PMT-H																																				
Weight gain																																				
Swelling of extremities																																				
Breast tenderness																																				
Abdominal bloating																																				
V. PMT-P																																				
General aches/pains																																				
Itching																																				
VI. DYSMENORRHEA																																				
Cramps (abdominal)																																				
Hot flushes																																				
Nausea/vomiting																																				
Diarrhea																																				
Backache																																				
Chest pain																																				
VII.																																				
Basal body temperature																																				
VIII.																																				
Basal Weight																																				

Fig. 11-2. Dysmenorrhea and PMT symptomatology.

daily during the menstrual cycle to observe significant changes during the luteal phase. Patients are also asked to take their weight and basal body temperature (BBT) daily upon awakening. Because of Vollman's[53] extensive studies, I prefer the rectal temperature, which is apparently more precise and consistent than the oral temperature. If the oral temperature is preferred by the patient, the temperature must be taken for a minimum of 10 minutes to improve reliability. The BBT intercept method of Vollman[53] is used as a demarcation between the follicular and the luteal phases. In cases in which the BBT curve is equivocal, the luteal phase is defined as the last 14 days of the cycle.

Criteria for inclusion in a PMT subgroup are: (1) The mean daily score from the MDQ for that subgroup must be significantly higher ($p < 0.05$) during the luteal phase compared with the follicular phase, (excluding the menstrual phase), or the daily score of at least 3 days during the luteal phase must be significantly higher ($p < 0.05$) than the mean daily score of the follicular phase, and (2) the severity of PMT must be more than mild. It is graded by the daily score of at least 3 days during the luteal phase:

1. Mild — if daily score is between 1 and 4 for PMT-A and PMT-H, between 1 and 5 for PMT-D, and between 1 and 6 for PMT-C.
2. Moderate — if daily score is between 5 and 8 for PMT-A and PMT-H, between 6 and 10 for PMT-D and between 7 and 12 for PMT-C.
3. Severe — if daily score is between 9 and 12 for PMT-A and PMT-H, between 11 and 15 for PMT-D, and between 13 and 16 for PMT-C.

Mild PMT is considered premenstrual molimina. A patient would therefore have PMT if she fulfills the criteria for one or more subgroups and if the severity is rated as moderate or severe.

At the present time, hormonal evaluation of PMT patients is still at an experimental stage and has no practical value in the management of PMT patients.

TREATMENT OF PMT

Treatment of PMT can be applied at different etiologic levels. The following treatments were tested on open trials. Double-blind longitudinal studies are currently being designed to assess the placebo effect of some of these therapies.

Nutrition

In my opinion, this approach tackles the PMT problem at the highest etiologic level. Research in nutrition has increased significantly over the past 10 years. However, the findings derived from such studies are not usually common knowledge among practicing physicians and nurses.

There is compelling evidence that neurotransmitters present in high concentrations in certain parts of the brain play a major role in mood and behavior.[43] Table 11-4 outlines various neurotransmitters and their believed effects on mood. Table 11-5 outlines some dietary precursors of these neurotransmitters. A very important enzyme in the conversion of these amino acids to biologically active compounds is called decarboxylase. Vitamin B_6 is a required cofactor for this enzyme. Under chronic stress,[7] decarboxylase may become rate limiting in the conversion of these amino acids to neurotransmitters (Fig. 11-3). Dietary tryptophan and choline have an acute and significant effect on brain neurotransmitters.[56] High carbohydrate–low protein diet favors transfer of tryptophan from serum to the central nervous system.[56] This may result in a CNS serotonin dominance and relative dopamine deficiency.

180 Selected Ob/Gyn problems and issues

1. Tyrosine hydroxylase
2. Dopa decarboxylase
3. Dopamine β-hydroxylase

Normal

Tyrosine $\xrightarrow{1}$ Dopa $\xrightarrow{2}$ Dopamine $\xrightarrow{3}$ N.E.

Chronic stress

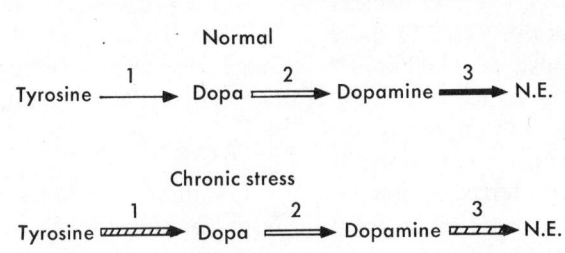

Tyrosine $\xrightarrow{1}$ Dopa $\xrightarrow{2}$ Dopamine $\xrightarrow{3}$ N.E.

Fig. 11-3. Effect of chronic stress on the synthesis of catecholamines. Chronic stress increases enzymes 1 and 3, but not 2. Normally, enzyme 1 is rate limiting, but under chronic stress, enzyme 2, for which vitamin B_6 is a cofactor, may become rate limiting, causing a relative dopamine deficiency.

Table 11-4. Effects of biogenic amines on mood and behavior

Biogenic amine	Effect
Norepinephrine	Aggression
Epinephrine	Anxiety, arousal
Dopamine	Relaxation, sedation
Serotonin	Stimulation, tension
γ-Aminobutyric acid	Sedation, anticonvulsant
Acetylcholine	CNS motor function memory

Table 11-5. Dietary precursors of neurotransmitters

Dietary precursor	Neurotransmitter
Tyrosine	Dopamine, norepinephrine, epinephrine
Tryptophan	Serotonin, metatonin
Glutamic acid	γ-Aminobutyric acid
Choline	Acetylcholine

The interplay of neurotransmitters in their influence on mood and behavior is still poorly understood. Nevertheless, enough information is now available to strongly suggest a significant influence of nutrition on mood and behavior. The nutritional evaluation will give an idea about the patient's nutritional status. Education of the patient about the value of good nutrition in relation to total well being is an important step and may be performed by a well-trained nurse or dietician. High intake of refined carbohydrates should be discouraged in favor of fresh fruits and vegetables. Brewers' yeast, wheat germ, and molasses are recommended as a source of vitamins, minerals, and trace elements. Green vegetables and uncooked food should be the main bulk of the diet. Intake of red meat and dairy products should be limited in favor of fish and poultry as a source of protein. Herbal spices and kelp are recommended as an alternative to table salt (NaCl). The diet may be supplemented with vitamins and minerals.

Outdoor activities and sports are recommended to improve physical well being and as an outlet for tension and hostility.

Environmental stress

I have observed a complete disappearance of PMT symptoms in some patients when they are away from a stressful situation, such as quitting a job where there is a lot of interpersonal friction, or going away for a vacation. On the other hand, symptoms have worsened during periods of stress. It is important to educate the PMT patient on the role of stress as one of the causes of her symptoms. Being aware of potential sources for problems is part of the treatment. Understanding and compassion from friends and relatives has a positive effect in decreasing tension.

Susceptibility to stress

As mentioned previously, there is some evidence that PMT patients have an increased susceptibility to stress in interacting with others during the premenstrual phase.[16] This increased susceptibility is believed to be caused by increased estrogen levels, a CNS stimulant.[8] This increased estrogen level is believed to be caused by decreased liver clearance secondary to nutritional deficiencies, mainly in the vitamin B complex.[11] It seems logical therefore to give a therapeutic trial of vitamin B complex, which is also part of the nutritional approach. Among the vitamin B complex, pyridoxine (B_6) at doses of 200 to 800 mg per day has resulted in the best responses, at least in uncontrolled studies.[1,2] The patients volunteered the following information on the effect of B_6 therapy:

1. Marked decrease in tension and anxiety
2. Sedation and better sleep pattern
3. More energetic at work
4. Decreased susceptibility to stress, being better able to cope
5. Improvement of mastalgia, breast congestion, and fibrocystic masses (In some patients without evidence of premature weight gain but with symptoms of premenstrual bloating and edema of the facies and extremities, there has also been marked symptomatic improvement.)
6. Control of premenstrual weight gain
7. Decreased urgency and frequency with increased volume of urine per urination suggesting increased bladder capacity and increased diuresis
8. Improvement or absence of menstrual cramps
9. Midcycle leukorrhea suggesting increased secretion of cervical mucus

Table 11-6. Effect of vitamin B_6 on midluteal serum progesterone (P) and estradiol-17β (E_2) levels in PMT patients

Patient	P (ng/ml)	E_2 (ng/ml)
Control	7.0 ± 1.3	0.23 ± 0.06
	$p < 0.01$	N.S.
B_6 therapy	12. ± 1.9	0.22 ± 0.01
Control	10.7 ± 1.6	0.16 ± 0.006
	N.S.	N.S.
B_6 therapy	9.2 ± 0.09	0.15 ± 0.008
Control	11.3 ± 1.8	0.13 ± 0.03
	$p < 0.05$	$p < 0.01$
B_6 therapy	14. ± 1.0	0.1 ± 0.
Control	15.8 ± 2.5	0.17 ± 0.016
	N.S.	$p < 0.05$
B_6 therapy	14 ± 1.0	0.14 ± 0.005
Control	12.7 ± 1.5	0.25 ± 0.009
	$p < 0.01$	N.S.
B_6 therapy	26 ± 2.4	0.27 ± 0.05
Control	4.8 ± 0.5	0.19 ± 0.017
	$p < 0.01$	N N.S.
B_6 therapy	14.7 ± 2.2	0.21 ± 0.011
Control	11 ± 1.2	0.18 ± 0.011
	$p < 0.01$	N.S.
B_6 therapy	17 ± 2.6	0.2 ± 0.016

Of 14 PMT eumenorrheic patients suffering from undiagnosed infertility of many years' duration, 12 conceived during B_6 therapy.[26] In five out of seven PMT patients studied, midluteal serum progesterone levels were significantly higher during B_6 treatment, compared with the control group (Table 11-6). Serum estradiol-17β levels were lower during B_6 therapy in two patients. This luteotrophic effect of B_6 combined with its stimulating effect on cervical mucus may explain the good response observed in infertile PMT patients.

The only subgroup that did not respond to B_6 therapy was the PMT-D patients who complained of severe headache when taking B_6. The dose of B_6 is adjusted to prevent side effects of overdosage: headache, dizziness, and nausea. In most patients, the optimun dose varies from 200 to 800 mg per day.

The patients are given B_6 at the beginning of the menstrual cycle, and the daily dose is maintained for the whole cycle. The dose is increased at each cycle until there is marked improvement of symptoms. If side effects occur, the dose is lowered. A double-blind crossover longitudinal study is currently being designed to test the placebo effect of B_6 therapy.

Hormonal therapy

PMT-A patients usually respond well to progesterone administration, as recommended by Dalton.[15] However, the other subgroups show poor response and PMT-D patients worsen while taking progesterone.

The best therapeutic response in PMT-D patients is obtained when they receive estrogen therapy the last 2 weeks of the cycle. This response is observed even in the PMT-D patients with normal luteal estradial-17β levels suggesting a decreased availability of or sensitivity to estrogens in these patients. Estrone sulfate, 0.31 to 0.62 mg per day, is usually required. The patients are told to adjust the dose depending on their symptoms. Some PMT-D patients prefer to take a small dose (0.31 mg) throughout the cycle and to increase the dose to 0.62 mg on days when they are more depressed. This dose of estrogen does not interfere significantly with the menstrual cycle. Psychiatric consultation should be obtained in all PMT-D cases.

Symptomatic treatment

This kind of therapy tackles the PMT problem at the lowest etiologic level. Diuretics, sedatives, tranquilizers, analgesics, and narcotics have all been prescribed for the treatment of PMT. This approach is the least desirable and should be used as a last resort on a temporary basis.

Birth control

If PMT patients desire contraception and choose the hormonal form, the pill described depends on the subgroup of PMT. Women in the PMT-A subgroup should be given a progestogen-dominated combination pill,[14] while women in the PMT-D subgroup should receive an estrogen-dominated contraceptive pill. It is advisable to encourage patients on hormonal contraception to take vitamin B complex, mainly B_6, because of the recent evidence that synthetic estrogens deplete the body of some of the B vitamins.[3,4,32] Magnesium supplementation is also recommended for the same reason.[20]

REFERENCES

1. Abraham, G. E.: The normal menstrual cycle. In Givens, J. R., editor: Endocrine causes of menstrual disorders, Chicago, 1978, Year Book Medical Publishers, Inc., pp. 15-44.
2. Abraham, G. E.: Primary dysmenorrhea, Clin. Obstet. Gynecol. **21:**139-145, 1978.
3. Ahmed, F., and Bamji, M.: Vitamin supplements to women using oral contraceptives, Contraception **14:**309, 1976.
4. Anderson, K. E.: Effects of oral contraceptives on vitamin metabolism, Adv. Clin. Chem. **18:**.247, 1976.
5. Arcangeli, P., and Furian, R.: Perception of touch and pain in the various phases of the menstrual cycle, Rassegna di neurolgia vegetatie **14:**461-473, 1960.
6. Asso, D., and Beech, H. R.: Susceptibility to the acquisition of a conditioned response in relation to the menstrual cycle, J. Psychosom. Res. **19:** 337-344, 1975.
7. Axelrod, J.: Regulation of the synthesis, release, and actions of catecholamine neurotransmitters. In Dumont, J., and Nunez, J., editors: First European Symposium on Hormones and Cell Regulation, The Netherlands, 1977, North Holland Biomedical Press, pp. 137-155.

8. Backstrom, T., and Carstensen, H.: Estrogen and progesterone in plasma in relation to premenstrual tension, J. Steroid Biochem. **5:** 257-260, 1974.
9. Backstrom, T., Wide, L., Sodergard, R., et al.: FSH, LH, TeBG-capacity, estrogen and progesterone in women with premenstrual tension during the luteal phase, J. Steroid Biochem. **7:** 473-476, 1976.
10. Bardwick, J. M.: Psychological correlates of the menstrual cycle and oral contraceptive medication. In Sacher, E. J., editor: Hormones, behavior and psychopathologies, New York, 1976, Raven Press.
11. Biskin, M. S.: Nutritional deficiency in the etiology of menorrhagia, metrorrhagia, cystic mastitis and premenstrual tension; treatment with vitamin B complex, J. Clin. Endocrinol. Metab. **3:**227-234, 1943.
12. Buzzelli, G., Voegelin, M. R., and Bozza, P. G.: Modification i Della Soglia Del Dolore Cutaneo Durante II Ciclo Mestruale, Boll. Soc. Ital. Biol. **44:**235-236, 1968.
13. Chesley, L. C., and Hellman, L. M.: Variations in body weight and salivary sodium in the menstrual cycle, Am. J. Obstet. Gynecol. **74:**582-590, 1957.
14. Cullberg, J.: Mood changes and menstrual symptoms with different gestagen/estrogen combinations, Acta Psychiatr. Scand. Supp. 236, 1972.
15. Dalton, K.: The premenstrual syndrome, Springfield, Ill., 1964, Charles C Thomas, Publisher.
16. Englander-Golden, P., Willis, K. A., and Dienstbier, R. A.: Stability of perceived tension as a function of the menstrual cycle, J. Hum. Stress **3:**14-17, 1977.
17. Ferdman, J.: Survey of recent literature on the menstrual cycle and behavior, J. Asthma Res. **11:**27-35, 1973.
18. Frank, R. T.: The hormonal causes of premenstrual tension, Arch. Neurol. Psychiatry **26:** 1053-1057, 1931.
19. Gilbert, C., and Gillman, J.: The changing pattern of food intake and appetite during the menstrual cycle of the baboon *(Papio Ursinus)* with a consideration of some of the controlling endocrine factors, S. Afr. J. Med. Sci. **21:**75-88, 1956.
20. Goldsmith, N. F.: Physiologic relationship between magnesium and the female reproductive apparatus. In Durlach, J., editor: First international symposium on magnesium deficiency in human pathology, Paris, 1971, Springer-Verlag.
21. Golub, L. J., Menduke, H., and Conly, S. S.: Weight changes in college women during the menstrual cycle, Am. J. Obstet. Gynecol. **91:**89-94, 1965.
22. Golub, S.: The effect of premenstrual anxiety and depression on cognitive function, J. Pers. Soc. Psychol. **34:**99-104, 1976.
23. Golub, S.: The magnitude of premenstrual anxiety and depression, Psychosom. Med. **38:**4-12, 1976.
24. Grant, E. C., and Pryse-Davies, J.: Effect of oral contraceptives on depressive mood changes and on endometrial monamine oxidase and phosphatases, Br. Med. J. **3:**777-780, 1968.
25. Halbreich, U., Ben-David, M., Assael, M., et al.: Serum-prolactin in women with premenstrual syndrome, Lancet **1:**654-655, 1976.
26. Hargrove, J. T., and Abraham, G. E.: J. Fertil. In press.
27. Herren, R. Y.: The effect of high and low female sex hormone concentration on the two-point threshold of pain and touch and upon tactile sensitivity, J. Exp. Psychol. **16:**324-327, 1933.
28. Janiger, O., Riffenburgh, R., and Kersh, R.: Cross cultural study of premenstrual symptoms, Psychosomatics **13:**226-235, 1972.
29. Kashiwagi, T., McClure, J. N., and Wetzel, R. D.: Premenstrual affective syndrome and psychiatric disorder, Dis. Nerv. Syst. **37:**116-119, 1976.
30. Kerr, G. D.: The management of the premenstrual syndrome, Curr. Med. Res. Opin. **4:**29-34, 1977.
31. Krohn, P., and Zuckerman, S.: Water metabolism in relation to the menstrual cycle, J. Physiol. **88:**369-387, 1937.
32. Larsson-Cohn, U.: Oral contraceptives and vitamins: a review, Am. J. Obstet. Gynecol. **121:** 84, 1975.
33. Lunde, D. T., and Hamburg, D. A.: Techniques for assessing the effects of sex hormones on affect, arousal and aggression in humans, Recent Prog. Horm. Res. **28:**627-663, 1972.
34. Mertz, W.: Human requirements: basic and optimal, Ann. N.Y. Acad. Sci. **199:**191, 1972.
35. Moos, R. H., Kopell, B. S., Melges, F. T., et al.: Fluctuations in symptoms and moods during the menstrual cycle, J. Psychosom. Res. **13:**37-44, 1969.
36. Morton, J. H.: Premenstrual tension, Am. J. Obstet. Gynecol. **60:**343-352, 1950.
37. Morton, J. H.: Symposium on premenstrual tension, editorial, Int. Record Med. **166:**463-510, 1953.
38. Muggeo, M., Bar, R. S., and Roth, J.: Change in affinity of insulin receptors following oral glucose in normal adults, J. Clin. Endocrinol. Metab. **44:**1206, 1977.

39. Nicholas, A.: Traitement du syndrome pre-menstruel et de la dysmenorrhee par l'ion magnesium. In Durlach, J., editor: First international symposium on magnesium deficiency in human pathology, Paris, 1973, Springer-Verlag.
40. Parlee, M. B.: The premenstrual syndrome, Psychol. Bull. **80**:454-465, 1973.
41. Persky, H.: Reproductive hormones, moods, and the menstrual cycle. In Friedman, R. C., Richart, R. M., and Vande Wiele, R. L., editors: Hormones and moods, New York, 1974, John Wiley & Sons, Inc.
42. Rees, L.: Psychosomatic aspects of the premenstrual tension syndrome, J. Ment. Sci. **99**:62-73, 1953.
43. Schildkraut, J. J., and Kety, S. S.: Biogenic amines and emotions, Science **156**:21-30, 1967.
44. Schwartz, U. D., and Abraham, G. E.: Corticosterone and aldosterone levels during the menstrual cycle, Obstet. Gynecol. **45**:339-342, 1975.
45. Smith, S. L.: Mood and the menstrual cycle. In Sacher, E. J., editor: Topics on psychoendocrinology, New York,. 1975, Grune & Stratton, Inc.
46. Sommer, B.: The effect of menstruation on cognitive and perceptual-motor behavior: a review, Psychosom. Med. **35**:515-534, 1972.
47. Spellacy, W. N., Carlson, K. L., and Schade, S. L.: Menstrual cycle carbohydrate metabolism, Am. J. Obstet. Gynecol. **99**:382-386, 1967.
48. Steiner, M., and Carroll, B. J.: The psychobiology of premenstrual dysphoria: review of theories and treatments, Psychoneuroendocrinol. **2**:321-335, 1977.
49. Sternbach, R. A.: Pain patients: traits and treatment, New York, 1974, Academic Press, Inc.
50. Stokes, J., and Mendels, J.: Pyridoxine and premenstrual tension, Lancet **1**:1177-1178, 1972.
51. Sweeney, J. S.: Menstrual edema, preliminary report, J.A.M.A. **103**:234-236, 1934.
52. Tonks, C. M.: Premenstrual tension. In Silverston, T., and Barraclough, B., editors: Br. J. Psychiat. Special Publication No. **9**:399-408, 1975.
53. Vollman, R. F.: The menstrual cycle, major problems in obstetrics and gynecology, vol. 7, Philadelphia, 1977, W. B. Saunders Co.
54. Winston, F.: Oral contraceptives and depression, Lancet **1**:1209, 1969.
55. Winston, F.: Oral contraceptives, pyridoxine and depression, Am. J. Psychiatry **130**:1217-1221, 1973.
56. Wurtman, R. J.: Control of neurotransmitter synthesis by precursor availability and food consumption. In Naftolin, F., Ryan, K. J., and Davies, I. J., editors: Subcellular mechanisms in reproductive neuroendocrinology, New York, 1976, Elsevier Scientific Publishing Co., pp. 149-166.

CHAPTER 12

Diagnosis of vulvovaginitis in the adult female

Loretta Ivory

INTRODUCTION

Long before Döderlein's description of *Lactobacillus* in 1892, women and their health care providers have pondered the source, cause, cure, and sequelae of vaginal discharge. Often the cures were as imaginative (and possibly as harmful) as the belief of the cause. Religion, politics, and magic often played a greater part in diagnosis and treatment than did science.

Women and their normal functions have long been a mystery to men, even to men of science. The reason and cause of normal menstruation were wonderful enough let alone the abnormal conditions of disease. Women were often accused of the sins of sexual perversion, witchcraft, or demonic possession to account for pain and foul discharge. Since cures fit the "crime," it is little wonder that many women suffered without seeking assistance. Not that help would, necessarily, have been available, even if sought.

Not only were women reluctant to seek help if they thought they had a problem, but many women believed discomfort and pain were normal and part of their "lot in life." This erroneous attitude is still prevalent in many parts of the country, especially among women 30 years of age and older. Many women have had chronic discharge with discomfort and have never sought help. If they were questioned, they often denied discomfort.

The purpose of this chapter is to aid the nurse-practitioner in the assessment, diagnosis, and treatment of vulvovaginitis.

ANATOMY

The vulvar area of the adult female consists of the external and internal generative organs. Internally these organs include the uterus with the ovaries and fallopian tubes and the uterine cervix, which protrudes into the posterior vault of the vagina. Externally, these organs include the escutcheon covering the mons veneris (mons pubis), labia majora, labia minora, clitoris, and vestibule. The urethra, vaginal opening, and ducts of the Bartholin glands all penetrate the vestibule and are all obvious when the client's in the lithotomy position. The urinary bladder and rectum are also of concern because of their proximity and the possibility of cross contamination.

The vaginal opening is located in the

lower half of the vestibule. It varies considerably in length and shape depending on age and parity. The hymen covers the lower third of the vaginal opening in a crescent-shaped membrane that may obstruct the opening until it is ruptured by intercourse or obliterated during childbirth. The vagina itself is a musculomembranous tube that represents the excretory duct of the uterus through which menstrual discharge and uterine and vaginal secretions flow. It is also used for sexual intercourse and forms the birth canal during late labor prior to expulsion of the fetus.

Normally the anterior and posterior walls of the vagina lie close to each other in a narrow-sided H shape, with little space between the sides. The upper end of the vagina forms a blind vault into which the uterine cervix protrudes. This vault is subdivided, for clinical convenience, into four fornices; the anterior, posterior, right, and left fornix. Of the four, the posterior fornix is the longest because of the attachment of the vagina on the anterior segment of the cervix. The entire length of the vagina is lined with transverse folds or pleats called rugae which develop after puberty, gradually become obliterated with each succeeding childbirth, and decrease with menopause.

The vaginal mucosa is composed of nonconified, stratified, squamous epithelium. Under this outer layer is a thin layer of connective tissue and occasional small lymphoid nodules. This layer has many blood vessels. Throughout most of a woman's life the cells of this superficial mucosa contain glycogen, the exact amount depending on age, health status, endocrine activity, and reproductive status.

When a woman is not pregnant, the vagina is kept moist by small amounts of secretions. During pregnancy, there is a marked increase in the amount of vaginal secretions. These secretions include vulvar sebaceous and sweat gland secretions, Bartholin gland secretions, transudate through the vaginal wall during sexual arousal, microscopically desquamated, vagina, epithelial cells, large numbers of Döderlein's bacilli, and cervical mucus.

Flora of the vagina probably represents pooling of bacteria from various anatomic sites, that is, vagina, endocervical mucus glands, urethra, and rectum. It is important for the nurse-practitioner to know the difference between normal appearing vaginal discharge and that which is suspicious for pathology. Normal secretions are of a nonhomogeneous floccular consistence. They contain visible aggregates of cells suspended in clear mucus that is white or whitish and has a pH of 4 to 5. There is also a normal musty odor that is not unpleasant. Depending on the time in the menstrual cycle, the secretions are thin and slippery or thick and viscous. They are not usually noted at the introitus and tend to pool, along with the cervicovaginal mucus, in the posterior fornix and posterior rugae.

Abnormal secretions on the other hand are homogeneous in appearance, have low to normal viscosity, and are yellowish in color. The pH is greater than 5, and the secretions, usually present at the introitus, are uniformly adherent to the vaginal wall. There is a disagreeable to foul odor that may be described as amine (fishy) when 10% potassium hydroxide (KOH) is added to the wet mount. The normal acidity (4.0) of the vagina is probably maintained by the action of lactobacilli breaking down the glycogen in the cells. (At least six species of lactobacilli have been identified.)

Many researchers believe that the acidity prevents colonization of the vagina and introitus by gram-negative organisms. If there is a rise in vaginal pH to 4.5, an error in the number of gram-negative organisms can be identified. These organisms are believed responsible for recurrent urinary tract infections. Although pathogenic organisms can be found in the discharge of healthy women, their numbers are insufficient to cause infection among the bacteria that commonly make up the indigenous flora, including diphtheroids, *Staphylococcus aureus,* streptococci (B-hemolytic, A-hemolytic, and nonhemolytic), *Escherichia coli, Klebsiella,* enterobacteria, *Proteus,* lactobacilli, and *Candida albicans.*

Some of these bacteria are considered opportunistic pathogens, those which strike a balance with the last organism to gain access to the environment, that is, as long as the last organism remains healthy, the pathogens will stay in check and will not cause an infection. Many factors cause an organism to grow rapidly, and these can best be explained by the concept of "niche." Microorganisms gain access to a particular microenvironment (niche) and will fill that space to the maximum extent possible, given the physical and chemical properties of the environment. This concept further dictates that endocrine-mediated changes will result in alterations in the resident microflora.

Bacteria will also proliferate under the following conditions or changes: vaginal acidity, glycogen level, hormonal activity and its effect on mucus production, vaginal vascularity, cellular composition, and systemic antibiotics. Of the hormonal changes, estrogen is responsible for the periodic expansion of bacterial counts, and progesterone suppresses flora, especially during the first trimester of pregnancy. Age also plays a factor, since age-dependent alterations of the indigenous flora are clearly evident in the mean numbers of anaerobic bacteria that can be identified.

Although this chapter will deal primarily with childbearing women, the nurse-practitioner may be asked to see a pubescent or prepubescent female. It should be remembered that vulvovaginitis in children is often caused by foreign bodies and by toxic or allergic reactions, especially from bubble baths. When there is a vague history, negative culture, and no definitive diagnosis, the nurse-practitioner should remember that purulent vaginitis will usually respond to systemic penicillin and that nonpurulent vaginitis will most likely respond to improvement in general hygiene.

To aid the nurse-practitioner in identifying microscopic findings and making a differential diagnosis, I have included illustrations of red blood cells, white blood cells, vaginal epithelial cells, Döderlein's bacillus, streptococci chains, and sperm (Figs. 12-1 to 12-6).

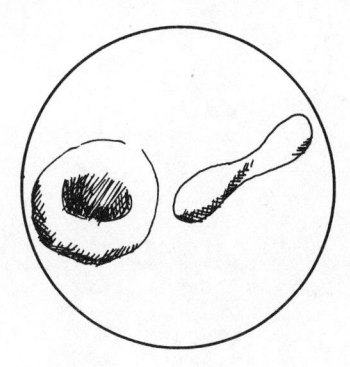

Fig. 12-1. Red blood cell.

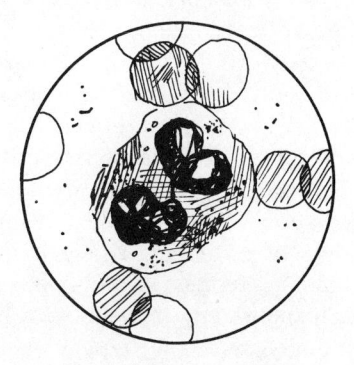

Fig. 12-2. White blood cell.

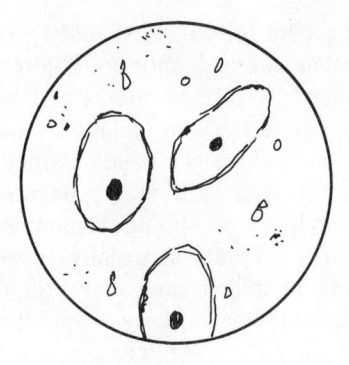

Fig. 12-3. Vaginal epithelial cells.

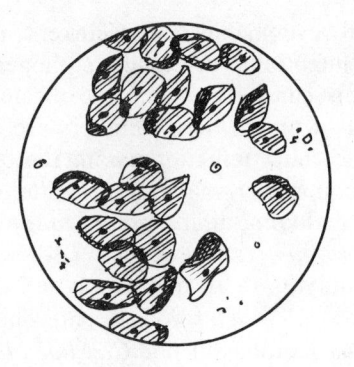

Fig. 12-4. Döderlein's bacillus.

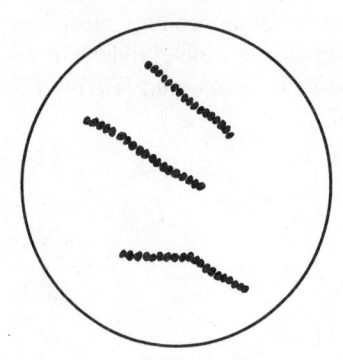

Fig. 12-5. Streptococci chains.

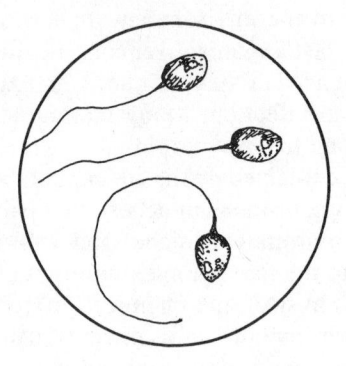

Fig. 12-6. Sperm—live and dead.

TYPES OF VULVOVAGINITIS
Monilia

Yeast is the most common cause of the nonsexually transmitted diseases. Otherwise known as *Oidium albicans, Endomyces albicans, Syringospora albicans, Monilia psiloses, Monilia albicans,* and *Candida albicans,* these fungal organisms are often found as a saprophyte in vaginal flora. The fungus reproduces asexually by the formation of blastospores, which are the result of a definitive process called *budding.* The fungus is monophasic, and the blastospores may appear with hyphae or pseudomycelia. The hyphae will show well-defined organelles, including a denticulate cytoplasmic membrane, nuclei, cristate mitochondria (slender microscopic filaments or rods), rough and smooth endoplasmic reticulum, and some storage granules. Fungus does not necessarily require living tissue to survive; it may be found on any usually wet surface such as plastic shower curtains, bathing caps, and bathing suits. It is also fairly resistant to antimicrobial substances, has been cultured from hexachlorophene soaps, and is not an unusual occurrence in the hospital bedding of both pediatric and adult patients.

Presenting symptomatology. Dysuria, itching, vulvar edema, dyspareunia, and heavy discharge are the symptoms of acute onset that generally cause the client to seek medical attention.

Pertinent history. Pruritus* is acute in onset usually prior to onset of menstruation. The history should include review of mitigating factors such as diabetes, hyperthyroidism, hypothyroidism, cell-mediated defects, antibiotics, chemotherapy, antibacterial agents, sulfonamides, corticosteroids, immunosuppressives, IUDs, indwelling catheters, recent intravenous transfusions, and any debilitating disease or terminal illness. Other factors that cause disturbances in the vaginal flora and that encourage fungal growth include pregnancy, endocrine disorders, blood dysuria, obesity, malignant disease, cytotoxic agents, heroin addiction, high-estrogen birth control pills, hypoparathyroidism, hypersensitivity, and poor genital hygiene.

Clinical course. With the client in the lithotomy position, the nurse-practitioner first inspects the vulvar area. (In acute monilial infections, the introitus may be so severely edematous that speculum examination may be difficult, if not impossible.) The vulva may be erythematous, edematous, and excoriated. The erythematous area may extend down the inner aspects of the thighs. There is a discharge that is easily seen when labia minora is parted. After gentle insertion of the bivalve speculum, the nurse-practitioner should assess the character of the vaginal discharge. Typically it will appear as a creamy, whitish, thick discharge that adheres to the side walls. Patches of thrush may be present and are easily dislodged from the vaginal wall. A typical discharge may appear as a thin, watery liquid producing a sheen on the vulva and labia. (The adherent film is probably caused by pseudomycelium and spores.) In severe cases there may be marked erythema (raw beefy appearance) with profuse discharge, while in chronic cases little discharge is seen and few organisms can be cultured. The client may have other associated lesions of the fingernails (onychia and paronychia), axillae, inguinal folds, nipples, toes, folds of the navel, conjunctiva, mouth and perlèche (mouth corners), and the anorectum, occasionally with diarrhea and stomatitis. It is presumed that the infection is carried from the vulva by the fingers from scratching in an attempt to relieve the intense itching. Some sensitive individuals may develop dermatophytids, that is, small, tense vesicles occurring in groups particularly along the sides of the fingers and hands. These are sterile and intensely sensitive.

Diabetic patients should especially be protected against monilial infections. The excoriations in the skin can serve as portals for pathogenic bacteria that, if untreated, could develop cellulitis and lymphangitis in tissue that may already be compromised by vascular disease.

The pregnant client also needs special attention. Moniliasis is the most common disease during pregnancy, being 10% to 20% higher in pregnant women than in nonpregnant women, and some studies report 56% of pregnant women have the disease. Chances of contracting the disease increase as the length of gestation increases. This may be a result of the higher glycogen levels during pregnancy and the direct effect of the estrogens to stimulate fungal growth. It is also important to note that up to 50% of babies born to mothers with untreated moniliasis at delivery will develop oral thrush or monilial diaper rash.

Microscopic examination. When taking a specimen for examination or culture, the nurse-practitioner should remember that

---

*Pruritus is probably caused by acetaldehyde acetic acid and pyruvic acid, which results from the fermentation of carbohydrates.

fungus is microaerophilic and may be more easily found in quantity at the introitus than in the vaginal pool.

To prepare a wet prep, the specimen is collected with a cotton- or rayon-tipped applicator and mixed with 10% KOH on a glass slide, and a cover slip is applied. Diagnosis is confirmed when either budding yeast or pseudomycelia are seen (Figs. 12-7 and 12-8). Some researchers insist that the diagnosis of moniliasis cannot be made unless the pseudomycelia are seen. (Serum factus stimulates the formation of the pseudomycelia probably because of the inflamed tissue "weeping" serum into the vaginal pool.) However, if the clinical symptoms and signs are present, the client is symptomatic and, only budding yeast is demonstrated, I believe that the client should be treated. This is especially true during pregnancy when the client needs to be treated even if she is not symptomatic but has clinical manifestations with microscopic support.

Unfortunately for the nurse-practitioner, direct microscopic examination of a wet prep may produce discouraging results — 40% to 80% are positive. Even with the substage condenser turned down to allow for maximum contrast, the organism may not be visualized. It may be necessary to use a Gram stain on the smear. With a Gram stain, the organism appears as a dense, gram-positive (blue), ovoid body. The pseudohyphae are long, gram-positive tubes of about the same diameter as the yeast form and can be seen to have dense, gram-positive dots. Accuracy of diagnosis using the gram stain increases to 70% to 100%. If the gram stain is negative and the clinical course is not predictive of moniliasis, the nurse-practitioner should do a culture. The recommended medium is Nicherson's medium on which the yeast will show up as chocolate brown or jet black colonies after 48 to 72 hours incubation at body temperature (37° C).

Treatment. Treatment regimens change as organisms become resistive and new products are made available. Current therapy includes monistator mycostin. For recurrent or unresponsive cases, the nurse-practitioner may wish to consider treatment of the sexual partner, especially if he is uncircumcised.

I have had success in treating extremely resistant cases with 1% gentian violet. The vault, cervix, and both posterior and anterior fornices and side walls of the vagina are carefully painted with cotton balls held by a ring forceps. The labia minora may also be

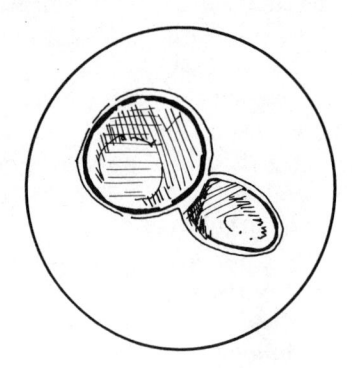

Fig. 12-7. Budding yeast.

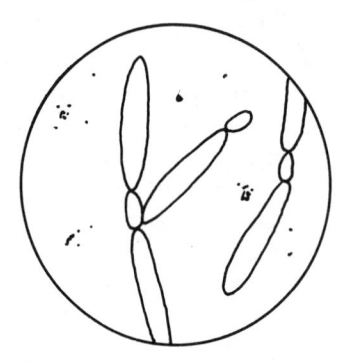

Fig. 12-8. Yeast in pseudomycelia (pseudohyphae) form.

treated. The client is asked to wear old panties (that she does not mind getting permanently stained) and a dress or skirt. She should also bring a sanitary napkin to protect against drainage. The client is counseled to shower, not bathe, and to refrain from intercourse until all the dye is gone.

As in all cases of vulvovaginitis, the client is requested to refrain from sexual intercourse until the vagina is healed. The small thrush spots (clumps) that are found harbor large numbers of organisms that are dislodged and broken up during intercourse and may spread the disease or prolong the treatment. Having the male wear a condom does not make any difference in this instance.

Trichomonas vaginalis

Trichomoniasis is the most common sexually transmitted cause of vulvovaginitis in the United States. The offending organism is a pear-shaped protozoan that is slightly larger than a polymorphonuclear leucocyte. The protozoan has four flagella at the curved "head," an undulating membrane along the right side with a single large flagellum or tail at the pointed end (Fig. 12-9).

The infection will persist indefinitely in the female until eradicated by proper treatment. In the male, the organism usually dies in 3 weeks unless continually reinfected, the infection has spread to the seminal vesicle or prostate (40%), or a urethral structure has been infected. *Trichomonas* is a fragile organism that will survive for only several hours outside the host, although it may survive up to 24 hours in urine. It is, therefore, theoretically possible for the infection to be acquired from public toilets where urine containing the organism is left on the seat or from droplets of urine sprayed onto the vulva when flushing contaminated urine down the toilet. However, no such cases have been documented.

Incubation time for the organism is 4 to 28 days from contact. Women whose sexual partners are infected have a 50% chance of contacting the disease, but male partners will contact the disease from infected females 100% of the time. Research has shown that up to 76% of women have some anti-trichomoniasis antibodies, but not in sufficient quantities to prohibit infection.

There are two phases to a trichomoniasis infection, the first phase being the florid phase that is associated with acute clinical symptoms. The organism is usually seen on wet mount and there are cellular disturbances, but permanent evidence of the bizzarre epithelial nuclear changes is seen in the latent or cleaner phase.

The latent phase occurs when the patient is asymptomatic and the organism is usually absent from wet mount but may be found in cellular spreads (Pap smears) of cervical material. The epithelial changes in the endocervix are produced by the very strong inflammatory reaction of the cells to the protozoan. Cellular, morphologic characteristics are so altered as to make the nature of the underlying epithelium obscure, thus the cells lose their diagnostic criteria. Trichomoniasis is the only infectious process known to be capable of producing reversible changes in the cytologic evaluation

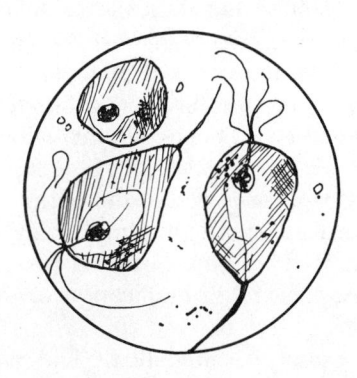

Fig. 12-9. *Trichomonas.*

of an endocervical smear. Within 2 weeks after initiation of treatment, the cytologic changes should be completely reversed if the treatment was successful. Of the women who have chronic trichomoniasis infections, 90% had cervicitis that may predispose them to malignant transformation. Chronic trichomoniasis infections in pregnancy may have two sequelae: (1) twice as many women who have trichomoniasis infections at the time of delivery have fever, prolonged discharge, or frank endometriosis than those who are not infected and (2) the newborn female may (but fortunately rarely does) contact the disease.

It is important to note that trichomoniasis is found not only in the vaginal pool (98.4%), but also in the urethra (82.5%) and paraurethral glands (97.8%) and the endocervix (13.1%). However, the organisms should be culled from the vaginal pool and not the endocervix in acute infections. These extravaginal sites also account for the poor cure rate with the use of topical vaginal therapy alone, since systemic treatment is really necessary for treatment of the extravaginal sites. Trichomoniasis is a frequent infection in women who have other venereal disease, and assessing and treating one does not treat the others. The cautious nurse-practitioner will be alert for and evaluate evidence of other venereal diseases so as not to delay proper treatment of the others.

Presenting symptomatology. The client with trichomoniasis vaginitis may complain of severe itching, dysuria, frequency, urgency, vulvar swelling, and foul-smelling discharge that stains the underpants brown. The pruritus and discharge often coincide with or immediately follow menstruation. A chronic condition may also be more symptomatic at this time because of the rise in vaginal pH associated with a higher pH of the menstrual flow (6.0 to 6.5), which in turn facilitates the protozoan proliferation.

The patient may be confused as to the exact end of her menstrual period as the brownish discharge may mimic the last day of menstrual flow. Clients with chronic infection may also complain of infertility. Trichomoniasis may indeed cause a temporary sterility since the toxins produced by the parasite may inhibit sperm mobility. The client may experience generalized lower abdominal pain with or without accompanying vaginal adenopathy as the chief complaint. The nurse-practitioner should always screen for pelvic inflammatory disease (P.I.D.) and a positive Chandelier's sign in these women.

Clinical course. The vulva appears edematous and reddened, often with excoriations that may have become secondarily infected with opportunistic bacteria. Speculum examination (the vagina is often very sore and the examination may be painful) reveals a characteristic thin, watery, often purulent, bubbly, or frothy discharge (likened to slightly beaten egg whites) of greenish or greenish yellow color and characteristic foul odor. Redness may extend down the inner thighs. One of the most striking characteristics of trichomoniasis infections is the large number of red punctations seen in groups on the surface of the cervix that may extend to the lateral walls of the vagina, the so-called "strawberry marks." These punctations are caused by the large number of parasites that affect the vaginal and cervical epithelia as demonstrated in the area of the terminal blood vessels. The hyperemia of the inflamed surface renders the coiling of the looped capillaries within the dermal papillae more apparent, thus producing a red-pink spot. The strawberry spots will fade and disappear with eradication of the disease.

Microscopic examination. The parasite appears as a motile, pear-shaped object with the caudal flagella more apparent than the four small "cephalic" flagella. Since trichomonads are fairly fragile, they can only be found on wet mount within 1 to 2 hours after sampling. After they die, the cell wall rounds out and the parasite is indistinguishable from a white blood cell.

Other methods of detecting trichomoniasis include pap smear (considered unreliable by some and acridine orange stain, although the latter requires an ultraviolet light adaptor on the microscope. Giemsa stain is also helpful especially if the wet mount is difficult to interpret. To use a Giemsa stain, a slide is prepared and heat-fixed with a Bunsen burner or an electric light bulb. The stain is allowed to "set" the slide for 20 seconds followed by a gentle tap water rinse. Using high power and with the substage condenser turned down to allow for maximum contrast, the nurse-practitioner will note the parasite by the characteristic shape and dense blue cytoplasm with reddish colored nuclei and flagella.

Treatment. Metronidazole (Flagyl) is still the treatment of choice in trichomoniasis although different treatment regimens are in current use. Treatment of the woman alone will effect a cure rate of 60% to 80%. If the sexual partner(s) is (are) treated concomitantly, the cure rate increases to 95%. The patient is counseled to abstain from sexual intercourse until cured, usually in 48 hours. Since dyspareunia may be present, most couples readily comply. The couple is also cautioned against taking any form of alcoholic beverage the day that metronidazole is used because this will cause mild to severe nausea. As in other cases of vulvovaginitis, the client should not douche or insert a tampon for 24 to 48 hours prior to examination because this will obscure results.

Corynebacterium vaginalis

Corynebacterium vaginalis and *Hemophilus vaginalis* are two names for the same bacteria. Its clinical significance is disputed by many researchers because it can readily be cultured from the vaginas of up to 52% of healthy women. However, it has also been the only isolate in symptomatic women and may indeed constitute indigenous flow for many women until influencing factors cause the organism to proliferate. Unfortunately these causative factors are not known.

Corynebacterium is a tiny, pleomorphic, gram-negative or gram-variable coccobacillus that adheres to the vaginal epithelial cell, sometimes covering the entire surface (Fig. 12-10). This is the so-called "clue" cell (Fig. 12-11), and the cell is commonly referred to as having a "ground glass" appearance. The organisms may also be ar-

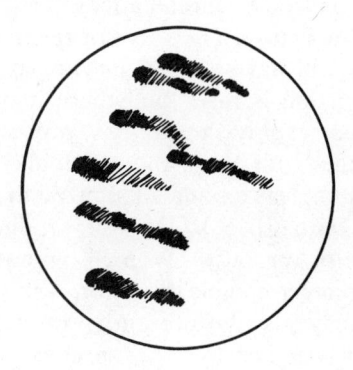

Fig. 12-10. *Corynebacterium.*

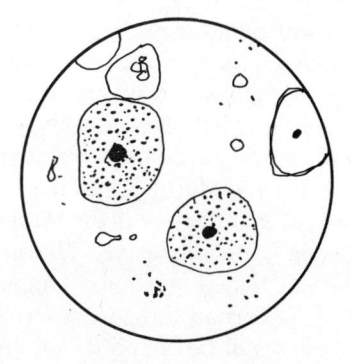

Fig. 12-11. Clue cell.

ranged at angles to each other or parallel with each other in groups. This is generally referred to as the "school of fish." Further findings include few, if any, leucocytes in the smear. Evidence favors sexual transmission, since 90% of males will demonstrate the organism if their female sex partner is infected.

Presenting symptomatology. The client may be asymptomatic or may complain of a foul odor. There may be cramps with or without mild, vague, diffuse abdominal pain. Pruritus and burning are the primary complaints in less than 50% of women. Onset does not seem to be related to menstruation. It is important to note that when *Corynebacterium* is the only bacteria present, the client is almost always symptomatic; whereas the client with a mixed infection may be asymptomatic.

Clinical course. The vulva of the infected woman will have a slight erythema (gross inflammation is rare), and there may be a thin watery, grayish to yellow-gray colored discharge with or without bubbles. The odor is unpleasant and alkalinization of the smear with 10% KOH will produce an amine (fishy) odor. Women without infection never exhibit this odor. Strawberry spots may also be present, however it is unclear whether this is a process of the *Corynebacterium* or a concomitant trichomoniasis infection.

Microsopic examination. Wet mount is usually insufficient for proper identification of *Corynebacterium,* the clue cell seen on Gram stain is almost always more accurate, and the characteristic ground glass appearance of the epithelial cell will be clear. Culture with Thayer-Martin or chocolate agar medium is often effective if the Gram stain is confusing or inconclusive. The medium must be incubated at body temperature (37° C) in a carbon dioxide environment. The colonies will be round (0.5 mm), convex, and translucent and will not produce greening on the chocolate agar after 48 hours.

Treatment. Treatment regimens vary; topical sulfa and systemic ampicillin are probably the most common. However, Pheifer showed a high failure rate (66%) with ampicillin and recommends metronidazole as for trichomoniasis.

Herpes simplex virus type II

Herpes genitalis is considered the fastest rising venereal disease in the United States and is the most common cause of genital lesions. The disease has spontaneous remissions and exacerbations usually precipitated by mental or physical stress of debilitation. The lesions often reappear during pregnancy in susceptible women. If the lesions are present at delivery or if viral cultures or Pap smear can demonstrate the virus, the fetus must be delivered by cesarean section. Infants who contact herpes can develop herpes meningitis, which may cause severe mental retardation or death.

Women seem to be more symptomatic then men who may not seek assistance, especially if the case is a mild one. In such instances, men are at greater risk to spread the disease since the discomfort is not sufficient for them to refrain from intercourse.

Presenting symptomatology. The typical complaint is of painful, single or grouped vesicles that later break down to form shallow, superficial, painful ulcers. Dyspareunia and often dysuria accompany the disease. Iliac glands are often involved, and complaints of lower abdominal pain are not uncommon. Cervical lesions are not necessarily painful, and there may or may not be complaints of a purulent discharge.

Microscopic examination. Since the infecting organism is a virus, there is no real evidence of the disease to be found on a wet mount. Viral cultures of the ulcerative lesion or material from the vaginal pool are diagnostic, as is a Pap smear. The nurse-practitioner is well advised to screen the client for other venereal diseases, especially if there is a suspicious history or if vaginal discharge is present.

Treatment. Unfortunately there is no known treatment for herpes. Red dye with ultraviolet light and inoculation with smallpox vaccine have failed to produce the desired results. Wet, warm, tea bags applied to the lesions appear to be of palliative help to reduce the pain, and some nurse-practitioners use a topical steroid cream to effect pain relief. If secondary bacterial infections develop from contamination of the lesions from scratching, they should be treated as needed. Needless to say, the client is counseled to abstain from sexual intercourse until the disease has run its course. Condoms will not necessarily provide protection.

Syphilis

Syphilis will be mentioned only briefly since it is a well-known clinical entity. It is difficult to diagnose clinically because of the multitude of secondary symptoms and the fragile nature of the spirochete, *Treponema,* which is rarely is ever found in a wet mount (Fig. 12-12). Often called the great mime, syphilis is best screened for by blood agglutination or rapid plasma reagin tests. The Communicable Disease Control Center in Atlanta, Georgia publishes periodic updates on recommended therapy. The nurse-practitioner must remember that syphilis is a reported disease and every known contact needs to be found and treated.

Gonorrhea

Neisseria gonorrhea, the causative organism in gonorrhea, is a fragile organism, readily killed by exposure and drying, thus wet mount is of no use in accurate diagnosis (Fig. 12-13). Even Gram stain is of questionable value for diagnosing gonorrhea in the female, thus cultures provide the only reliable diagnosis. Gonococcus will attack the columnar epithelium of the urethra, paraurethral ducts and glands, and the endocervix, from which it may travel up to the endometrium and thus the fallopian tubes. The peritoneum and anorectal canal may also become involved. True gonorrheal vaginitis is seen only in prepubescent females, as a result of a thickening of the mucosa under the influence of estrogen at puberty, and in postmenopausal women. For this reason, gonococcus is rarely found in the vaginal pool.

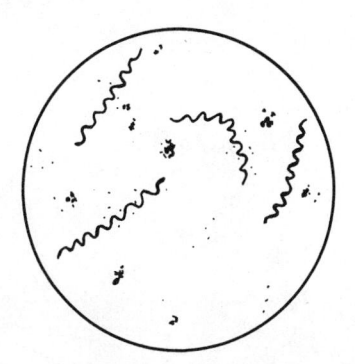

Fig. 12-12. Spirochetes.

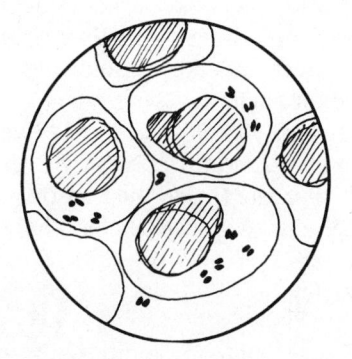

Fig. 12-13. *Neisseria gonorrhea.*

Presenting symptomatology. Although only 25% of women infected with gonorrhea are symptomatic, these symptoms may include dysuria, dyspareunia, and generalized lower abdominal pain. If the Bartholin or Skene glands are involved, the complaint will be of a hard, tender, sometimes reddened cyst, either posteriorly and laterally to the fourchette as seen with Bartholin cysts or similar complaints at or along the urethra. Purulent material may or may not be present at the duct opening. If the disease is untreated in the female, fallopian tube scaring leading to sterility may result. Other sequelae include monoarticular or polyarticular suppurative arthritis, meningitis, or endocarditis.

Clinical course. Most women seek medical attention because their male sex partner suspects or has been diagnosed as having gonorrhea. Routine examination may reveal few signs or symptoms. However, the urethra should be stripped and the Bartholin glands carefully palpated to elicit the characteristic greenish yellow, purulent discharge.

Microscopic examination. Cultures should be taken of the urethra, rectum, and endocervix and plated onto Thayer-Martin medium for incubation in a carbon dioxide environment. Positive results will increase by 2% to 4% if the endocervical swab is plated onto chocolate agar. Since more than one type of veneral disease may be present, wet mounts should always be checked for vaginitis.

Treatment. Patients with positive contacts and those with positive cultures should be treated according to the Contagious Disease Control Center's latest protocols.

Crabs—pediculus pubis

Pediculus pubis, or pubic lice, are six-legged, crablike, wingless insects. They are obligate parasites that live on skin and feed on blood (Fig. 12-14). The louse is approximately 3 mm in length and breadth and moves slowly. It is usually found hanging on the pubic hair shaft with its mouth parts buried in the pubic skin. The insect is gray and semitranslucent in appearance. Sometimes the egg capsules can be seen as dark spots or dots attached near the base of the individual hair shafts. The insects may spread to other areas of body hair, and infestation appears to be related to hair density. The nits (eggs) hatch 1 week after laying and mature in another 3 weeks. This sexually transmitted disease has a high association with other venereal diseases.

Primary complaint. The overwhelming complaint is severe pruritis.

Clinical course. The nurse-practitioner should always take a complete history and examine the client for signs of other vulvovaginitis causes. Itching is usually so intense that excoriation and secondary infection may result and should be treated accordingly.

Microscopic examination. The insects or nits are trapped between the edges of two slides, and the hair follicle is usually sacrificed when pulling the insect off for inspection. The louse is usually visible to the

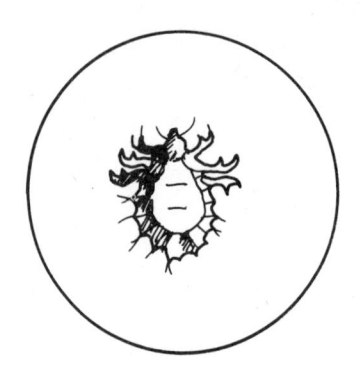

Fig. 12-14. Pubic crab.

naked eye when the slides are held in strong light. The insect is clearly seen under the microscope.

Treatment. Kwell lotion is the most current treatment. Usually the infected hair may be left intact, but if the infection is resistant to treatment, the affected area may need to be shaved.

Scabies

Sarcoptes scabiei (the itch mite) is a skin-living parasite. The female is seen as a minute white dot only 0.3 mm in diameter at the end of a burrow. The female burrows horizontally in the horny layer of the epidermis laying eggs behind her as she goes. Sometimes a small vesicle is noted in the burros behind her. The larvae hatch after 3 days, migrate to a hair follicle, and mature in about 2 weeks.

Presenting symptomatology. Itching is again the primary complaint. It begins with the maturing of the first larvae and is worse at night and in warm weather. Erythematous patches and follicular patches will be found near the burrows, and excoriation with secondary infection is common.

Clinical course. Scabies are extremely contagious and may be acquired sexually as well as from infected clothing, bed sheets, and the like. All members of the client's family need to be carefully inspected and treated if necessary.

Microscopic examination. Diagnosis may be made from the typical appearance of the lesion. The larvae is also excised for examination under the microscope (Fig. 12-15).

Treatment. Recommended treatment is Kwell lotion.

The remainder of this chapter will discuss care and/or unusual conditions as reported in the literature that may account for vulvovaginitis and its symptoms. Ridley described a tuberculosis-caused ulcer of the vulva with an accompanying sinus of the groin causing elephantiasis of the vulva. The basic problem in this rare manifestation is one of missed diagnosis. Referral to the gynecologist or dermatologist is recommended.

Threadworm vaginitis can occur in any female with rectal threadworm. The nurse-practitioner should suspect threadworms in cases of recurrent or intractable vaginitis that does not respond to the usual treatment.

Meningococcal infection of the genitourinary tract is rare but not unknown.

Shigella flexneri has been isolated from the vagina of clients with a history of bloody, purulent discharge that responds poorly or not at all to topical applications of sulfa preparations usually used to treat bacterial vaginitis. Especially in pediatrics, the nurse-practitioner should consider *Shigella* when there is a history of a *Shigella* dysentery or an epidemic of *Shigella* in the community. It is important to remember that the vaginitis will be manifested as a chronic condition that may remain after the dysentery has disappeared.

One of the most unusual cases reported was of a family (mother and two daughters) who were all diagnosed as having allergic seminal vulvovaginitis. Their collective history was of stinging, burning pain in the va-

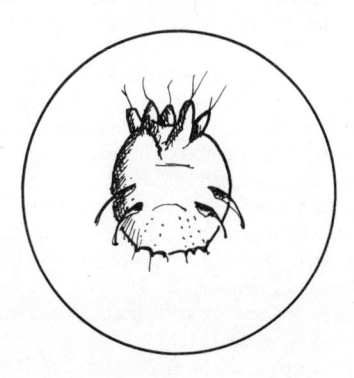

Fig. 12-15. Scabies — mites.

gina immediately after or during intercourse that lasted several hours or until the woman douched. One woman reported that she had had cessation of symptoms when her husband used a condom. Clinical signs were erythema and edema of the vulva and vagina with urticarial lesions on the vulva and any skin exposed to the ejaculate.

Allergic salivary vulvitis has been reported in the literature as has psychosomatic vulvovaginitis. The former should be suspected if symptoms arise following oral/vaginal intercourse and include pain, burning, itching, and general discomfort. In the case of psychosomatic vulvovaginitis, the primary symptoms are those of most other genital infections plus a history of mild dyspareunia up to complete loss of sexual functioning, chronic failure to cure, negative wet mounts, and negative cultures. The client will also resist the suggestion that her symptoms are of psychological origin. It is not uncommon for the client to be emotionally labile and very dependent. One of the frustrating aspects of this situation is that the client is often "allergic" to the topical/vaginal preparations.

Intrauterine contraceptive devices are also indicated in vaginal infections. In one patient, a long (5 cm), untrimmed IUD string had knotted and trapped a small piece of what had been a vaginal tampon. The menstrual flow had become suppurative and caused an exceedingly foul smelling discharge that cleared readily when the string was trimmed.

Finally, the influence of antibiotics on the development of vaginitis must be considered. In a study by Hall and Lupton, tetracycline was used to treat acne in teenage girls. Of the girls in the study, 5% reported vaginal infections. Hall and Lupton also quoted infection rates as high as 33% in general practice.

SUMMARY

In researching the literature, it became apparent that almost any bacterial infection, virus, or allergen that can cause infection in the body may also be a potential source of genital infection or vulvovaginitis. The most important message for the nurse-practitioner is: (1) take a very careful history, information gained in history taking can lead to a diagnosis or eliminate a number of possible diagnoses, thus saving valuable time, (2) listen to what the client is saying, faulty or misinformation about general hygiene and normal physiology is often the culprit, (3) note and record all clinical signs even if the signs do not "fit" the clinical diagnosis, (4) take material for microscopic examination or culture from the site most likely to yield results, (5) obtain a consultation in recurrent cases that resist treatment or when the clinical findings are incompatible, (6) treat the client and her sexual partner or partners, (7) always screen for additional disease, a client with one venereal disease often has another, and (8) remember that mental and physical disease, especially metabolic diseases, and bacterial infections and their cures can reduce the host defense mechanisms and allow or even promote a pathogenic state.

BIBLIOGRAPHY

Adam, E., Decker, D., Herbst, A., et al.: Vaginal and cervical cancers and other abnormalities associated with exposure in utero to diethylstilbestrol and related synthetic hormones, Cancer Res. **37**:1249-1251, 1977.

Akerlund, M., Anderson, K., Bengston, L., et al.: Uterine activity in diabetes insipidus, Acta Obstet. Gynecol. Scan. **56**:381-385, 1977.

Blechner, J., Vincent, S., and Prystowsky, H.: Blood flow to the human uterus during maternal metabolic acidosis, Am. J. Obstet. Gynecol. **34**:789-794, 1975.

Borten, M., and Friedman, E.: Duration of colposcopic changes associated with trichomonas vaginitis, Obstet. Gynecol. **51**:111-113, 1978.

Bracey, D.: Fringe benefit, Br. Med. J. **2**:1072, 1976.

Braverman, R.: Cutaneous manifestations of diabetes

mellitus, Med. Clin. North Am. **55:**1019-1025, 1971.

Brehm, H., and Albrecht, I.: Contraceptive efficacy determination by postcoital testing, Fertil. Steril. **29:** 144-147, 1978.

Chang, T.: Familial allergic seminal vulvovaginitis, Am. J. Obstet. Gynecol. **126:**442-444, 1976.

Coope, J., Thomson, J., and Poller, I.: Effects of natural oestrogen replacement therapy on menopausal symptoms and blood clotting, Br. Med. J. **14:**139-143, 1975.

Daus, A., and Hafez, E.: *Candida albicans* in women, Nurs. Res. **24:**430-431, 1975.

Davis, T.: Chronic vulvovaginitis in children due to *Shigella flexneri,* Pediatrics **56:**41-43, 1975.

Dodson, M., and Friedrich, E.: Psychosomatic vulvovaginitis, Obstet. Gynecol. **51:**23-25, 1978.

Donlan, C., and Scutero, J.: Transient eosinophilic pneumonia secondary to use of a vaginal cream, Chest **67:**232-233, 1975.

Dunlop, E.: Sexually transmitted diseases, Clin. Obstet. Gynecol. **4:**350-364, 1977.

Fong, R.: Vaginal discharge, Nurs. Times **73:**1256-1257, 1977.

Fowler, J., and Stamey, T.: Studies of introital colonization in women with recurrent urinary infections, J. Urol. **117:**472-476, 1977.

Galask, R., Larsen, B., and Ohm, M.: Vaginal flora and its role in disease entities, Clin. Obstet. Gynecol. **19:**61-68, 1976.

Jones, R., Slepack, J., and Eades, A.: Fatal neonatal meningococcal meningitis, J.A.M.A. **236:**2652-2653, 1976.

Katzman, E.: Common disorders of female genitals from birth to older years: implications for nursing intervention, J. Obstet. Gynecol. Nurs. **3:**19-21, 1977.

Komaroff, A., Cohen, A., and McCue, J.: Alternatives to metronidazole, J.A.M.A. **235:**2081-2082, 1976.

Nagamani, M., Lin, T., McDonough, P., et al.: Clinical and endocrine studies in menopausal women after estradiol pellet implantation, Obstet. Gynecol. **50:**541-547, 1977.

Parsons, C., Lofland, S., and Mulholland, S.: The effect of trichomonal vaginitis on vaginal pH, J. Urol. **118:**621-622, 1977.

Pierog, S., Nigam, S., Marasigan, D., et al.: Gonococcal ophthalmia neonatorum: relationship of maternal factors and delivery room practices to effective control measures, Am. J. Obstet. Gynecol. **122:**589-592, 1975.

Plavidal, F., and Werch, J.: Gonococcal fetal scalp abscess: a case report, Am. J. Obstet. Gynecol. **127:** 437-438, 1977.

Rein, M., and Chapel, T.: Trichomoniasis, candidiasis and the minor venereal diseases, Clin. Obstet. Gynecol. **18:**73-88, 1975.

Rich, O.: The sociogram: a tool for depicting support in pregnancy, Matern. Child Nurs. J. **7:**1-9, 1978.

Smith, R., Rodgers, H., Hines, P., et al.: Comparisons between direct microscopic and cultural methods for recognition of corynebacterium vaginale in women with vaginitis, J. Clin. Microbiol. **15(5):** 268-272, 1977.

Stone, S., Micka, A., and Rye, P.: Postmenopausal symptomatology, maturation index, and plasma estrogen levels, Obstet. Gynecol. **46:**625-627, 1975.

Wallenburg, H., and Wladimiroff, J.: Recurrence of vulvovaginal candidiasis during pregnancy, Obstet. Gynecol. **48:**491-493, 1976.

CHAPTER 13

Differential diagnosis of cervical pathology

Thomas F. Rocereto

Anatomically the cervix is the lower aspect of the uterus. In the adult female, it is approximately 2.5 cm in length and 2 to 3 cm in diameter. It is composed of two anatomic parts—the endocervix and the exocerivx. The *endocervix* is lined by a mucus-producing columnar epithelium and, except for the lower few millimeters, is usually not visible on examination. The *exocervix* is easily seen during the pelvic examination. It extends from the external os, which is the inferior opening of the endocervical canal, to the vaginal fornix. With some exceptions, most of the exocervix is lined by a squamous cell–type of epithelium. The area on the cervix where squamous cell epithelium and columnar epithelium meet is known as the *squamocolumnar junction*. This junction does not necessarily correspond to the anatomic external os. In the early reproductive age group, this junction may be on the exocervix; while in the postmenopausal age group, it is generally in the endocervical canal.

Abnormalities of the cervix in many cases will produce a vaginal discharge and in some cases abnormal bleeding. Some symptomatic abnormalities are readily seen on examination, but abnormalities that are asymptomatic may be seen also. The purpose of this chapter is to discuss the many pathologic and, in some cases, nonpathologic changes that may occur in the cervix and the approach to their diagnosis and treatment.

The cervix is easy to visualize and reach without anesthesia or analgesia in most females. It is not as sensitive to pain as other surfaces of the body and is one part of the female body from which a small biopsy specimen can be taken in the office without much discomfort. Since it is so accessible and easily biopsied, a lesion on the cervix should always be sampled when first seen. As will be discussed later in this chapter, a cervical carcinoma can be present even if the results of a Pap smear are normal and waiting for the results of a Pap smear when an abnormal growth is present is a waste of time.

ACUTE CERVICITIS

A cervix that is acutely infected is usually reddened and edematous and bleeds easily when touched by the speculum or when taking a specimen for a Pap smear. The appearance is usually the same regardless of the causative agent, except that white patches are generally present with moniliasis. Trichomoniasis is one of the most common infections, but infections caused by gonorrhea are increasing. Other bacteria can be the causative agent.

The patient with acute cervicitis may be asymptomatic but usually has a vaginal discharge. She may experience pelvic pressure and/or pain especially if the cervix becomes congested and an associated parametritis occurs. In the latter case, any elective surgery should be postponed until the infection is treated and the parametritis and congestion disappear.

Trichomoniasis is usually diagnosed easily with the aid of a saline wet prep and normally does not require a culture. Gonorrhea can be suggested when gram-negative intracellular diplococci are seen on a gram stain, but a culture is necessary for definitive diagnosis. The Thayer-Martin medium is probably the best selective medium for culturing the gonorrhea organism. With proper care in the laboratory, *N. gonorrhoeae* can be cultured from the endocervix of patients with such infection in about 80% of the cases.[10] Nongonorrheal bacterial cultures are not usually very helpful since the vagina and cervix normally contain many bacteria that are not necessarily pathogens.

Trichomoniasis is easily treated with metronidazole (Flagyl). The treatment course has been either 2 gm orally at one time or 250 mg orally, three times a day for 7 days. More recently 1 gm orally, twice a day for 1 day has been found to be just as effective as the 7-day course. It is important to treat both the patient and her sexual partner(s) at the same time with the same dose. Metronidazole (Flagyl) should not be used in the first trimester of pregnancy.

The recommended treatment for gonorrhea is 1 gm of probenecid orally, followed by 4.8 to 6.0 million units of procaine penicillin G intramuscularly. Patients who are allergic to penicillin can be treated with 1.5 gm of tetracycline orally, followed by 500 mg four times a day for 5 days. The patient's sexual partner(s) should be treated at the same time. Spectinomycin is a relatively new drug, and its use should be restricted to resistant gonorrheal organisms. However, in the pregnant patient who is allergic to penicillin, its use is preferred over tetracycline. The dose is 4 gm intramuscularly.

Vaginal sulfa may be sufficient as treatment for mild, acute cervicitis secondary to nongonorrheal bacteria. However, a wide-spectrum antibiotic should be used for a moderate to severe infection. The common ones are ampicillin and tetracycline at doses of 500 mg orally, four times a day for 10 days.

CHRONIC CERVICITIS

Chronic cervicitis is the most frequently encountered gynecologic problem and the most common cause of leukorrhea. The discharge is usually thick and mucopurulent and often malodorous and irritating. Other symptoms may include intermenstrual bleeding and pelvic pain. The bleeding is usually a contact type such as after douching or intercourse. With increasing severity, a degree of pelvic cellulitis may occur, possibly causing pelvic pain, dyspareunia, and/or dysmenorrhea.

Pathologically chronic cervicitis may be found in a majority of hysterectomy specimens from parous women. The process usually begins with a pregnancy-related cervical laceration. With the laceration, the endocervical mucosa is usually everted. This everted mucosa and devitalized tissue, which may be present at the lacerated site, are subject to infection from the normal vaginal flora. The bacteria eventually lie deep in the tissue continuing the infection process.

Grossly, the cervix is usually hypertrophied and congested. It may appear hyperemic because of the increased vascularity. Numerous retention cysts, known as Nabothian cysts, are present in many cases. These cysts are essentially gland openings that have been covered with metaplastic epithelium. The mucopurulent material in the closed glands usually builds to a point at which the covering epithelium is pushed out from the surface becoming cystic in appearance.

Microscopically, there is usually an extensive subepithelial inflammatory process consisting mostly of plasma cells with a considerable number of polymorphonucleocytes being present in the subacute stage.[21]

Prior to treatment, a Pap smear should be performed. If the results of the smear show nothing worse than inflammation and there are no questionable lesions on the cervix, treatment may be started. Antibiotics may be used as primary treatment in mild cases but should be used as adjunctive therapy in moderate to severe infections. Hot cauterization or cryosurgery can also be used and is easily performed in the office. The cryosurgery may have to be repeated depending on the degree and depth of the infection. Some hot cauterization can be performed in the office, but the amount needed to treat moderate to severe infection usually requires an anesthetic. This type of cauterization can be performed by using a hot iron or a special hot wire that will cone out the inflamed cervix. The hot wire should not be used when performing a cone biopsy for an abnormal Pap because the tissue is burned and is a poor specimen for pathologic diagnosis.

Chronic cervicitis may possibly be prevented by treating vaginitis and acute cervicitis vigorously. Mild cauterization of eversions and lacerations at the 6-week postpartum visit may aid in prevention.

POLYPS

A polyp is an outgrowth of epithelial tissue. Polyps on the cervix are usually asymptomatic and appear as a bud of red tissue. When symptoms do occur, they are usually in the form of bleeding, either postmenopausal spotting or intermenstrual spotting of the contact type. They are more commonly seen in women over 40 years of age than in younger women.[17]

The etiology for cervical polyps is uncertain, but they probably arise from the columnar epithelium since most are covered by that type of epithelium, although squamous metaplasia may occur. They are usually attached to the endocervical canal by a slender pedicle, but occasionally have a broad base. Some may be from the endometrial cavity, but only rarely is the attachment on the exocervix. In most cases, they are easily removed by simple torsion of the stalk. Although malignancy is rare, they should be sent for pathologic evaluation. When bleeding is a symptom, a Pap smear and sampling of the endometrial cavity should be done to exclude other pathology.

CERVICAL EROSION

Two types of erosion are seen on the cervix—congenital and acquired. The so-called congenital erosion is not a true lesion, but rather is an area of columnar tissue on the exocervix. It may be an eversion secondary to a laceration or an ectopy, which is commonly seen in females exposed to diethylstilbestrol in utero.

A true or acquired erosion is secondary to trauma or cancer. The epithelium in a traumatic erosion is lacking and is replaced by granulation tissue while new epithelium grows back. In a carcinoma, the center of the erosion is usually replaced by necrotic tissue. Even if the results of a Pap smear are normal, a biopsy of all true erosions should be performed with the specimen taken from the edge of the lesion.

The carcinomatous ulcer is the only erosion that needs treatment. The traumatic ulcer should heal by itself in 3 to 4 weeks. If it does not heal, another biopsy should be performed and the etiology for the trauma investigated.

CONDYLOMA ACUMINATUM

This warty lesion, commonly seen on the vulva, can occur on the cervix. Its appearance is the same as on the vulva. Although malignancy is rare, a biopsy should be performed to rule out a verrucous carcinoma. The condylomata are stimulated by pregnancy as are those of the vagina and vulva. Cryosurgery can easily be used to irradicate the lesion except during pregnancy.

LEIOMYOMA

Leiomyomata of the lower aspect of the uterus are usually found in the isthmus. Rarely do they occur on the exocervix, but as in any other lesion on the cervix, a biopsy should be performed prior to treatment. If they are diagnosed when small, simple excision may be possible; however, larger ones may require removal of the entire cervix or uterus.

Diethylstilbestrol

Just after World War II, obstetricians began to use the drug diethylstilbestrol (DES), a synthetic estrogen, in patients who had complications during pregnancy. These complications included diabetes, previous abortion, and threatened abortion. The peak of its use was between 1950 and 1955. In 1971 Dr. Arthur Herbst[15] of the Harvard Medical School reported on eight patients with a clear cell carcinoma of the vagina and/or cervix referred to him for treatment. Until this time, clear cell carcinoma of the vagina or cervix was a rare occurrence. An epidemiologic study on these patients discovered that in seven of the eight cases their mothers had been treated with DES while pregnant with the patient.

Just over 300 cases of clear cell carcinoma of the vagina and/or cervix have been reported to the Registry of Clear Cell Adenocarcinoma of the Genital Tract in Young Females as of February 1976.[13] The age of peak incidence is reported as 19 with almost all cases diagnosed between 14 and 23 years of age. Since it is not known how many females were exposed to DES, the incidence of carcinoma can only be estimated at around 1 per 1000 females exposed. These lesions are usually on the cervix or in the upper vagina, and although they were not all diagnosed when the patient was first examined, retrospectively they were present. They are usually exophytic and polypoid-like, but in some cases are well-indurated ulcerative lesions.

The treatment for clear cell carcinoma of the cervix or vagina is the same as that for squamous cell carcinoma. There is, however, a tendency to attempt a radical hysterectomy and partial or total vaginectomy on patients with a Stage IIA lesion rather than using radiotherapy because of their young age. A vaginal graft can be placed at the same operation if needed.

More commonly, changes of the cervix and upper vagina, so far non-malignant, have been noted in many of these patients. The most common change is known as ectopy,[14] in which columnar epithelium covers a wide area of the portio of the cervix resembling an erosion. The vaginal fornix and, in some cases, a good portion of the vagina may also be covered by columnar epithelium. The latter change is known as *adenosis*. Because of the extensive amount of mucus-producing glandular epithelium, these women may experience a fair amount of mucoid discharge, especially at the time of ovulation.

The other major changes are a vaginal or cervical hood, either partially or entirely surrounding the cervix, and a configuration of the anterior lip of the cervix, which is called a cockscomb because it resembles that of a rooster. The hood may surround the cervix so well that it itself resembles a cervix and the true cervix resembles a polyp. This latter change is called a *cervical pseudopolyp*. All these changes are easily seen during a pelvic examination and so far are considered benign. They do not seem to have any effect on the workings of the female genital organs.

The degree of adenosis and other changes have been correlated with the time during pregnancy that DES was used.[14] Use prior to the thirteenth week of pregnancy is associated with a high incidence of changes. The incidence decreases thereafter, and changes are rare if DES was started after the eighteenth week. These changes can occur without exposure to DES or other synthetic estrogens, but occur more commonly with DES exposure.

As stated above, these are all benign changes. The present concern with the exposed females, especially those with extensive adenosis, is that they have a wider transitional zone and therefore may possibly have an increased chance of cervical intraepithelial neoplasia (CIN) and/or squamous cell carcinoma of the cervix. At present, there has been no indication of such an increase. The significance of the transitional zone will be discussed in the section on colposcopy. Colposcopy has made it easy to follow these changes. The suggested frequency of colposcopy varies from every 3 months to yearly depending on the degree of adenosis and the metaplastic changes. The follow-up of a large number of these patients has been 5 to 6 years, and only a few cases with dysplastic changes have been noted.[25] Results of the progress of these changes will not be known for some time, but it is believed that once a normal metaplastic epithelium covers the areas of adenosis and ectopy the follow-up can be as for any patient not exposed to DES. At present, there is no indication for surgical correction of these changes. The method of birth control does not seem to adversely affect the patient nor does pregnancy.

WORKUP OF THE ABNORMAL PAP SMEAR

The cervical Pap smear is a very simple procedure to perform, but sometimes its results are misinterpreted. It must be remembered that the Pap smear does not yield a final diagnosis, but only the hint of a diagnosis. The quality of the results are only as good as the quality of the smear, the staining technique, and the cytologist or/and pathologist who read the smear. An adequate specimen is easy to obtain if the person performing the smear remembers two important points. First, the specimen must contain cells. If the cervix is dry, then few, if any, cells will be present in the specimen. This can be prevented by soaking the cotton tip in normal saline prior to taking the specimen. Second, to prevent drying on the slide, the specimen should be fixed immediately after being placed on the slide.

It is important to understand what the results of a Pap smear mean. If the results of a Pap smear are reported as normal (Class I), the procedure need not be repeated for at least 1 year, assuming the patient has not had a Pap smear with abnormal results in the past. When the results are reported as inflammatory (Class II), an infection should be looked for and treated. It is common today for the cytologist to report the type of infection. One to 2 months after treatment for the infection has been completed, the Pap smear should be repeated, preferably within 6 months of the previous inflammatory smear. If the smears continue to be inflammatory and the cause cannot be found, a colposcopic examination should be done.

Once a patient has a Pap smear reported as having cells typical of dysplasia or worse (Class III, IV, V), investigation should be conducted to determine the reason for the abnormal smear regardless of what a repeat smear shows. There are essentially three ways to evaluate an abnormal Pap smear: (1) random biopsy, (2) colposcopy, and (3) cone biopsy of the cervix.

Random biopsy

Prior to the popularity of colposcopy, random biopsies were commonly performed in the office with the aid of an iodine stain, either Lugol's iodine or Schiller's solution. This procedure is still acceptable, but unless the biopsy specimen shows invasive carcinoma, further diagnostic procedures must be done since a Pap smear specimen with mild to moderate dysplasia may have come from an area near an invasive carcinoma. The basis for using an iodine stain to help in directing the biopsy is that normal squamous epithelium is rich in glycogen and glycogen stains a dark mahogany color with iodine. However, some areas of normal squamous epithelium may not contain glycogen and thus not stain with the iodine as they should, while some dysplastic epithelium may contain glycogen. A recent report of Rubio and Thomassen[27] using Schiller's solution to stain the cervix prior to a cone biopsy showed a 31% false positive test, that is nonstaining quadrants of the cone had normal squamous epithelium, and a 64% false negative test, that is, stained quadrants contained an area of dysplasia and/or carcinoma in situ. Although these iodine solutions should not be discarded, their limitation must be understood.

Colposcopy

The use of a colposcope in the evaluation of the abnormal Pap smear specimens has been available for over 50 years, but it is only in the last decade that it has gained popularity in the United States. Its use has helped to decrease the use of the cervical cone biopsy so that approximately 90% of all patients with cervical intraepithelial neoplasia (CIN) are now treated on the basis of the colposcopic diagnosis.[9] By eliminating the cone biopsy, the complications of the anesthetic and the surgery are also eliminated and the problems with infertility may decrease in these patients. This is important since there are more abnormal Pap smears in females in the teens and early twenties than previously.

The colposcope essentially is a microscopic instrument that allows a more thorough examination of the surface contour and terminal vascular pattern of the cervix than can be done with the naked eye. Colposcopy need not be done by a physician. In many teaching institutions nurse colposcopists perform the examination. The most important qualification for a colposcopist is experience.

The colposcopist is most concerned with the examination of the transitional zone since this is the area in which CIN develops.[9] Simply stated, the transitional zone is that area that was once covered by columnar epithelium, but because of a process of metaplasia, is now covered with squamous epithelium. This metaplastic process occurs to a greater extent in the teenage years, and with the increase in sexual activity in these years, there may be an increased chance of developing CIN.[9]

Certain criteria must be met prior to

treating a patient on the basis of the colposcopically directed biopsy.

1. The colposcopist must be experienced. Experience is gained by doing colposcopy frequently and by correlating the biopsies of the first 100 or so patients with cone biopsies done on the same patients.
2. The experienced colposcopist must believe that the examination was adequate.
3. The squamocolumnar junction (SCJ) must be seen in its entirety.
4. The endocervical curettage (ECC) must be negative for dysplastic cells.
5. A biopsy must be done on the worst area of abnormality.
6. The diagnosis must be other than microinvasive carcinoma. For reasons that will be apparent later in this chapter, microinvasive carcinoma can only be diagnosed on a cervical cone biopsy.
7. The colposcopic biopsy must answer the reason for the abnormality in the Pap smear. The biopsy pathology must not be more than one degree less than the Pap smear.

If these criteria are not met, a cone biopsy should be performed.

Cone biopsy

Prior to the introduction of colposcopy, the cervical cone biopsy was used routinely for the diagnosis of the cause of a Pap smear that had abnormal results. Today when the cone biopsy is performed, its borders can be tailored with the help of the colposcope. Since it is important to evaluate the entire transitional zone, a narrow, cylinder-type cone biopsy can be performed when the exocervix is normal, the SCJ cannot be seen adequately, and/or the ECC is abnormal. On the other hand when the SCJ is seen in its entirety and the ECC is negative, a deep cone biopsy need not be done, but only the transitional zone on the exocervix removed.

CERVICAL INTRAEPITHELIAL NEOPLASIA

The term *cervical intraepithelial neoplasia* (CIN) is replacing dysplasia and carcinoma in situ because it better describes the disease process. There are three degrees of CIN: CIN I is equivalent to mild dysplasia, CIN II is equivalent to moderate dysplasia, and CIN III is equivalent to severe dysplasia and carcinoma in situ. The main difference among the degrees of CIN is the degree of lack of maturation of the epithelial cells in squamous epithelium from the basal layer to the surface. In CIN III, there is essentially no maturation to the surface. CIN is only rarely seen by the naked eye. A keratotic area (leukoplakia) may be seen on examination of the cervix and occasionally may be covering CIN. Otherwise the lesion is diagnosed from the workup of an abnormal Pap smear.

CIN I

CIN I (mild dysplasia) is an early cervical intraepithelial change. In almost half the cases the abnormality disappears and the Pap smear reverts to normal.[11,31] Whether this is a result of excisional biopsy or a true regression is debated, but it is probably a little of each. With this in mind, the question arises as to whether or not any specific treatment is needed and, if so, how drastic the treatment need be. In most cases, treatment is not necessary. However, it must be remembered that women have been told that an abnormal Pap smear can mean that a cancerous lesion may be present. When a patient is told that an abnormality is present, but she does not need treatment, she may become anxious. It is my policy to perform cryosurgery on all patients with multiple focal areas of mild dysplasia and on patients with unifocal areas who are anxious or have completed their childbearing.

Once an adequate diagnosis is made, treatment by a cone biopsy or hysterectomy is considered inappropriate. This is not to say that a cone biopsy should not be performed for diagnosis if it is necessary. Treatment with hot cauterization can be used, but cryosurgery seems much simpler and more comfortable for the patient.

CIN II

CIN II (moderate dysplasia) is essentially that degree of cervical intraepithelial abnormality that is not severe enough to be called CIN III, but is more severe than CIN I. Once diagnosed, this abnormality should be treated. If a cone biopsy has been done for diagnosis, no further treatment is necessary. If the diagnosis has been made by colposcopically directed biopsy, cryosurgery is usually the easiest mode of therapy. Once again, hysterectomy is not indicated for treatment.

CIN III

CIN III includes both severe dysplasia and carcinoma in situ. These lesions are included under one heading because of the small degree of difference between them histologically. The definitions of carcinoma in situ and severe dysplasia differ among pathologists, and most gynecologic oncologists now treat them in the same manner.

CIN III is considered to be a precancerous disease. It is known that a patient with CIN III can develop an invasive carcinoma of the cervix. Because the peak age of carcinoma in situ was 35 and that of invasive carcinoma of the cervix was 45, it was generally believed that it took about 10 years to progress from carcinoma in situ to invasive carcinoma. In truth, it is not known how long it takes that progression to occur, if indeed it does,[31] because in most cases the initial diagnostic methods, the methods of follow-up, and the results differ widely. Some cases of carcinoma in situ, if untreated, will progress to invasive carcinoma. In cases treated by less than a hysterectomy, there may be some progression to invasive carcinoma, but with adequate treatment and follow-up these will be very few in number.

The diagnosis of CIN III can be made from colposcopic examination alone. It is important that the criteria for an adequate colposcopy be met and that, if there is any doubt, a cone biopsy be performed. It is my belief that, if on colposcopy, the lesion covers a wide area of the exocervix, a cone biopsy should be performed.

In the past, the generally accepted treatment for CIN III has been a simple hysterectomy, either transvaginally or transabdominally. This is still the generally accepted treatment; however, with the increase in the number of patients in the younger age group who have not had children or who want more children, other methods of treatment are being used.

The cervical cone biopsy may be adequate treatment. In a recent report from Sweden,[1] 343 patients suspected of having carcinoma in situ were reviewed. Cone biopsy was done on all patients, and in a 1 to 5-year follow-up of just over 300 of these patients, the cervical cytology returned to negative in 93% of the patients. All were alive at the time of the report without evidence of invasive carcinoma. The same report stated that those patients whose cone biopsies had negative margins had a much better success than those patients whose biopsies had margins with carcinoma in situ.

Those patients who have negative margins on cone biopsy should have an adequate Pap smear performed at 3-month intervals for the first year starting 3 months from the biopsy and then, if continued negative, twice yearly. The question arises whether or not those patients with positive margins on cone biopsy should have some further therapy. Although there are no reports in the literature on its success or failure, I suggest that these patients have cryosurgery performed 3 months after the cone biopsy. They can then be followed in the same manner as those with negative margins.

Cryosurgery is becoming more popular for treatment of CIN III. It should not be done during pregnancy. It is suggested that nitrous oxide or carbon dioxide and a freeze-thaw-freeze technique be used. Reports in large series are few.[8,24,33] Townsend[33] has reported a 90% success rate in patients with carcinoma in situ. More large series and longer follow-ups are required before the success of cryosurgery can be adequately evaluated.

Cryosurgery has many advantages over cone biopsy. No anesthesia is required, blood loss is negligible, hospitalization is not required, and there is no loss of work time. Although not proved as yet, there is probably no problem with infertility after cryosurgery.[8,24] Cryosurgery tends to allow continued follow-up with the colposcope as the squamocolumnar junction is usually still visible. With a cone biopsy, the squamocolumnar junction may end up in the endocervical canal and out of view.

Follow-up after cryosurgery is the same as for cone biopsy. When a colposcope is available, it should be added to the examination. At present, the patient should be advised to have a hysterectomy when she has completed her childbearing. If, in the future, studies show an adequate success rate with cryosurgery, hysterectomy may not be necessary.

Simple hysterectomy has been and still is the generally accepted definitive treatment for CIN III. The procedure may be done either transvaginally or transabdominally and does not require that a vaginal cuff be taken. Removal of the ovaries is not part of this procedure. Obviously since removal of the uterus precludes further childbirth, it is done when no further pregnancies are wanted.

The advantage of hysterectomy over other treatments is that the cervix is removed in its entirety and, in the vast majority of cases, CIN totally removed. This is not to say that there is no chance of recurrent disease. In fact, the success rate of hysterectomy for CIN III is slightly less than 100%. Most series report a recurrence rate of carcinoma in situ or invasive carcinoma in the vaginal cuff of 0% to 2%.[32]

All patients should have continued pelvic exams and vaginal Pap smears following a hysterectomy for any reason, but it is even more important when the reason for the procedure was CIN III. The Pap smear should be performed at least twice yearly for the first 2 to 3 years and then at least yearly thereafter. If one smear is taken from the cuff and a second from the upper vaginal walls, any new or persistent abnormality should be found.

Another therapy that is being used in the treatment of CIN is the laser beam. This is purely experimental at present and may never come into general use because of economic factors.

MICROINVASIVE CARCINOMA

Microinvasive carcinoma of the cervix is diagnosed mainly in terms of the depth of penetration of tumor cells into the submucosal tissue. When the International Federation of Obstetricians and Gynecologists added this to the staging system, they did not elaborate on a definition for microinvasion. Some oncologists use a depth of penetration up to 1 mm only,[3] some up to 5 mm,[6,16] but most at present are using a depth of 3 mm as has been suggested by the Society of Gynecological Oncologists.[7,29] My definition of microinvasive carcinoma of the cervix includes any penetration of tumor cells below the basement membrane of the surface epithelium up to 3 mm.

The diagnosis of microinvasive carcinoma of the cervix must be confirmed on a cervical cone biopsy for two reasons: (1) the colposcopically directed biopsy may not be deep enough to totally rule out further invasion, and (2) other areas of the cervix may contain deeper invasion. On gross inspection of the cervix no lesion is obvious. Colposcopically there may be marked mosaicism, punctation, and/or large, irregular vessels. The area involved may bleed easily.

Until 1970, the routine treatment for microinvasive carcinoma of the cervix was a radical hysterectomy and pelvic lymph node dissection. A review of all cases in which the depth of penetration was less than 5 mm revealed only an occasional lymph node with tumor and cases in which penetration was less than 3 mm revealed that no nodes were involved in most series.[16,28,29] With few exceptions, when modified radical hysterectomy is being used, the routine treatment since then has been a simple hysterectomy without removal of lymph nodes performed transvaginally or transabdominally. Cases in which a lymph node is discovered to have a tumor and/or recurrence are reportable.

Until recently, the presence or absence of lymphatic involvement on the cone biopsy did influence the type of treatment. The incidence of node metastases and/or recurrent tumor with lymphatic involvement in the cervical tissue is so small that such involvement no longer influences the type of treatment.[26] What does influence the type of therapy—simple versus radical hysterectomy—is the bulk of the tumor. The definition of microinvasion is limited only to depth of invasion, but the width and length of the area is important.

Radiotherapy does have a role in the treatment of microinvasive carcinoma, especially in the patient who is not a candidate for an operation. The patient in whom a radical procedure is believed to be the treatment of choice should have the option of treatment with radiotherapy. When simple hysterectomy is believed to be the treatment of choice, radiotherapy should be used only if it is believed that the patient cannot undergo an operation.

INVASIVE CARCINOMA

Invasive carcinoma of the uterine cervix is one of the few tumors in the human body that has had fairly good standardization of treatment for many years. Some of these tumors may be occult and only diagnosed during the workup following a Pap smear with abnormal results. The majority, however, are either ulcerative, exophytic, or endophytic.

The ulcerative and exophytic lesions are usually symptomatic. In the beginning, there may be a contact-type bleeding such as after intercourse or douching, which may become intermenstrual spotting without contact along with a foul-smelling discharge. A Pap smear is usually not necessary for diagnosis and, in fact, may have normal results with the ulcerative type of lesion. As stated above, a biopsy should be performed on any ulcer that does not heal and/or is suspicious regardless of the results of the Pap smear. The biopsy specimen should be taken from the edge of the ulcer. The exophytic lesion may not be obvious in its early stage, but can be identified by a good colposcopist. When it is obvious, there is no reason to wait for the results of a Pap smear to perform a biopsy. It is best to take the biopsy specimen from areas that do not look necrotic.

Unfortunately, the endophytic or infiltrating lesion may not produce early symptoms. This type of tumor generally starts in the endocervical canal and infiltrates throughout the cervix prior to producing abnormal bleeding and/or foul-smelling discharge. It is usually diagnosed during the workup for a Pap smear with abnormal results. It must be remembered that if the diagnosis is made on a punch biopsy, there is no reason for any further biopsy of the cervix such as a cone biopsy. The nonpalpable pathologic extent within the cervix itself does not influence the treatment. If carcinoma is suspected, but the results of the first set of biopsies are not diagnostic, an endocervical curettage may help to make the diagnosis without performing a cone biopsy.

Ninety percent to 95% of all cervical carcinomas are of the squamous cell variety,[12] between 5% and 10% may be adenocarcinoma, and about 1% are a mixed adenosquamous cell carcinoma. The latter has a poorer prognosis stage for stage.

The workup for a patient prior to treatment varies among oncologists. It is generally agreed that these patients should have at the least a complete blood count and an intravenous pyelogram (IVP). If radical surgery is to be performed, the location, number, and configuration of the ureters is important, and an abnormal IVP may influence the stage of the disease. Some oncologists believe that in addition to these studies, a barium enema, bone scan, lymphangiogram, cystoscopy, and proctoscopy should also be done. Others believe that these latter studies need to be done depending on the stage of disease.

Staging

The staging of cervical cancer is easy to understand and should be included in any discussion of this disease. It is a clinical staging system using any radiologic or pathologic studies that are available in most communities. In this respect a lymphangiogram, CT scan, and exploratory surgery cannot be used for staging purposes. The staging system for carcinoma of the cervix set up by the International Federation of Obstetricians and Gynecologists is as follows:

Stage I — Carcinoma confined to the cervix
  IA — Microinvasive carcinoma
  IB — All other cases of Stage I with occult cancer mark "occ"
Stage II — Carcinoma is beyond the cervix, but has not extended to the pelvic wall or lower third of the vagina
  IIA — Vaginal, but not parametrial involvement
  IIB — Parametrial involvement
Stage III — Carcinoma is on the pelvic wall or involves the lower third of the vagina
  IIIA — Lower vaginal involvement with pelvic wall free of tumor
  IIIB — Tumor is on the pelvic wall; also, any ureteral obstruction or hydronephrosis that is believed to be secondary to tumor
Stage IV — Tumor has spread beyond the true pelvis and/or involves the mucosa of the bladder or rectum; positive results of biopsy of bladder or rectum are required for this stage. Although cytology and bullous edema of the bladder mucosa suggest involvement by tumor, they are not acceptable without biopsy.

The basic purpose of clinical staging for this disease is to evaluate statistically to some extent the outcome of treatment and to compare that outcome with the results of other institutions. This staging is not used in all cases to determine treatment modality. Some institutions are performing an exploratory laparotomy on some or all patients with carcinoma of the cervix to further evaluate the tumor and its possible metastases, especially to the lymph nodes. This may be important in the earlier stages. In Stage IB, 15% to 25% of patients may have positive pelvic lymph nodes.[5,23] In small series[2,30] (40 patients each), the incidence of extrapelvic node metastases in Stage IB has been reported as high as 12%. The pelvic nodes are included in the normal fields of radiation, but it might be better to remove a 3- to 4-cm node prior to radiotherapy since the therapy may not irradicate such a large node. The upper, common, iliac nodes are not included in the normal fields, but if these and/or the para-aortic nodes are positive, extended fields of radiation should be used. It is not yet known whether the use of these extended fields increases the survival rate of these patients. The perfection of the CT scan may decrease the need for pretreatment exploratory surgery. This pretreatment surgery does increase the morbidity from radiotherapy, especially when extended fields are used.[22] Some institutions are investigating the use of a long, 23-gauge needle for transperitoneal biopsy of suspicious nodes on lymphangiogram. The morbidity from this is minimal, and the placement of a needle of this size through the bowel and/or major vessels produces no sequelae. I have had some experience with this technique and have been able to prevent surgery in patients with a positive result. At present if the result is negative, surgery is performed.

Treatment

The treatment of Stage IA (microinvasive) carcinoma has been discussed previously. There is no significant difference in the survival rate of patients with Stage IB carcinoma whether treatment is by radical surgery or radiotherapy when large series are reviewed.[19,20] The choice of treatment usually depends on the training background and expertise in the surgical treatment of the physician and the preference of the patient. Both treatment modalities, along with their complications and availability, should be presented to the patient so that she may take part in the choice of her therapy.

The basis behind radical surgery for a cancerous tumor is to remove a specific amount of tissue surrounding the gross tumor so that nonpalpable malignant cells that may be surrounding that tumor are also removed. The radical hysterectomy involves the removal of the upper one third of the vagina, the cervix and corpus of the uterus, and the parametrial and paravaginal tissue attached to these structures. The procedure is done en bloc, that is, as one specimen. Along with this, the lymph nodes along the external iliac arteries and veins, the hypogastric arteries and veins, the common iliac arteries and veins, and the lower 2 to 3 cm of the aorta, vena cava, and obturator space are removed. If any of the lymph nodes or margins of resection show tumor, supplemental radiation is usually suggested. If any lymph node contains tumor at surgery or if the tumor is found to be more extensive, the surgery is not performed.

There are four major complications of a radical hysterectomy. In all cases, there is dysfunction of the bladder that requires some type of urinary drainage for at least 10 days. The majority of patients are able to urinate well with low residues at that time. A few patients must continue drainage from a few weeks to a few months, but only rarely does a patient need continued drainage after 6 months. The amount of blood loss during a radical hysterectomy is usually greater than during a simple hysterectomy, and the patient may require blood intraoperatively and/or postoperatively. Infection has been a problem in the past, but its incidence seems to have been decreased with the use of prophylactic antibiotics.

The fourth major complication is fistula formation. In its natural course, the ureter runs under the uterine artery close to the cervix. During the operation, the lower 4 to 6 cm of the ureter must be dissected out of the parametrial tissue. During this dissection, the blood supply to that portion of the ureter may be decreased and the ureter may be damaged. If this occurs, especially in association with a partial or complete obstruction of that ureter below the damaged area, a fistula may occur in the retroperitoneal space or vagina. The incidence of this fistulization occurring when this operation is performed by surgeons well trained in the procedure is about 2% to 5%.[9] If the fistula does not close by itself, reimplantation of the ureter is usually performed 6 to 8 weeks postoperatively.

The length of hospitalization for a patient undergoing a radical hysterectomy, including preoperative x-ray examinations, is about 14 days. Complete recovery at home, return to full, normal activity, is another 5 to 6 weeks. Compared with a simple hysterectomy, the hospital stay is about 1 week longer and the posthospital recuperation is 2 weeks longer.

Radiotherapy is given in two phases. The first phase is usually external irradiation by means of a Cobalt 60 machine or a Linear Excellerator. In most cases, the total dose will be 5000 rads and is given over 25 to 30 working days depending on the daily dose. One to 2 weeks after the completion of the external therapy, an apparatus containing cesium (radium is rarely used anymore because of the danger of radon gas) is placed into the cervical canal and upper vagina to give a larger dose to the tumor in the cervix and the parametrial tissue. The external beam gives most of the treatment to the nodal tissue. Some institutions give the dose of the internal system in two separate applications 2 weeks apart, while others use only one application.

The activity of the patient during radiotherapy varies. Although very little, if any, discomfort is felt during the external irradiation, the patients usually become tired more easily and may have to decrease their normal activity. Complete recuperation usually takes about 4 weeks after the insertion of the cesium.

Complications following a radical hysterectomy usually occur at the time of the operation or within 15 days and, in the vast majority of cases, are repairable and not permanent. The initial complications from radiotherapy are usually temporary, but the delayed complications, usually occurring from 6 months to 2 years or more after the completion of therapy, are generally permanent. The initial complications are diarrhea, bladder irritation, and weakness. The diarrhea usually begins after 3 weeks of therapy and is generally controllable with medication without the interruption of therapy. In most cases, the diarrhea usually disappears without the aid of medication 4 weeks after the completion of therapy. The bladder irritation is less frequent and is easily controlled with analgesics, antispasmodics, and/or antibiotics.

The major delayed complications are bowel and urinary fistulae and radiation proctitis. Vesicovaginal, ureterovaginal, and rectovaginal fistulae usually occur more than 6 months after radiotherapy if they are from the radiation alone. Fistulae that occur during radiotherapy are usually secondary to tumor breakdown in that area. Fistulae secondary to radiation therapy are very difficult to close. In most instances they require some type of diversion, either a colostomy in the case of a rectovaginal fistula or a ureteroileostomy in the case of a vesicovaginal fistula. Ureterovaginal fistulae can be corrected by means of a ureteral reimplantation.

Radiation proctitis may be mild, causing increased frequency of soft stools with occasional diarrhea, or severe, causing bloody diarrhea that may require blood transfusions. Except for the severest type, this complication can usually be controlled with hydrocortisone retention enemas and low-residue diet.

Sexual function is better following radical surgery and is very important in helping to maintain a patient's vagina after radiotherapy. Although surgery shortens the vagina, it should not be enough to cause a problem with intercourse, unless problems had previously existed. Following radiotherapy, the upper vagina may become fibrotic and stenotic and may cause some dyspareunia. These women should be treated with estrogen cream per vagina and encouraged to continue an active sex life.

In the young patient with an early Stage IIA lesion, a radical hysterectomy may be attempted. If there is any evidence of nodal involvement, radiotherapy should be the choice of treatment. In all other lesions of Stage II, III, and IV, radiotherapy is the choice of therapy. If an exploratory laparotomy is done to evaluate the tumor prior to therapy, the ovary can be suspended near the iliac crest and possibly kept out of the field of irradiation, thus preventing a radiation-induced menopause and the use of exogenous hormones.

Follow-up

The follow-up for a patient with invasive carcinoma of the cervix is very important. The majority of recurrences are within 2 years of therapy, but a recurrence can occur after 5 years.[9] The main symptoms are bleeding per vagina, foul-smelling discharge, leg edema, leg pain of a nerve root type, weakness, and weight loss.

At the follow-up examinations, a hematocrit should be performed because anemia may be the first sign of recurrence. The examination itself should include the neck, breasts, abdomen, and pelvis. Any nodule in the neck region, especially supraclavicular, is abnormal and needs a biopsy. Patients with cancer of the genital organs have an increased risk of cancer of the breast, thus, examination of this organ is important.

Following radiotherapy, a smooth sheet of radiation fibrosis may develop from side wall to side wall in the area of the upper rectum. This is normally called a *radiation shelf*. It is important to note that this is smooth and not nodular. Nodularity in this area of fibrosis and/or an enlarging mass in the pelvis is suggestive of recurrent or persistent tumor.

The frequency of the follow-up examinations are suggested as follows: every 6 to 8 weeks for the first 6 months, every 3 months for the next 1½ to 2 years, and twice yearly thereafter. At each examination, a Pap smear should be done. Six months after treatment and yearly thereafter it is advisable to perform an x-ray film of the chest and an IVP.

Recurrence

If there is a recurrence the treatment depends on the type of initial treatment and the site of the recurrence. A recurrence outside the pelvis can be treated but is rarely cured. A recurrence within the pelvis after radical surgery has a greater chance for cure than after radiotherapy.[20] A full course of irradiation may be given to the pelvis following radical surgery, but, except in rare cases, once radiotherapy has been given, no further irradiation can be delivered to the same area without serious complications.

For a pelvic recurrence after radiotherapy, surgery is the best treatment. Occasionally a radical hysterectomy can be performed, but the fibrosis that occurs following radiotherapy creates poor tissue plains and the incidence of major complications, especially fistula formation, is increased.[18] In many cases, a radical hysterectomy will not remove all the tumor.

The usual surgical treatment for recurrence is pelvic exenteration, which involves the removal of the uterus, vagina, bladder, rectum, and all the parametrial and paravaginal tissue to the pelvic side wall. Because the mortality from the operation is high (10% to 20%), it is not performed if there is any evidence of tumor outside the pelvis, if any lymph nodes have metastatic tumor, or if all the tumor in the pelvis cannot be removed. Depending on the location of the tumor, it may be possible to leave either the rectum or the bladder in place. This operation can be devastating to the patient, both physically and psychologically, and she must be well prepared for it. The 5-year cure rate is only 25% to 40%.[9]

The results of chemotherapy in carcinoma of the cervix are very poor. It is never used as primary therapy and is used for recurrence only after treatment by surgery and radiotherapy have been exhausted. When discussing its success, response rate, that is, decrease in the size of tumor by more than 50% for 3 months, not cure rate is referred to. From 0% to 30% response can be expected from chemotherapy with a better chance of success when the tumor is outside the previously radiated field, and less when in the field. The length of the response varies. There are rare reports in the literature of 5-year survival after chemotherapy.

REFERENCES

1. Ahlgren, M., Ingemarsson, I., Lindberg, L. G., et al.: Conization as treatment of carcinoma in situ of the uterine cavity, Obstet. Gynecol. **46:**135-140, 1975.
2. Averette, H. E., Dudan, R. C., and Ford, J. H., Jr.: Exploratory celiotomy for surgical staging of cervical cancer, Am. J. Obstet. Gynecol. **113:**1090-1096, 1972.
3. Averette, H. E., Nelson, J. H., Jr., Ng, A. B. P., et al.: Diagnosis and management of microinvasive (Stage IA) carcinoma of the uterine cervix, Cancer **38:**414-425, 1976.
4. Averette, H. E., Weinstein, G. D., Ford, J. H., Jr., et al.: Cell kinetics and programmed chemotherapy for gynecologic cancer, Am. J. Obstet. Gynecol. **124:**912-923, 1976.
5. Boronow, R. C.: Stage I cervix cancer and pelvic node metastasis: special reference to the implications of the new and the recently replaced FIGO classifications on Stage IA, Am. J. Obstet. Gynecol. **127:**135-137, 1977.
6. Boutselis, J. G., Ullery, J. C., and Charme, L.: Diagnosis and management of Stage IA (microinvasive) carcinoma of the cervix, Am. J. Obstet. Gynecol. **110:**984-989, 1971.
7. Creasman, W. T., and Parker, R. T.: Management of early cervical neoplasia, Clin. Obstet. Gynecol. **18:**233-245, 1975.
8. Crisp, W. E.: Cryosurgical treatment of neoplasia of the uterine cervix, Obstet. Gynecol. **39:**495-499, 1972.
9. DiSaia, P. J., Morrow, C. P., and Townsend, D. E.: Synopsis of gynecologic oncology, New York, 1975, John Wiley & Sons, Inc.
10. Eschenbach, D. A.: Acute pelvic inflammatory disease: etiology, risk factors and pathogenesis, Clin. Obstet. Gynecol. **19:**147-166, 1976.
11. Fox, C. H.: Time necessary for conversion of normal to dysplastic cervical epithelium, Obstet. Gynecol. **31:**749-754, 1968.
12. Gompel, C., and Silverberg, S. G.: Pathology in gynecology and obstetrics, ed. 2, Philadelphia, 1977, J. B. Lippincott Co.
13. Herbst, A. L., Cole, P., Colton, T., et al.: Age-incidence and risks of diethylstilbestrol-related clear cell adenocarcinoma of the vagina and cervix, Am. J. Obstet. Gynecol. **128:**43-50, 1977.
14. Herbst, A. L., Poskanzer, D. C., Robboy, S. J., et al.: Prenatal exposure to stilbestrol: a prospective comparison of exposed female offspring with unexposed controls, N. Engl. J. Med. **292:**334-339, 1975.
15. Herbst, A. L., Ulfelder, H., and Poskanzer, D. C.: Adenocarcinoma of the vagina: association of maternal stilbestrol therapy with tumor appearance in young women, N. Engl. J. Med. **284:**878-881, 1971.
16. Lehman, M. H., Jr., Benson, W. L., Kurman, R. J., et al.: Microinvasive carcinoma of the cervix, Obstet. Gynecol. **48:**571-578, 1976.
17. McLaren, H.: The management of benign cervical abnormalities. In Jordan, J. A., and Singer,

A., editors: The cervix, Philadelphia, 1976, W. B. Saunders Co.
18. Mikuta, J. J., Guintoli, R. L., Rubin, E. L., et al.: The problem radical hysterectomy, Am. J. Obstet. Gynecol. **128:**119-127, 1977.
19. Morley, G. W., and Seski, J. C.: Radical pelvic surgery versus radiation therapy for Stage I carcinoma of the cervix (exclusive of microinvasion), Am. J. Obstet. Gynecol. **126:**785-798, 1976.
20. Newton, M.: Radical hysterectomy or radiotherapy for the Stage I cervical cancer, Am. J. Obstet. Gynecol. **123:**535-542, 1975.
21. Novak, E. R., and Woodruff, J. D.: Novak's Gynecologic and obstetric pathology, ed. 6, Philadelphia, 1967, W. B. Saunders Co.
22. Piver, M. S., and Barlow, J. J.: High dose irradiation to biopsy confirmed aortic node metastasis from carcinoma of the uterine cervix, Cancer **39:**1243-1246, 1977.
23. Plentl, A. A., and Friedman, E. A.: Lymphatic system of the female genitalia: the morphologic basis of oncologic diagnosis and therapy, Philadelphia, 1971, W. B. Saunders Co.
24. Popkin, D. R., Scali, V., and Ahmed, M. N.: Cryosurgery for the treatment of cervical intraepithelial neoplasia, Am. J. Obstet. Gynecol. **130:**551-554, 1978.
25. Robboy, S. J., Keh, P. C., Nickerson, R. J., et al.: Squamous cell dysplasia and carcinoma in situ of the cervix and vagina after prenatal exposure to diethylstilbestrol, Obstet. Gynecol. **51:**528-535, 1978.
26. Roche, W. D., and Norris, H. J.: Microinvasive carcinoma of the cervix: the significance of lymphatic invasion and confluent patterns of stromal growth, Cancer **36:**180-186, 1975.
27. Rubio, C. A., and Thomassen, P.: A critical evaluation of the schiller test in patients before conization, Am. J. Obstet. Gynecol. **125:**96-99, 1976.
28. Ruch, R. M., Pitcock, J. A., and Ruch, W. A., Jr.: Microinvasive carcinoma of the cervix, Am. J. Obstet. Gynecol. **125:**87-92, 1976.
29. Savage, E. W.: Microinvasive carcinoma of the cervix, Am. J. Obstet. Gynecol. **113:**708-717, 1972.
30. Sedlacek, T. V., Mangan, C. E., Giuntoli, R. L., et al.: Exploratory celiotomy for cervical carcinoma: the role of histologic grading, Gynecol. Oncol. **6:**138-144, 1978.
31. Sedlis, A., Cohen, A., and Sall, S.: The fate of cervical dysplasia, Am. J. Obstet. Gynecol. **107:**1065-1070, 1970.
32. Selim, M. A., So-Bosita, J. L., and Neuman, M. R.: Carcinoma in situ of the cervix uteri, Surg. Gynecol. Obstet. **139:**697-700, 1974.
33. Townsend, D. E.: Cryosurgery in gynecology. In Taymor, M. L., and Green, T. H., Jr., editors: Progress in gynecology, vol. 6, New York, 1975, Grune & Stratton, Inc.

CHAPTER 14

A guide to a healthy pubococcygeus muscle: kegeling, not cutting*

Salee Berman and Victor M. Berman

Approximately one third of all women suffer to some degree from the effects of genital relaxation.[5] Young female children may show bladder weakness and a need to urinate too frequently, perhaps become bedwetters. The female beginning sexual activity may experience bladder discomfort or a lack of sensation during intercourse. A woman giving birth may feel unusual pain or tightness and have a prolonged second stage of labor. The children are spanked for their "naughtiness." Females are dubbed "frigid" and embark on a lifetime of sexual dissatisfaction. The woman in labor is drugged and her perineum is cut to avoid tears; with each subsequent labor, the damage increases. By middle age, the condition may have deteriorated to the point that surgical repair seems imperative.

What causes genital relaxation? Is it the inevitable price a woman must pay for motherhood? Is surgery the answer?

The cause is self-evident, if not too widely understood. The genital muscles, for any one of several reasons, show a loss of tone or even atrophy. In the very young, the condition is probably congenital. But in the maturing adult, it may occur because there is a lack of awareness of the deeply hidden musculature that supports the lower organs. With each successive childbirth, the stretching of these birth canal muscles creates further neuromuscular damage. In the young, active mother, their function may be self-restoring. As she ages, however, repeated trauma coupled with absence of understanding about the physiologic nature of the phenomenon will result in chronically injured muscles throughout the pelvic floor. The ensuing urinary incontinence, loss of vaginal sensation, herniations, or even more severe injury can create a lifetime of misery that the woman will, indeed, attribute to childbirth. She may discover that after bearing several children, she can

---

*We are indebted to Georgia Kline-Graber, R. N. and Benjamin Graber, M.D., for stimulating our interests in pelvic and pubococcygeus muscle evaluation and for their demonstration of the examination, particularly the technique for intravaginal palpation of the muscle. Furthermore, the Grabers' instructions for some of the exercises described were the basis for the expanded regimen developed at NACHIS/Natural Childbirth Institute. We also thank our editor, Jean D. Radler, for her assistance throughout the writing of this chapter.

no longer hold a tampon or diaphragm securely. She and her physician might accept this as the inevitable price of motherhood and proceed with plans for an anteroposterior colporrhaphy.

Yet surgery is not the only answer. Surgery may repair torn fasciae or restore a prolapsed uterus to its proper position. Nevertheless, it is not enough to suture torn and lacerated muscle into place. The apparent form will be restored, but not the function. "In some way," writes one concerned physician, "reinnervation of muscle cells must be accomplished and the injured muscle cells must again be educated to function."[9]

Medical history is full of facts and lore about physicians who, as long ago as Hippocrates, were aware that this problem occurred in women after childbirth. Centuries of remedies included oils, massage, and packing the vagina. In recent years, anthropologic studies have discovered that exercises and instruction were passed from the older women to the young primiparous women.[9]

This chapter reviews the physiology and degeneration of the muscles that have been a source of much distress for women and describes the historical research leading to simple, physiologic methods for restoring muscle function or initiating the function in some women who have never had it. The thorough pelvic examination necessary to evaluate genitourinary health and muscle tonus is outlined. Step-by-step instructions are given for teaching exercises designed to compensate for congenital weakness or injury sustained during childbirth, surgery, or menopause. The stretching process of childbirth will be shown to be a precipitating factor in genital relaxation, but it should not be considered the primary or only cause, not is it the inescapable price that women must pay for bearing children.

THE PUBOCOCCYGEUS MUSCLE

The pelvic diaphragm lies above the superficial muscle and fascia of the urogenital diaphragm and anal triangle that together make up the perineal floor. Composed of five great muscle groups, this pelvic diaphragm between the pubis and the coccyx provides a firm platform supporting the pelvic organs. The greatest part of the platform comprises the levator ani, a trio of large, smooth muscles called the coccygeus, the iliococcygeus, and the pubococcygeus. The two remaining muscles, the obturatorius internus and the piriformis, arise in the lateral pelvic arch and the sacrum, respectively, and extend downward through the sciatic notch to terminate at the femur. Both lie at the periphery of the pelvis. Their function is primarily to assist the movement of the hip and only secondarily to support the pelvic organs.

On the other hand, the levator ani form a broad three-part band filling the pelvic floor. The posterior muscle, the coccygeus, is a triangle with the apex arising from the ischial spine of the pelvis and the base attached to the lateral sacrum and the coccyx. Forward of the coccygeus is the iliococcygeus, which also arises from the ischial spine and inserts into the last two segments of the coccyx, below the base of the coccygeus. Anterior to the insertion, the iliococcygeus fibers from each side meet to form a "seam" and intermesh with fibers from the sphincter ani externus and the transverse perineal muscles.

Most important of the three muscles is the pubococcygeus, which occupies the critical position and provides a sling of longitudinal fibers as well as a network that interlocks with the intrinsic musculature of the urogenital and rectal openings. It arises from the pubis on either side of the urethra, vagina, and rectum to join behind the rectal canal and continue to the terminating seg-

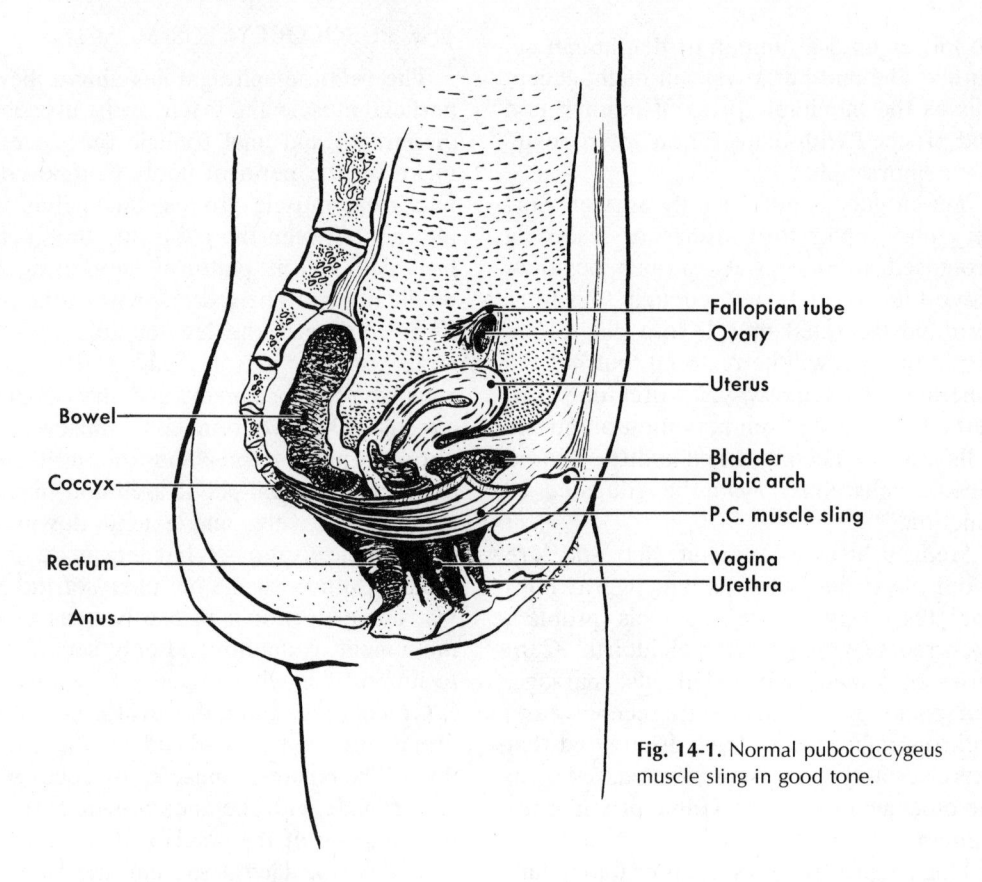

Fig. 14-1. Normal pubococcygeus muscle sling in good tone.

ments of the coccyx. The gap between the anterior segments at the pubis is filled with the urogenital diaphragm. However, lateral fibers of the two pubococcygeal segments extend to insert in the muscular fibers of the urethra, vagina, rectum, and urogenital diaphragm itself.

In normal tone, the pubococcygeus muscle (P.C. muscle) is a firm sling supporting the uterus, ovaries, fallopian tubes, lower bowel, bladder, and vagina in a high position. The fibrous network surrounding the canals also acts as a sphincter, able to constrict the rectum, vagina, and urethra or to relax completely during defecation, parturition, and micturition.

If the muscle is healthy, it is a flexible, powerful structure that prevents urinary incontinence, squeezes firmly to increase sexual arousal and climax, and relaxes to open the birth canal during labor. For these reasons, the P.C. muscle is considered "the key muscle of the pelvis, the longest and strongest of the female pelvic floor."[8]

What happens when the muscle tone is poor or the muscle structure itself has been damaged? A myriad of distresses can afflict women from childhood to old age as the result of genital relaxation. The various signs and symptoms that may manifest themselves at different life stages are the following:*

---
*Adapted from Kegel, A. H.: Early genital relaxation, Obstet. Gynecol. 8(5):54, 1966.

Toddler thru adolescence
  Bladder weakness
  Bedwetting
Beginning sexual activity
  Sexual difficulties related to sensory disturbances in the vagina
  Lack of awareness of function of the pubococcygeus muscle
  Occasional bladder discomfort
During pregnancy
  Poor tone of the soft (neuromusculofascial) pelvic tissues
  Lack of awareness of function of the pubococcygeus muscle
  Inability to contract perivaginal muscles
  Incontinence
During birth
  Increased pain
  Prolonged second stage
  Contribution to muscle damage and episiotomy
In the postpartum period
  Persistent subinvolution, with or without bleeding
  Incomplete recovery of pelvic muscle tone as revealed by relaxation of the middle third of the vagina and poor support of bladder, rectum, and uterus
  Pelvic fatigue, "falling-out" sensations with or without cystocele, rectocele, and prolapsed uterus*
  Failure to recover sexual sensory perceptions in the vagina, painful intercourse, and the inability to reach orgasm
During menopause
  Loss of tone of tissues of urogenital tract
  Loss of libido
  Decline of sexual sensory perception in the vagina
  Cystocele, rectocele, and prolapsed uterus
In old age
  Annoying bladder disturbances such as recurrent nocturia, urgency, and frequency
  Stress incontinence (may be early sign of degenerative process)
  Cystocele, rectocele, and prolapsed uterus

*Herniation of bladder, rectum, or uterus into the vaginal canal.

Although many physicians have suspected that the pelvic muscles were vital to a woman's well-being, almost none have known how to correct loss of muscular function. As recently as 1944, Bergler reported that women have no conscious control over the pelvic and perineal muscles. Further, Dickinson stated that most women were unaware of the muscle and "certainly had no voluntary control over it."[4]

THE HISTORICAL RESEARCH

In the early 1940s, a pioneering California surgeon who specialized in female disorders became interested in finding a more satisfactory method than surgery to deal with urinary stress incontinence. Many of his patients were referred to Dr. Arnold H. Kegel for relief of this little understood but embarrassing affliction. A cough, a sneeze, even hearty laughter, caused them to urinate involuntarily—often so heavily that they were constrained to wear pads.

Kegel conducted investigations directed particularly to the muscles of the pelvic floor, which he thought might be the key. Eventually satisfied that these structures, when weakened, would relax urinary control, he began to search for methods of exercising and strengthening the hidden muscles. He discovered that many women had what he called a "lack of awareness of function."[11] In other words, they were unaware that the muscles existed and were totally unable to control them.

He also learned that passive and stimulative exercises, such as massage and hydrotherapy, had been attempted in the past century but had failed to restore muscle strength. It was clear to Kegel that only active effort on the part of the patient against progressively increasing resistance "could thicken and strengthen the fibers and reinnervate the muscle."[6] Eventually, he developed a device (described later) that could be inserted in the vagina and activated to "push" with increasing force against the vaginal walls and the part of the P.C. muscle fibers interlaced in the musculature of the vaginal canal as a woman contracted her P.C. muscle against the device.

Among the discoveries made in Kegel's investigation of the P.C. muscle was that the stretching process of childbirth should not be considered the primary or only cause of genital relaxation. During delivery, a normal, relaxed muscle lies high in the pelvis and retracts behind the pelvic bones—the ischial rami—where the P.C. muscle is fairly well protected against injury. However, some injury in the immediate vaginal area may occur because of the extremes of pressure and dilation. Kegel notes that "in any region where tissues become overstretched, even through lacerations of muscles or fascias are not visible, nerve injury is inevitable."[9] Such injury is usually self-repairing in the woman with firm and elastic musculature. If she is adequately prepared to handle her contractions during labor, she will be able to relax her perineum provided she is not too drugged to remain in control. She should also be instructed and encouraged in the necessary restorative exercises during the postpartum period. However, a poorly developed P.C. muscle lies at a low level and is pushed down by the fetus, where it may be impinged against the bones and injured laterally. In other instances, a fibrous muscle may be pushed down so far that it tears posteriorly or it may be included in a mediolateral episiotomy, which causes irreparable damage.

Over the years, Kegel began to work out simple exercises that strengthened the P.C. muscle and could, if the patient were persistent, restore almost total function. Deutsch relates the story of one patient who came to Kegel in desperation after 2 long years of wearing pads for urinary incontinence.[11] Skeptical, but willing to try anything, she began the exercises. Within 2 months, her problem was gone.

There was one serious problem, however, in teaching the women where the muscle lay and how it felt and that they could indeed control it. Even when they began to understand the feeling of contraction, it was difficult to motivate them. There was no day-to-day measurement of improvement, Kegel believed that a visual aid that could help the patient make an immediate connection between effort and result would create the psychologic encouragement necessary to stimulate the patient's continuing efforts.

Eventually, he developed an instrument with which to measure her contractions, an instrument simple enough for the patient to use at home in conjunction with her exercises. By keeping a record of her progress, she was able to see clearly that her efforts were succeeding. This instrument, the perineometer, is described later. Unfortunately, it is not always accurate and can also discourage a patient if she believes she is progressing too slowly. It is possible to get a false reading unless the perineometer is used with care. Nevertheless, it has provided some women with the visual translation of effort necessary to their continuing belief in the efficacy of the exercises.

Kegel developed his special exercises to remedy urinary incontinence. To his amazement, his female patients not only achieved control of their bladder, but also began to report their first experiences of orgasm during intercourse. Women who had been unable to retain a contraceptive diaphragm could now do so. Others reported greater ease in childbirth, less pain, and simpler deliveries requiring fewer drugs.[10]

Nor was Kegel's success limited to women of childbearing age. He reports the case of a 61-year-old woman with second degree genital relaxation, cystocele, rectocele, and moderate senile atrophy.[8] She had had urinary stress incontinence for 4 years. An operation 6 months before she came to Kegel had not alleviated her condition. Measurement of her contractile strength by perineometer gave a reading of practically zero. She was instructed to exercise (using the perineometer) for three 20-minute periods a day. At the end of 2 weeks, her condition had greatly improved. After 3 weeks, she was remaining dry, and after the fourth week, she was able to discontinue all cognitive exericse.* Two years later, she showed no sign of recurrence.

By 1949, Kegel had successfully treated hundreds of women, from 26 to 79 years of age.[8] He was able to group his typical cases into urinary stress incontinence, poor tone and function of the genital muscles during the childbearing years, persistent postpartum relaxation of the genital muscles, and postmenopausal atrophy of the perivaginal muscles.[8]

By 1952, he had established that supportive function of the pelvic muscles was acquired about the time a child begins to stand and walk, and voluntary control of the bladder is a reflex acquired through childhood training. Sexual perception centered in the perivaginal tissues is also an acquired function. While some individuals may establish these functions readily, others may have great difficulty, may never gain control of the reflexes, or may be subject to loss of control and perception because of various influences such as childbirth, surgery, or menopause.[10] He also concluded that the P.C. muscle functions are rarely lost, only weakened or injured, and that "every case of genital relaxation, whether early or late, is benefited by physiologic therapy. . . ."[7]

Generally, a patient passed through four phases of restoration:[10]

Phase 1: Reestablishment of awareness of function and coordination

Phase 2: Transition period of exercise with no clear improvement

Phase 3: Regeneration period, with gradual restoration of resistance to satisfactory level

Phase 4: (If the patient wished to continue beyond Phase 3) A marked and steady increase to very high levels of control and muscular resistance

Whether the patient stopped after Phase 3 or continued through Phase 4, the tonus and control established were self-maintaining, unless interrupted by further birth traumas or surgery. Even then, damage was likely to be slight and easily overcome with a regimen of exercise.

Today, 30 years after Kegel began to publish his findings, his theories are just beginning to filter down to the lay public and a wider range of the helping professions. His exercises, called *kegeling*, are included in most popular manuals on feminine sexual response[1,4] and natural childbirth methodology.[3,12]

Thanks to the research of Kegel and others, we are now able to confirm genital relaxation and to provide instruction in exercises that will bring relief. A woman can, in fact, learn to explore and evaluate her own P.C. muscle and to teach herself the exercise routine. Both *Our Bodies, Ourselves*[2] and *The Well Body Book*[13] describe adequate self-examination techniques that will enlighten a woman about much of her bodily functions and state of health. They are

---

*Kegel makes the point in several of his studies that once the P.C. muscle is restored to normal function, the daily contractions that contribute to sphincteric action become almost involuntary and self-mobilizing. As long as no further damage is imposed, this is sufficient to maintain muscle contractile strength without conscious effort or exercise.

analogous to the breast examination women are urged to perform each month.

However, the thorough pelvic examination described must be made by medical personnel and should be considered mandatory annually for every woman of childbearing age or older. Genital relaxation may be a result solely of weakened pelvic musculature. But other conditions of the genitourinary system may also be present, contributing to complications that cannot be detected by the lay person.

THE PELVIC EXAMINATION

Diagnosis of the degree of genital relaxation is made by a thorough pelvic examination. Since almost any abnormality of the genitals can contribute to a loss of muscle control or sexual response or to painful labor, the entire genitourinary area should be carefully inspected for signs of infection, scars, herniations, benign tumors, and cancer. The exterior genitals should be evaluated for healthy color and absence or presence of surgical scars (particularly episiotomy scars) and their extent, location, and quantity. The clitoris and prepuce should be examined for possible adhesions. The presence of hemorrhoids, unusual pressures during pregnancy, or the patient's habit of "bearing down" because of constipation may signal inadequate control of the P.C. muscle. If the entry to the vagina is a "gaping introitus" two or three fingers wide, there is clearly a problem.

The internal examination is twofold: speculum and digital. The speculum will open the vagina for unhindered inspection of the vagina walls, cervical area, and pocket of the fornix where the vagina terminates. However, it may obscure the evidences of a sagging P.C. muscle. This must be searched for both digitally and visually. Kegel cautions that at this point only one finger should be used, since two or more will distort the shape of the vaginal canal and can even temporarily displace organs.[5] The false data will result in erroneous evaluation.

The internal examination should include a Pap smear for cancer and palpation of the uterus, bladder, rectum, and ovaries between the inserted fingers and the examiner's other hand as it exerts gentle pressure on the exterior abdominal wall. A partial examination limited to evaluation of muscular contraction should never be considered adequate if the woman has not had a total examination in the current year. Until the health of the entire genital region is evaluated, an optimal evaluation of the P.C. muscle cannot be made.

The pelvic examination begins with inspection of the external organs: labia majora and labia minora, vaginal introitus, remains of the hymen, perineum, urinary meatus, prepuce (a fold of tissue also known as the clitoral hood), and clitoris (Fig. 14-2). Signs of infection or abnormality should be looked for. It is particularly important to ascertain whether the prepuce is adhered to the clitoris, which, rather than a lax P.C. muscle, may be the cause of diminished sexual sensation.

Before proceeding with the internal examination, the episiotomy scar should be carefully evaluated. Has the incision been made at the midline through the perineum, or is it a mediolateral incision slanting across the area in a diagonal toward the thigh? How many scars are there? Is there an unusual aggregation of scar tissue? Are the labia firm and pink to brown, free of ulcerations, rash, or other abnormalities?

A speculum is then inserted into the vagina to facilitate visualization of the cervix and vaginal walls. The cervix should have a healthy pink color, and there should be no evidence of infection or undue discharge from the opening. Since the vagina is nor-

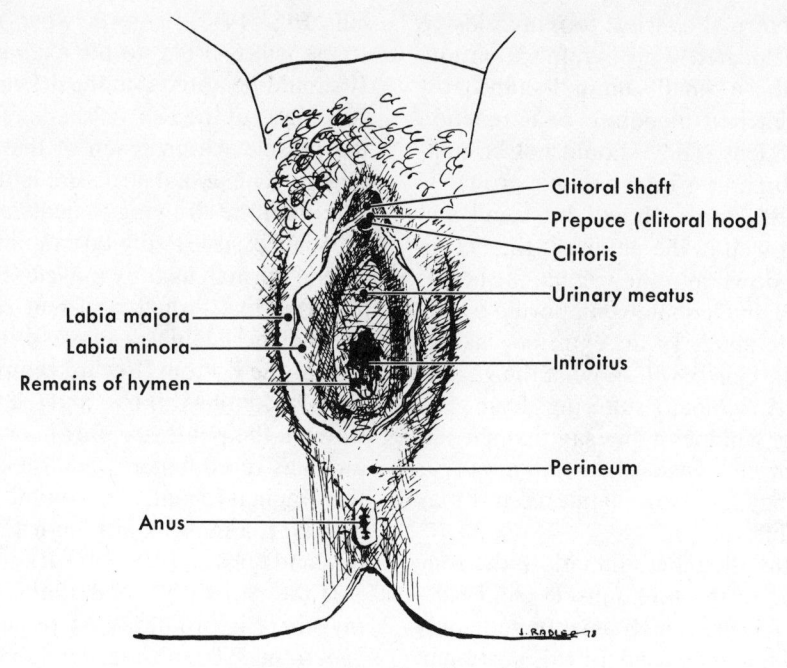

Fig. 14-2. External female genitalia.

mally self-cleaning, a strong, unpleasant odor may warn of infection or fungus.

If the cervical opening is shaped like a tiny circle, it may indicate that the woman is nulliparous (has never had a baby). The cervix of a multiparous woman, one who has had several children, will usually have an irregular opening or one that resembles a horizontal fissure. If the woman has had a cesarean section, the appearance of the cervix will most likely approximate that of the nulliparous woman.

As the speculum is partially removed, the patient is instructed to cough. A pouching or relaxation of the rectum into the vaginal walls could indicate a rectocele (herniation of the rectum into the vagina); a pouching of the bladder may be a cystocele (herniation of the bladder). When herniation occurs, the bowel or bladder may be unable to empty completely, causing feelings of fullness or irritation. Intercourse or labor may be painful. If either condition is severe, frequent infection is likely.

The digital examination is the more revealing in terms of genital relaxation, weakly developed abdominal musculature, and abnormal positioning of the uterus. It also reveals very early tendencies toward herniation that can elude the visual examination.

The examiner's gloved and lubricated fingers are gently inserted into the vagina, while the other hand probes and palpates the lower quadrants of the external abdomen. The organs thus felt between both hands can be fairly accurately evaluated for size, placement within the abdominal cavity, and extreme tenderness indicating infection or growths. Unusual masses are readily identified. Unless there is an infection, the fallopian tubes will probably escape detection. Normal ovaries, too, are elusive but can be located with careful attention. Touching these small, almond-shaped organs may elicit a moderate pain reaction from the patient. They should not be unusually painful unless infection or a growth is present. The uterus should be small and firm, sitting well in the pelvis. If the cervix has sagged down into the vagina, the uterus is prolapsed, inadequately supported by the P.C. muscle sling. In an extreme case of prolapse, the cervix will show at the vaginal introitus. A woman suffering from this abnormality will inevitably say that she has feelings that her "insides are falling out" — as indeed they are. Normal intercourse may be impossible.

During the digital examination, the tone and position of the P.C. muscle can be determined. As previously mentioned, only one finger should be used for this portion of the examination. In addition to any indirect indications of poor tone, such as the herniations described or a widely gaping vagina, the muscle can be felt by pushing laterally against the walls of the middle third of the vagina, that is, about one inch into the canal. Fig. 14-3 suggests what the muscle shape will feel like to the examining finger. It should be noted that the drawing is only a schematic of the *sensed* shape of the part of the muscle within reach of the examiner's fingers. The actual structure is more extensive than the drawing indicates. Parts of it are inaccessible to digital examination.

The normal, healthy muscle (Fig. 14-3,*A*) will feel like a thick and taut rubber band around the vaginal walls, and the broadest part at the bottom (toward the rectum), the sides becoming thinner, and the top tapered (toward the pubic area). It may measure as much as three fingers wide on each side of the vaginal canal. In genital relaxation, however, a muscle with poor tone will feel thin and fibrous. (Fig. 14-3,*B*).

If the patient has had a midline episiotomy, there is ordinarily no permanent damage to the P.C. muscle. There may, however, be a temporary loss of strength and control. But if the patient has had a mediolateral episiotomy, the muscle will have been included in the incision and the examining finger will feel a deep scar and a dip (Fig. 14-3,*C*), which are permanent.

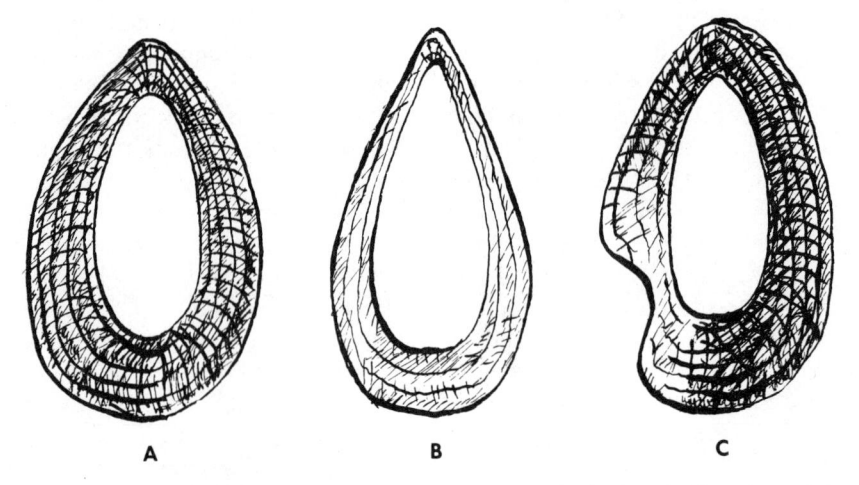

Fig. 14-3. Shape of pubococcygeus muscle as sensed by intravaginal palpation. **A,** Normal muscle in good tone. **B,** Poor, fibrous muscle. **C,** Muscle scarred by mediolateral episiotomy.

To complete the examination, one finger is again inserted about one inch into the vagina. Starting at the point on the vaginal wall nearest the rectum, the examiner's finger traces the circumference of the vagina clockwise in a series of short movements. As the finger stops at each position, the patient is instructed to contract and relax the muscle. This procedure should not be painful. Pain in any sector usually indicates a poor, fibrous portion.

Testing the strength of the contraction can be facilitated by the use of a perineometer (Fig. 14-4). This instrument was developed by Kegel to serve as a "medium between the sense of sight and the training of the perivaginal muscle."[8] The perineometer can be used as a training device for the resistive exercises, but begins service as a diagnostic evaluator of the patient's ability to control the P.C. muscle.

The perineometer is a long, truncated cone of rubber stretched over a rigid core that is flanged at both ends. At the base of the cone is a circular rubber shield about 3 inches in diameter that can be grasped to insert the cone in the vagina and pivoted for correct positioning. The core of the instrument is connected by rubber tubing to a simple pressure gauge measuring pressure equivalents of 0 to 100 mm Hg.[9] When the vaginal apparatus is in position, the patient is asked to contract her P.C. muscle. Strength of the contraction is read on the

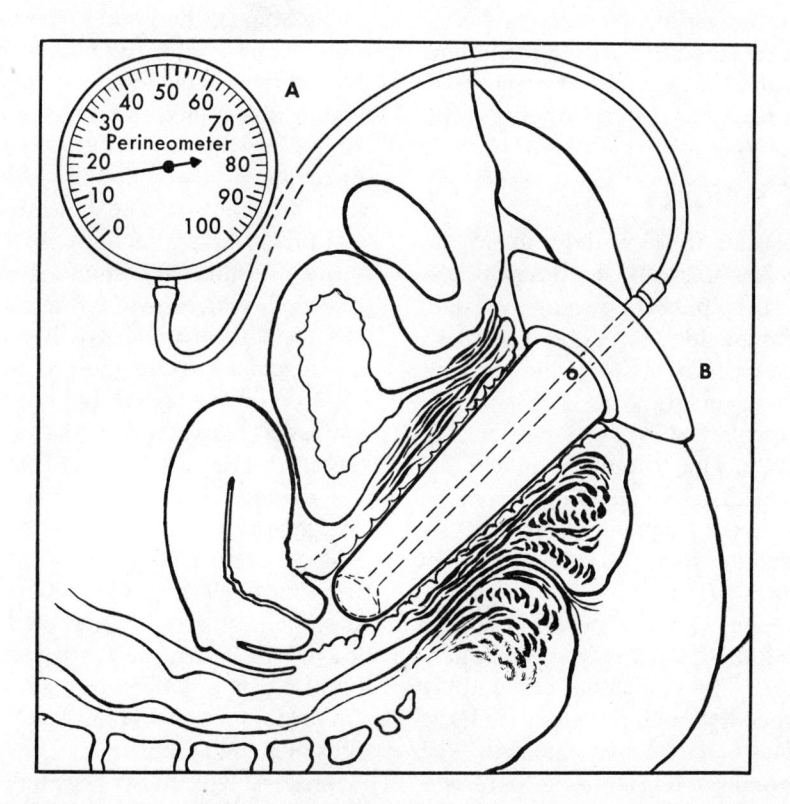

Fig. 14-4. Diagram of perineometer properly positioned. (From Kegel, A.: Progressive resistance exercise in the functional restoration of the perineal muscles, Am. J. Obstet. Gynecol. **56** (2):243, 1948.)

dial. A patient who is unaware of the muscle or who has very poor tone may only register from 0 to 15 mm Hg.

The perineometer can be useful in trained hands. However, on insertion the tubing could collapse and give an inaccurate reading. If the practitioner has not been taught to distinguish between a 1 to 10 mm reading resulting from a failed perineometer and a 1 to 10 reading resulting from the patient's inability to contract the muscle, an erroneous evaluation can be made. The qualitative digital examination is more reliable than dependence on the quantitative perineometer measurement.

When the pelvic examination has been completed and the patient's degree of muscle control evaluated, she will be given instructions in the series of exercises developed by Kegel to restore the function and elasticity of the P.C. muscle. Prompt treatment of any pathology should, of course, be started.

THE KEGEL EXERCISES

It is important to know how to do the Kegel exercises correctly to develop and strengthen the pubococcygeus muscle. Exercises can be done throughout the day: in the morning before arising, while driving the car, standing in line at the grocery store, talking on the telephone, and particularly while urinating. They should be done while lying down, sitting, and standing. Improvement occurs most frequently when the patient consistently does 100 or more Kegel contractions a day.

For someone who has never done the exercises before, the first step is the fluttering technique. The vagina is very quickly squeezed together and released, and the patient is instructed to continue until she feels a pronounced sensation of "contracting" in the vagina. For some, it may take several days to achieve this sensation, and the patient will need to be encouraged to continue. The novice may achieve Step 1 results more easily when lying down or sitting.

When she has felt the vagina contracting, the patient is ready for Step 2. She should place her hands on the lower part of the abdomen, just above her pubic bone, to feel whether the abdominal muscles move. When she has learned to keep the abdominal muscles immobile, she should cup her buttocks during a round of exercises to check that they, too, are not contracting. If any of these muscles become involved, the exercise is probably being done incorrectly. Not only will the woman tire easily and become sore or irritated, but the P.C. muscle is not being exercised and will not strengthen.

For Step 2, the patient stands with legs slightly apart and envisions drawing the sides of the vagina together. Starting at the rectum, she should slowly squeeze up, as if pulling up on a string, then continue squeezing up through the vagina and toward the clitoris. The tension should be held for at least 3 seconds. Just before relaxing the hold, she should try a "power squeeze," which is an extra hard contraction, then she should slowly relax, letting the imaginary string loosen, and taking a full 3 seconds to reach full relaxation. The controlled relaxing is as vital a part of the exercise as the contracting. It is imperative that a woman learn to relax the muscle during pregnancy to prepare for childbirth.

Steps 1 and 2 should be done five to ten times each session. The patient should be cautioned not to "push out" or "bear down," as when defecating or urinating forcefully, at any time during the exercises. This would inevitably aggravate the symptoms of genital relaxation.

Because women with genital relaxation frequently leak urine when they laugh or cough, learning how to stop the flow of urine is important. The anterior segment of the muscle nearest the bladder is usually the weakest and has often been damaged by the pressures exerted during pregnancy and birth. Step 3 should be practiced at each urination.

1. Sit on toilet with legs apart.
2. Begin to urinate and contract the muscle to stop the flow.
3. Allow some urine to pass and then contract again.

The contraction should close off the flow of urine, but may not be achieved completely in the beginning. When the goal of urinating 4 to 5 cc at a time has been attained, however, the pants-wetting symptoms will disappear.

It is not uncommon for a woman to feel sexually stimulated while doing the exercises. She should be advised that this may happen and is perfectly normal. Explaining to her that restoring the muscle to normal tone and health may very likely improve her sexual gratification is, in fact, a powerful motivator for patient adherence to the exercise routine.

The patient can check her progress in one of several ways. She can insert a finger in her vagina while practicing. In succeeding weeks of exercises, she will become aware of gradually increasing strength. A second effective evaluator is the woman's mate, whose subjective reaction during intercourse can provide perhaps the most encouraging test of improvement. The third method, particularly useful for women who are shy about touching themselves or not involved in a sexual relationship, is urination control described previously. Regarding the perineometer, it should be remembered that anyone interested in using it as an aid in the pelvic examination and evaluation would need training. Furthermore, the perineometer is quite an expensive investment for the patient, and the daily readings can cause her unnecessary discouragement if she believes that they are lower than some arbitrary numerical goal she has set for herself.

Foremost in the regimen is encouragement. The process of bringing the P.C. muscle to full function may require only a few weeks of exercise; but at times a woman with unusually extensive damage or total unawareness of function can need several months to reach her goal. Her mentor should watch for signs of discouragement or anxiety when improvement seems to come slowly.

In our own NACHIS/Natural Childbirth Institute, we have used the exercises as a teaching tool for pregnant clients and for women with gynecologic complaints such as those discussed. The positive results have demonstrated the successful application of the technique, particularly in two types of cases: (1) multiparous women who have reported their birth experience much improved over earlier deliveries, with fewer episiotomies and birth traumas and quick recovery of muscle tone after delivery, and (2) women with urinary stress incontinence as their chief complaint, whose improvement is sufficient to preclude formerly recommended surgical repair.

We are also convinced that primiparous women experience their first deliveries with greater ease and a shorter second state of labor then women who have not done the exercises during pregnancy. However, this conviction is the result of observation, not a controlled study. Nevertheless, the evidence is clear and positive. The function of the pubococcygeus muscle is rarely lost, only weakened or injured,[7] and women of all ages should be urged to practice the Kegel exercises.

SUMMARY

The pubococcygeus muscle, one of the five great muscle groups in the pelvic region, has been shown to be the major support of the pelvic organs and to provide necessary sphincteric action. The research of Kegel proved the important role of the pubococcygeus muscle and the restorative powers of exercises to counteract genital relaxation resulting from an underdeveloped, lax, or damaged muscle. A thorough pelvic examination of external and internal genitalia is necessary to evaluate the condition of the pubococcygeus muscle and any contributory pathology that might be causing urinary stress incontinence, lack of sexual response, painful and prolonged labor, or pelvic discomfort such as "falling out" sensations. If the muscle is in poor tone or damaged, the disorders yield to a dedicated regimen of exercise that restores function within a reasonable time and lessens or dispenses entirely with the need for surgical repair.

REFERENCES

1. Barbach, L. G.: For yourself: the fulfillment of female sexuality, Garden City, N.Y., 1976, Doubleday & Co., Inc.
2. The Boston Women's Health Book Collective: Our bodies, ourselves, ed. 2, New York, 1976, Simon & Schuster, Inc.
3. Bradley, R. A.: Husband-coached childbirth, New York, 1974, Harper & Row, Publishers.
4. Deutsch, R. M.: The key to feminine response in marriage, New York, 1968, Ballantine Books, Inc.
5. Kegel, A. H.: Early genital relaxation, Obstet. Gynecol. 8(5):545-550, 1955.
6. Kegel, A. H.: The nonsurgical treatment of genital relaxation, Ann. West. Med. Surg. 2(5):213-216, 1948.
7. Kegel, A. H.: Pathologic physiology of the pubococcygeus muscle in women (film).
8. Kegel, A. H.: The physiologic treatment of poor tone and function of the genital muscles and of urinary stress incontinence, West. J. Surg. Obstet. Gynecol., pp. 527-535, November 1949.
9. Kegel, A. H.: Progressive resistance exercise in the functional restoration of the perineal muscles, Am. J. Obstet. Gynecol. 56(2):238-248, 1948.
10. Kegel, A. H.: Sexual functions of the pubococcygeus muscle, West. J. Surg. Obstet. Gynecol. pp. 521-524, October 1952.
11. Kegel, A. H., and Powell, T. O.: The physiologic treatment of urinary stress incontinence, J. Urol. 63(5):808-813, 1950.
12. Lamaze, F.: Painless childbirth: psychoprophylactic method, New York, 1972, Simon & Schuster, Inc.
13. Samuels, M., and Bennett, H.: The well body book, New York, 1973, Random House, Inc.

BIBLIOGRAPHY

Brecher, R., and Brecher, E.: Sex during and after pregnancy. In Brecher, R., and Brecher, E., editors: An analysis of human sexual response, New York, 1966, The New American Library, Inc.

Chesler, P.: Women and madness, New York, 1972 Avon Books.

Comfort, A., editor: The joy of sex, New York, 1972, Crown Publishers. Inc.

"J": The sensuous woman, New York, 1969, Dell Publishing Co., Inc.

Kegel, A.: Physiologic therapy for urinary stress incontinence, J.A.M.A. 146:915-917, 1951.

Kegel, A.: Physiologic therapy for urinary stress incontinence. In Carter, B. N., editor: Monographs on surgery, Baltimore, 1952, The Williams & Wilkins. Co.

Kegel, A.: Stress incontinence of urine in women: physiologic treatment, J. Int. Coll. Surg. XXV:487-499, 1956.

Klein-Graber, G., and Graber, B.: The use of the pubococcygeus exercise to improve vaginal sensation, pelvic examination, from personal interviews, 1974-1975.

Klein-Graber, G., and Graber, B.: Woman's orgasm, New York, 1975, Popular Library.

Solberg, D. A., Butler, J., and Wagner, N. N.: Sexual behavior and pregnancy, N. Eng. J. Med. 288(21): 1098-1103, 1973.

Wharton, L.: The non-operative treatment of stress incontinence in women, J. Urol 69(4):511-519, 1953.

CHAPTER 15

Real-time ultrasound in obstetrics and gynecology

Louise Sipos, Lawrence D. Platt, and Frank A. Manning

This chapter will present a general introduction to the principles of ultrasound, the types of instruments used for scanning (with emphasis on the real-time B-scan [RTBS]), techniques of scanning, applications of ultrasound in obstetrics and gynecology, and the nursing responsibilities applicable to the use of ultrasound.

PRINCIPLES

When using equipment in any field of medical practice, it is essential to have a basic understanding of the principles relating to the functioning of that equipment so that it will be used safely and efficiently for the optimum benefit to both the operator and the patient. This is certainly important in the medical application of ultrasound to obtain accurate interpretations from the information provided and to fully understand the limitations of its applications. For that reason, a brief discussion of the principles of ultrasound follows.

Sound is defined as a mechanical vibration that is propagated through matter. The speed at which sound travels, its velocity, is a function of the properties of the material through which the sound passes and is independent of the manner in which the sound was produced. The more rigid the material, the greater the sound velocity. This principle of sound velocity holds true for various tissues of the body. The more rigid the tissue, for example, bone, the greater the sound velocity.

The molecular vibration, that is, sound, produces two types of waves—transverse and longitudinal. Transverse sound waves occur when molecular excitation occurs at right angles to the direction of propagation. Only solids can support transverse waves. Longitudinal sound waves occur when molecules vibrate to and fro in the same direction as the propagation of energy. All materials can support longitudinal waves. With the exception of bone, all the tissues of the body behave acoustically as though they were fluids. Consequently, longitudinal waves are predominant in medical applications.

As sound travels, it causes areas of unequal intermolecular spacing, which in turn cause variation in pressure since pressure is proportional to molecular concentration. The distance from one pressure peak to another is the wavelength of a sound wave.

The wavelength is important because it determines the theoretical limit of resolution (the ability to differentiate two separate structures). Under no circumstances are structures that are closer than one wavelength identifiable as two distinct entities. Therefore, ultrasound is unable to distinguish individual cells or the component layers of membranes. However, gross anatomic structures and their boundaries are well within the resolving capability of diagnostic ultrasound.

The frequency of a sound wave is defined as the number of peaks of the associated pressure wave that pass a given point in 1 second. The unit of measurement for frequency is the *hertz* (Hz). The human ear is sensitive to sonic frequencies from 16 to 20,000 Hz. Ultrasound has a frequency range that is greater than 20,000 Hz.

The choice of frequency used in any medical application is a compromise between resolving capability and penetration. The higher the frequency, the more rapidly the sound is absorbed and the smaller the distance it can penetrate into tissue. The lower the frequency, the poorer the resolving capability. In obstetrics and gynecology, the frequency used is generally equal to 2 to 5 million Hz, or 2 to 5 megahertz (MHz).

Ultrasound is produced through the use of piezoelectric crystals. These crystals respond to applied electrical signals at high frequencies to produce ultrasonic waves, and they are likewise able to accurately convert ultrasound waves into corresponding electronic signals. For medical uses, these crystals are cut wafer thin and mounted in a casing, the *transducer*. Transducers are made in a variety of shapes and sizes designed for their particular application. For example, transducers used with the linear array RTBS are oblong, and the transducer for the Doppler method is pencil shaped. The function of the transducer depends on electronic circuitry to: (1) stimulate the initiation of the ultrasonic pulse, (2) receive the returning echoes, and (3) process these echoes electronically for visual display.

Currently two types of ultrasound are being used for diagnostic purposes — continuous wave Doppler and pulsed ultrasound. The continuous wave form of energy is based on the Doppler effect — frequency of sound when reflected from a moving object will vary with the velocity of the object. Different types of sound patterns are discernible from different tissue interfaces. Therefore Doppler instruments are used in obstetrics to detect and monitor fetal heart activity. The pulsed ultrasound or "pulse-echo" system has a transducer that will transmit 0.1% of the time and listen 99.9% of the time. It therefore functions in two ways — transmits and then receives reflected echoes.

Reflected ultrasound signals can be displayed in a variety of ways. Briefly, the displays used in obstetrics and gynecology are:

1. Doppler — for detection of fetal heart. The Doppler produces an audio signal.
2. B-scan — for imaging of abdominal and pelvic organs, masses, and tumors. In this mode, echoes from within the body are converted to illuminated dots and recorded in a two-dimensional, cross-sectional representation of anatomic structures.
3. RTBS — for imaging abdominal and pelvic organs, masses, and tumors. Like the B-scan echoes are converted to illuminated dots that produce motion picture — like images of the two-dimensional, cross-sectional representation of anatomic structures.

TECHNIQUE OF SCANNING

The patient lies on her back with the abdomen exposed. Mineral oil or an aqueous gel is used to coat the abdomen to eliminate air between the transducer surface and the skin. When the B-scan mode is being used, the operator holds the transducer and slides it across the abdominal skin. As the transducer moves, lines of bright dots representing the echoes from the ultrasound beam appear on a display screen. The operator continues to sweep the transducer across the abdomen until a satisfactory picture is built up and a polaroid picture of the display screen is taken for a permanent record. Scans are repeated at 1- to 2-cm intervals both longitudinally and transversely. Each picture is a cross section in one thin plane necessitating multiple pictures to capture a composite that represents a three-dimensional structure.

In real-time scanning, the patient preparation is the same. Again the transducer is moved longitudinally, transversely, and at various angles across the abdomen. With real-time, an image is created rapidly enough to allow all the relevent motion in the organ being visualized to be presented. In this mode, the pictures presented on the display screen are two-dimensional moving pictures. To fully capture what is seen while scanning in this mode, videotaping of the display screen may be done. Polaroid pictures for such scans as biparietal diameters or placenta localization can also be taken from the real-time display screen for permanent records (Figs. 15-1 to 15-3).

RECORD KEEPING—NURSING RESPONSIBILITIES

Ultrasound scanning is becoming a frequently used diagnostic tool in the areas of gynecology and especially obstetrics. Along with this increased use comes the responsibility to thoroughly explain the procedure to the patient, advise her as to the safety of ultrasound, and what it can and cannot tell regarding diagnosis and fetal well-being.

For record keeping, and as a pattern for

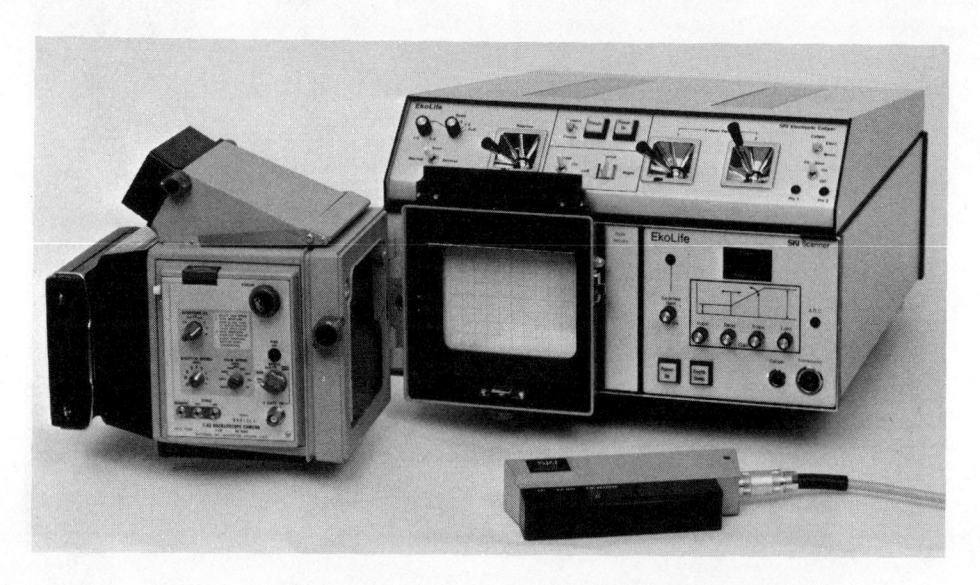

Fig. 15-1. Ekolife real-time ultrasound scanner. (Smith Kline Instruments, Inc.)

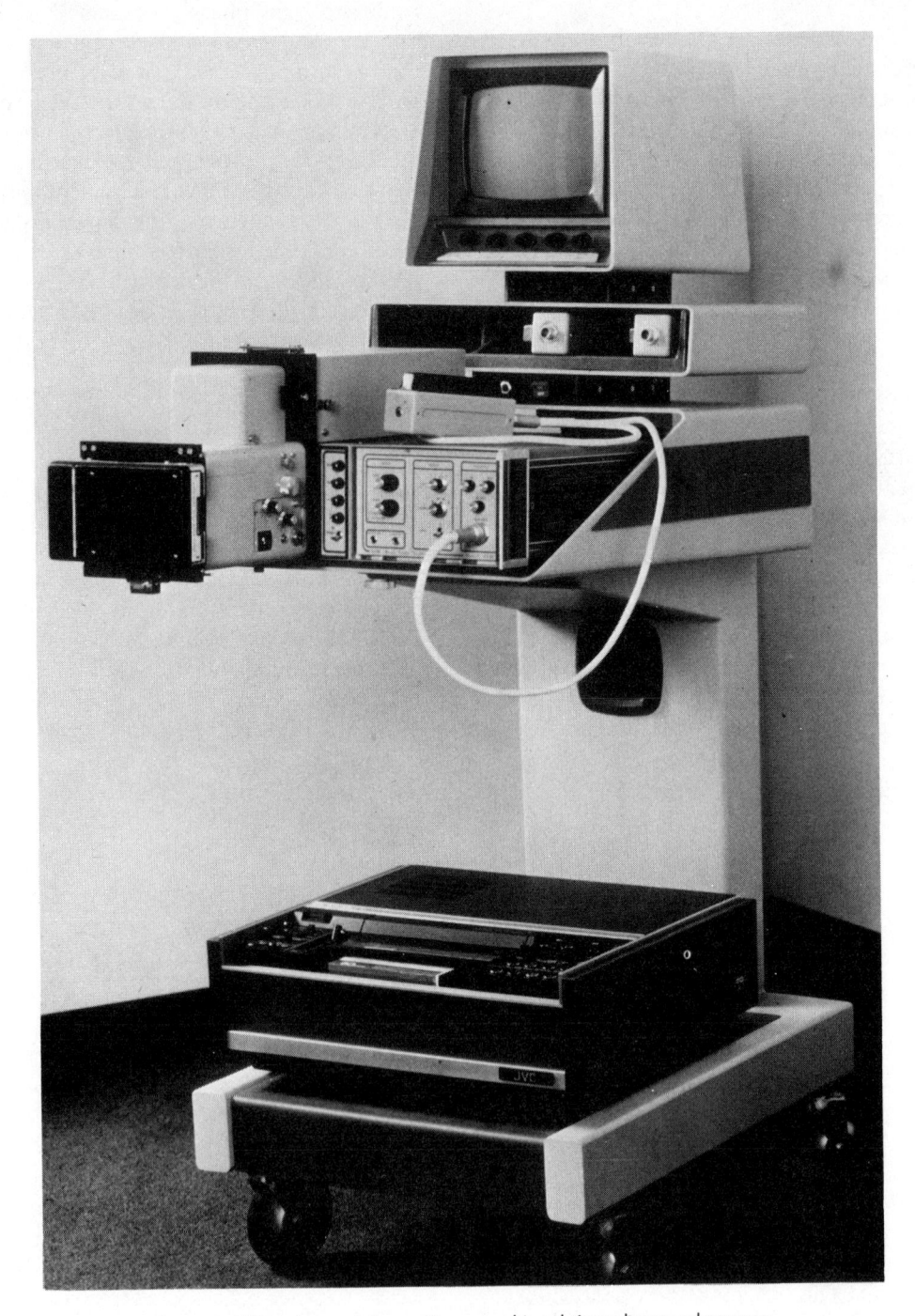

232 Selected Ob/Gyn problems and issues

Fig. 15-2. ADR (advanced diagnostic research) real-time ultrasound scanner.

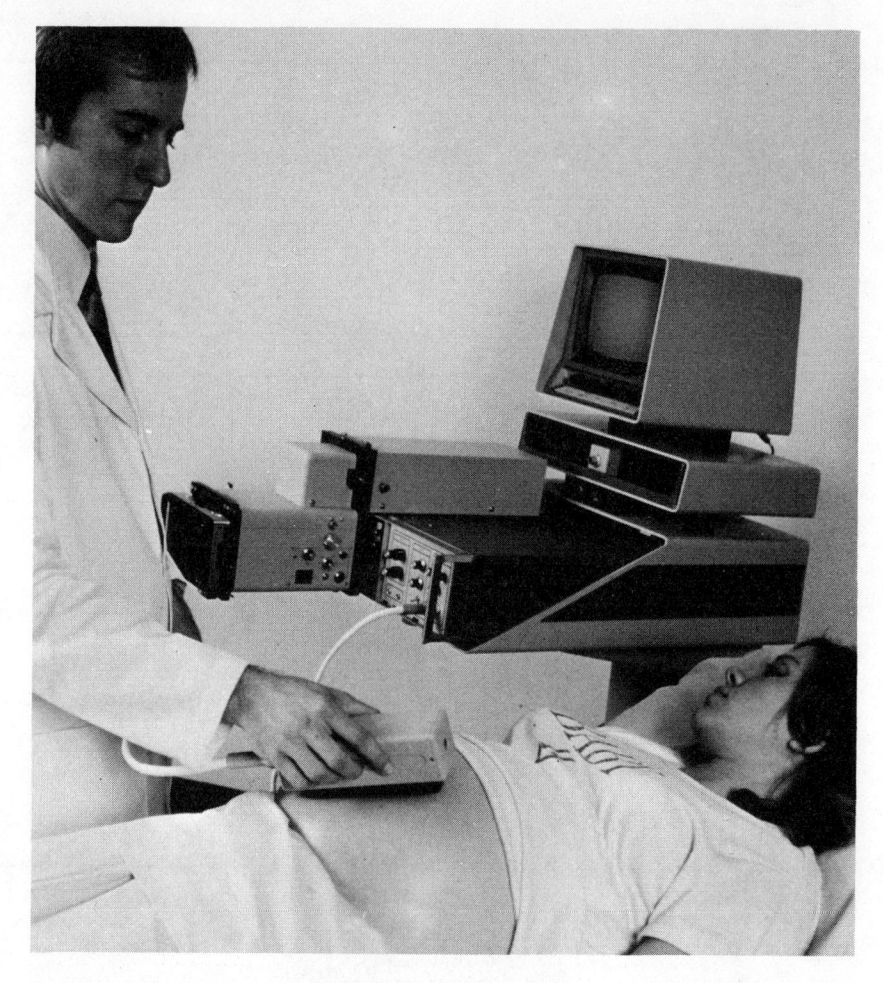

Fig. 15-3. Scanning with RTBS.

scanning, one can design and use a form that is a checklist on observations. Information included on such a checklist might include patient identification, reason for scanning, date, and what was observed. In the obstetric case, this might include more detailed information—gestational age at time of scan, location of the placenta, amniotic fluid volume, fetal position, biparietal diameter, fetal movement, details of fetal anatomy, and any other pertinent observations. These observations should be noted while scanning or immediately after so no detail is forgotten or overlooked (Fig. 15-4).

In addition to a written report, polaroid photographs should be taken as a permanent record of observation. For unusual cases and when equipment is available, videotaping of the scan is another form of record keeping. It is essential that the photographs and videotapes be accurately labeled and dated so that there is no confusion as to when and what patient was photographed.

234 Selected Ob/Gyn problems and issues

OB ULTRASOUND EXAM

Patient Name _____ Age _____ Date _____

Referring Physician _____ Exam No. _____ VTR _____

Exam Requested: Complete _____ BPD _____ PL _____ Other _____ Initial _____ Repeat _____

_____

_____

History: LMP _____ EDC _____ Fundal Hgt. _____ cm _____

_____

Comments: _____

_____

ANALYSIS

LIE	PRESENTATION	FETAL HEAD	
___ Longitudinal	___ Cephalic	___ LUS Above/Engaged	Biparietal Diameter _____ mm
___ Transverse	___ Breech	___ Corpus	Gestational Age _____ ± 2 weeks
___ Oblique	GESTATION	___ Fundus	Fetal Movement ___ Yes ___ No
	___ Multiple	___ Lateral R L	Cardiac Activity ___ Yes ___ No
	___ Single		

FETAL BODY

Location   Extremities
___ LUS   ___ LUS   R L
___ Corpus   ___ Corpus   R L
___ Fundus   ___ Fundus   R L

AMNIOTIC FLUID

___ Normal
___ Oligohydramnios
___ Polyhydramnios

PLACENTA

___ Anterior Wall
    ___ Right Lateral
    ___ Left Lateral
___ Posterior Wall
    ___ Right Lateral
    ___ Left Lateral
___ Upper Uterine Segment
___ Corpus
___ Lower Uterine Segment
___ Fundal
___ Previa
    ___ Marginal
    ___ Partial
    ___ Total

POSITION   PLACENTA LOCATION

Fig. 15-4. Sample of form used for record keeping of scans.

There are varying opinions as to whether a patient should be allowed to see the scan as it is being performed. The indication for scanning may influence this decision. When a mass, fetal anomaly, or fetal demise is suspected, one may be more comfortable if the patient does not see the scan. Even in these circumstances, however, the patient may desire to see for herself. In obstetric cases while scanning for location of placenta, crown-rump measurement, biparietal diameter, fetal position, and so forth, one may use this as an opportunity for patient teaching. Pointing out the placenta and umbilical cord and explaining their functions are generally of greater interest to the patient.

Recently there has been much discussion regarding the importance of early maternal-infant bonding. Listening to the fetal heart beat while at the physician's office and feeling the fetus move have been the only ways a mother could begin to relate to her baby. Now, through the use of real-time ultrasound, the fetus is no longer an unknown entity. A mother can see her baby moving about in her uterus and at times may even see the baby sucking its thumb. Through the use of real-time scanning, the maternal-infant bond is begun long before the baby is delivered. This is not an indication for ultrasound scanning, but it is one of the most pleasurable side benefits for the patient.

ULTRASOUND IN OBSTETRICS

Ultrasound scanning is a most widely used technique in obstetrics.[10,16] Ultrasonic beams penetrate fluids easily and are reflected from planes and surfaces within tissues. The fetus, a solid structure contained with the amniotic fluid sac, is easily and clearly imaged through ultrasound scanning (Fig. 15-5). There are a multitude of applications in both the normal and abnormal or high-risk pregnancy.

Fetal viability, fetal demise, missed abortion

When fetal heart sounds are unable to be detected with the use of the Doppler method and the mother does not feel fetal movement, real-time scanning can readily detect fetal movement and/or fetal cardiac motion to confirm viability. When a woman complains of decreasing or no fetal movement and fetal viability has been confirmed, it is helpful and reassuring to the mother to point out fetal movement while scanning and to observe her perception of these movements. When ruling out a fetal demise, one must not confuse passive movements of the fetus caused by maternal respiration or transmitted maternal aortic pulsation with active fetal movements.

When a pregnancy has been confirmed to be nonviable and the products of conception have not been expelled, the diagnosis of missed abortion can be made. Whereas biochemical pregnancy tests may remain positive for days after demise, real-time ultrasound will allow rapid and definitive diagnosis. In a series of 110 successive referrals to our service to rule out fetal demise (inaudible fetal heart tones, lack of uterine growth, and so forth), 44 of these fetuses (38%) were found to be viable and the pregnancies continued to term.[12]

Fetal position

In patients, such as the obese, in whom it is difficult to clinically determine the presentation of the fetus, ultrasound can make the diagnosis. One can readily determine whether the fetus is vertex, breech, or transverse. With increased expertise in scanning, one can develop the ability to diagnose the type of breech presentation. Differentiation of the incomplete breech from the complete breech is more difficult. Utilizing ultrasound in determining fetal

236 Selected Ob/Gyn problems and issues

Fetal body

Fetal head

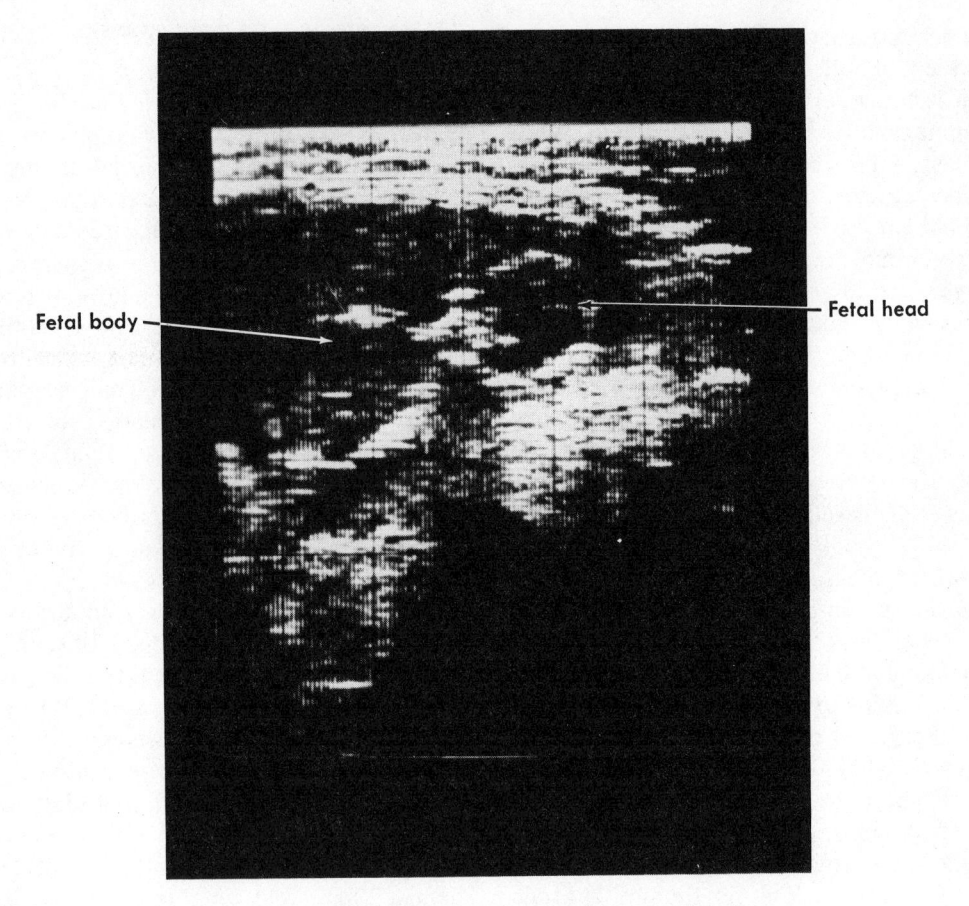

Fig. 15-5. Second trimester fetus.

position decreases the need for x-ray examination.

Multiple gestation

When multiple gestation is suspected, for example, in the patient who is large for dates, ultrasound scanning provides a rapid and accurate means of confirming or ruling out the diagnosis. In the singleton pregnancy, a single fetal head and thorax can be seen. In multiple pregnancy, with real-time scanning, two biparietal diameters can be determined and the transducer moved to trace the fetal thorax and cardiac motion in each of the fetuses (Fig. 15-6).

Gestational age

In determining gestational age, the crown-rump length measurement is most accurate in the gestation period from 8 to 12 weeks.[15] The fetus is very mobile at this time, which makes real-time scanning more useful for this measurement than static scanning. The crown-rump measurement is the longest demonstrable length of the fetus excluding the limbs (Fig. 15-7).

From 12 weeks on, the fetal head is more easily measured and the biparietal diameter (BPD) is then an excellent means for estimating gestational age.[10] The BPD is chosen because the diameter may be consis-

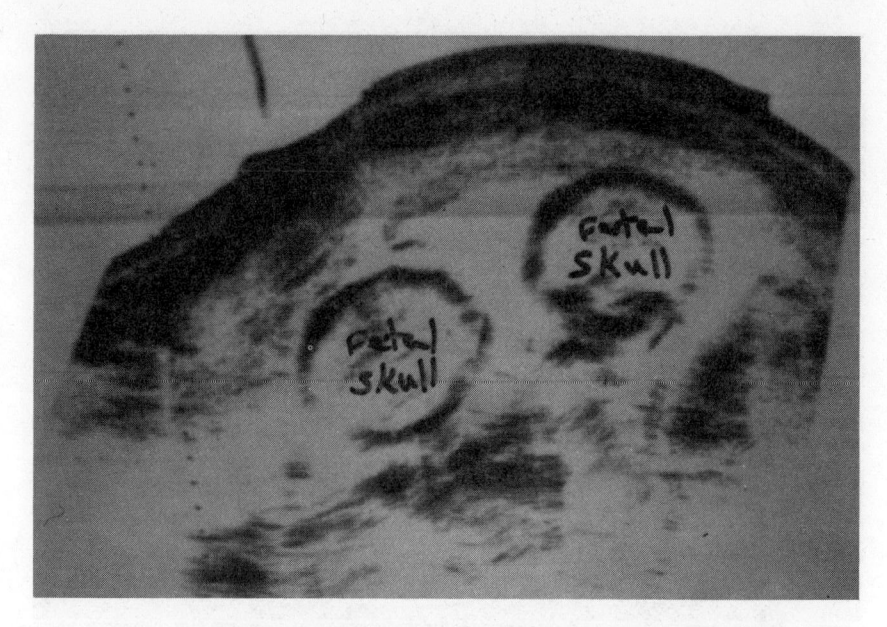

Fig. 15-6. Contact scan demonstrating twin gestation.

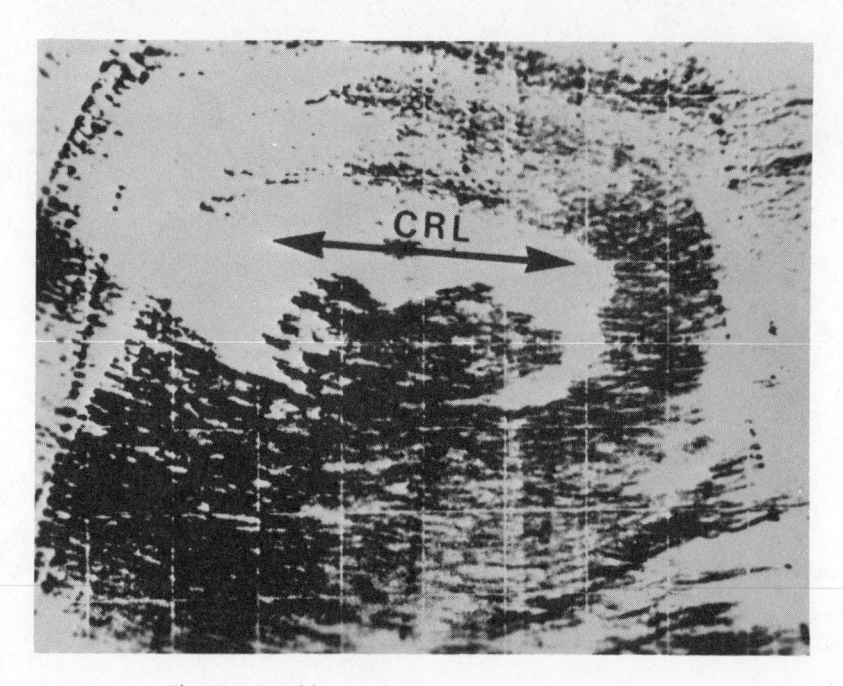

Fig. 15-7. Bistable scan demonstrating crown-rump length.

238 Selected Ob/Gyn problems and issues

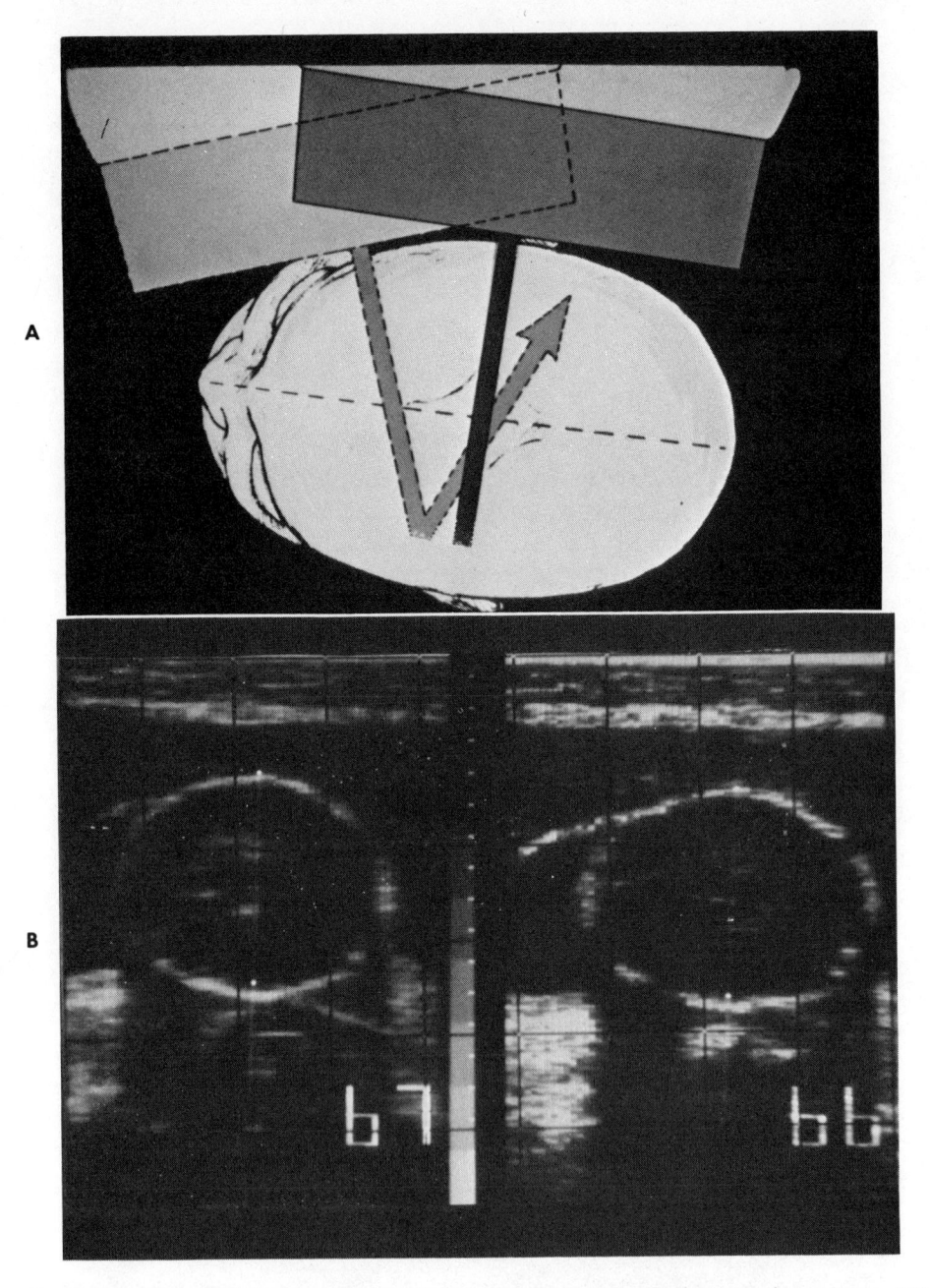

Fig. 15-8. A, Proper (dark line) and improper (light line) ways to obtain BPD. **B,** RTBS demonstrating BPD measurement.

tently identified in a given fetus and repeated measurements are therefore possible as pregnancy advances. The correlation between BPD and gestational age is closest during the second trimester.

The BPD requires skill and experience to obtain the correct axis and position of the sound beam through the fetal head. The correct plane is that which is perpendicular to the midline in the occipitofrontal axis and passes through the greatest biparietal diameter (Fig. 15-8, *A* and *B*). BPDs are helpful in diagnosing and following cases of intrauterine growth retardation (IUGR).[2]

In patients with suspected IUGR, the measurement of BPDs should begin in the second trimester. Growth retardation may be symmetrical, that is, the head and trunk are proportionate but are smaller than normal, or asymmetrical when the head size remains close to normal but the trunk is smaller. Measurements of both the BPD and abdominal circumferences are used in these cases.

Placenta localization

The placenta is readily located with both the static B-scan and the RTBS.[5,6] The pla-

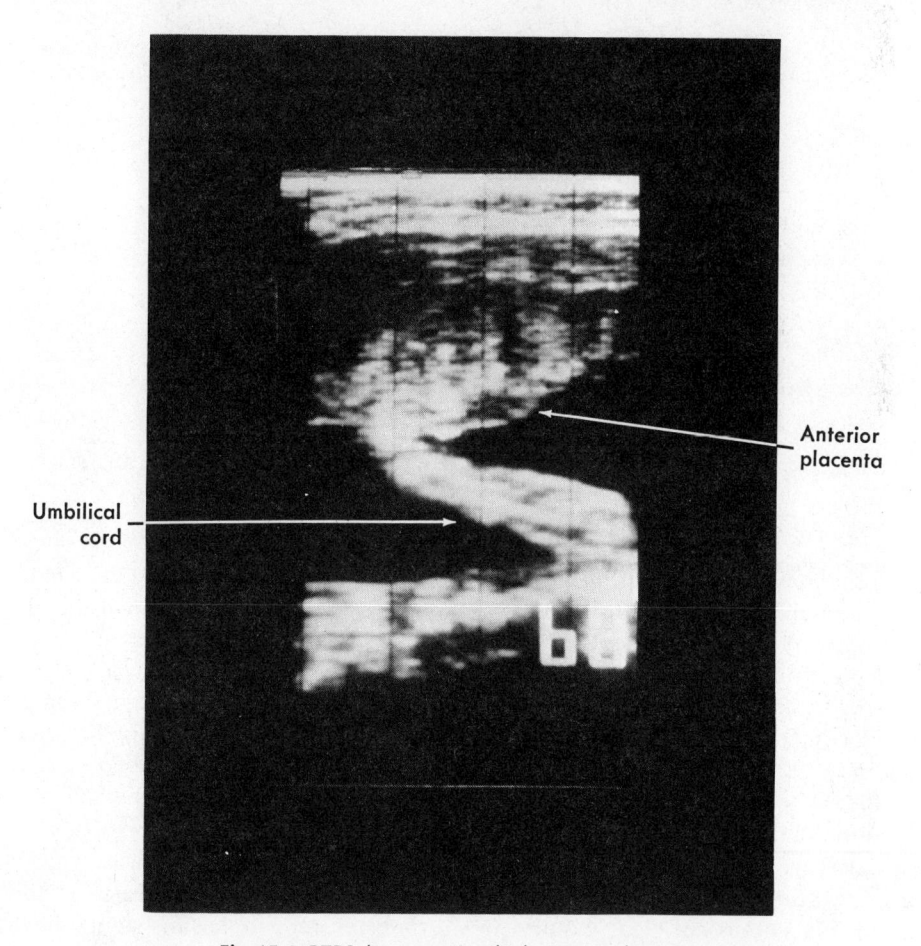

Fig. 15-9. RTBS demonstrating thick anterior placenta.

240 Selected Ob/Gyn problems and issues

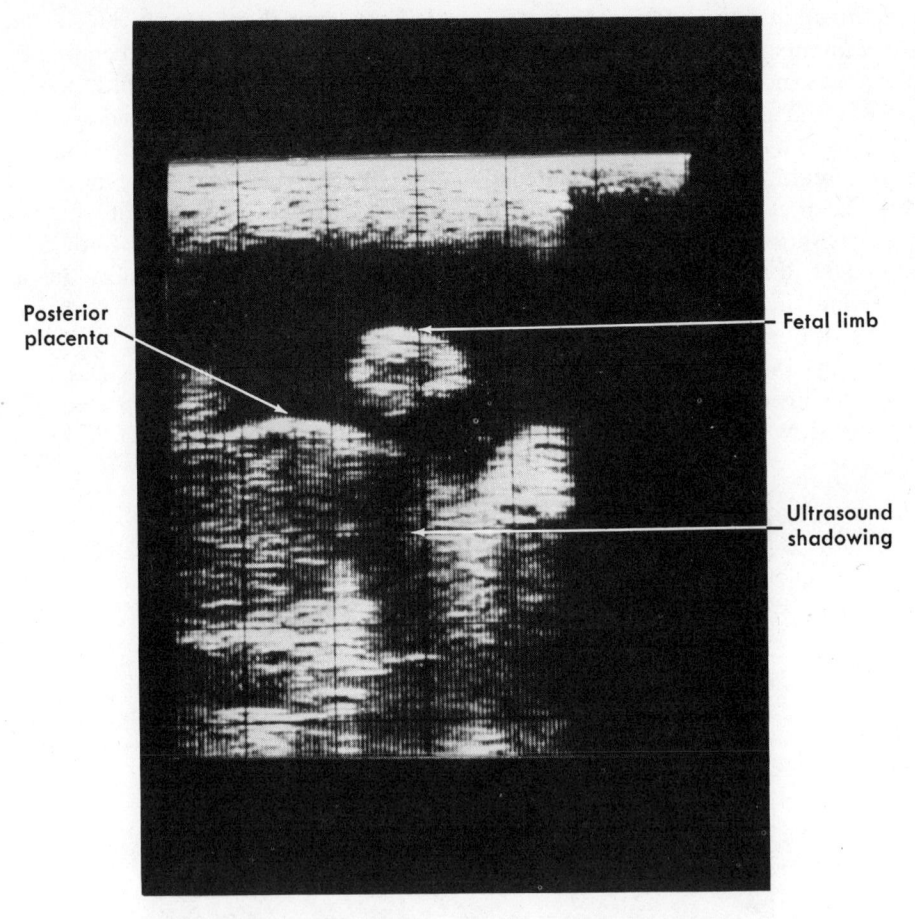

Fig. 15-10. RTBS of posterior placenta demonstrating ultrasound shadowing caused by fetal limb.

centa is relatively homogenous in texture until late in pregnancy (later than 36 weeks) and is outlined by the interface between the chorionic plate and amniotic fluid.[17] There is generally no difficulty in identifying the anterior placenta (Fig. 15-9). The posterior placenta may be more difficult to identify because the ultrasound beam may be attenuated by intervening fetal parts (ultrasound shadowing) (Fig. 15-10). When there is a decrease in the amount of amniotic fluid present, the placenta is not clearly outlined because of a lessening or absence of the interface between fluid and chorionic plate. When scanning for location of the placenta, the patient should have a full bladder so that a low-lying placenta can be differentiated from a placenta previa (Fig. 15-11). A full bladder aids in raising the uterus out of the pelvis toward the abdomen and also serves as an outline of the lower uterine segment.

When a placenta previa is diagnosed in the second trimester or early in the third trimester, repeated scans should be done at a later date since it is common that this

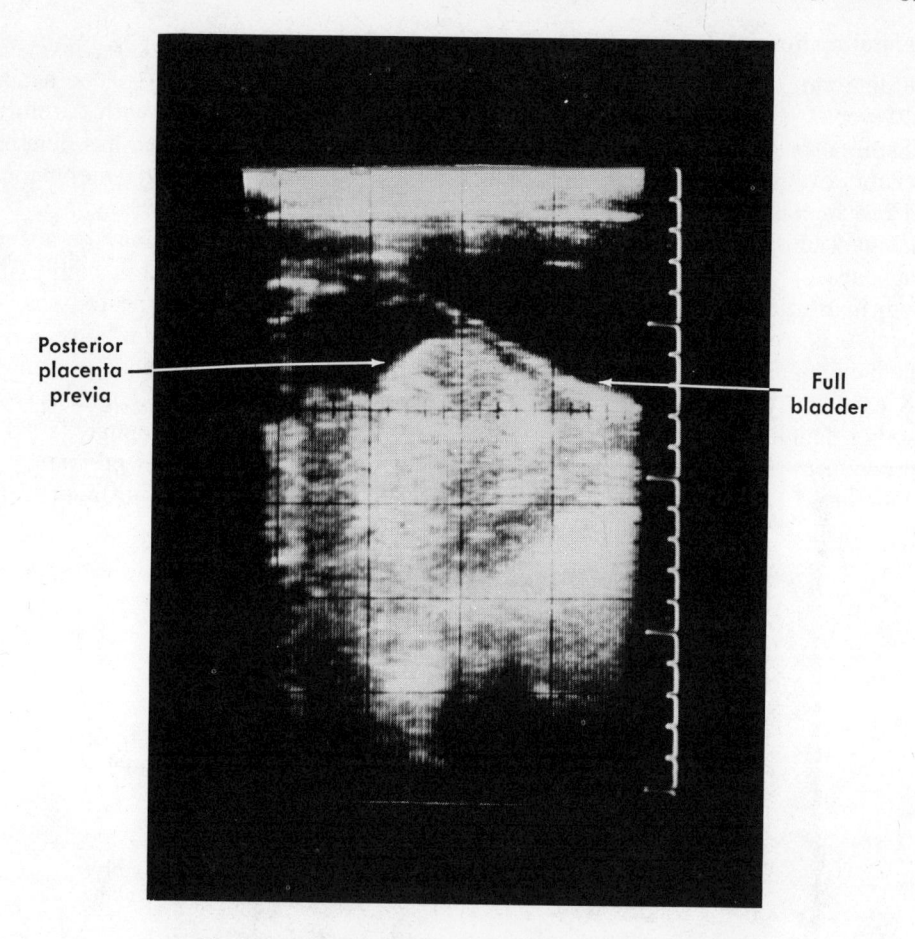

Fig. 15-11. RTBS demonstrating posterior placenta previa.

finding may change. This change in the position of the placenta may be caused by the lengthening of the lower uterine segment, with displacement away from the cervix as pregnancy progresses.[8]

Ultrasound examination has been helpful in reducing the incidence of complications with amniocentesis.[13] Scanning prior to amniocentesis not only locates the placenta but also identifies the areas of amniotic fluid that are accessible. The position of the fetus and umbilical cord in relationship to the tap site can be visualized, and the depth and angle of needle insertion can be calculated. Immediately following these procedures, the fetus is again scanned to observe for cardiac activity and fetal movements to ensure that there has been no fetal injury. For intrauterine transfusion, scanning also identifies the site of needle insertion into the fetal abdomen. Continuous scanning during transfusion is done for observation of fetal cardiac activity. With increased expertise in utilizing RTBS for transfusion procedures, the radiation exposure from fluoroscopy can be greatly reduced.[4,7,11]

242 Selected Ob/Gyn problems and issues

Congenital malformations

The detection of an abnormal fetus before 20 weeks gestation, while legal abortion is still permissible, is the goal of prenatal genetic evaluation. The use of ultrasound has become an integral part of the management of patients referred for prenatal diagnoses.

In our institution, all patients undergoing amniocentesis for chromosomal or biochemical evaluation are first screened by an RTBS examination. We have shown that ultrasound scanning immediately prior to the procedure reduces the incidence of traumatic taps.[8]

Campbell and co-workers have demonstrated that spina bifida can be accurately detected on ultrasound with careful scanning.[3] Similarly, Robinson has demonstrated a method of detecting meningomyelocele with reasonable accuracy.[14]

After 14 weeks gestation, the absence of a well-formed fetal head is highly suggestive of anencephaly. Repeated scans with definitive outline of a fetal body and facial bones, but without evidence of cranial formation, will confirm this diagnosis (Fig. 15-12). Conversely, hydrocephaly is a difficult diagnosis to make in early pregnancy. A reliable means of diagnosing hydrocephalus

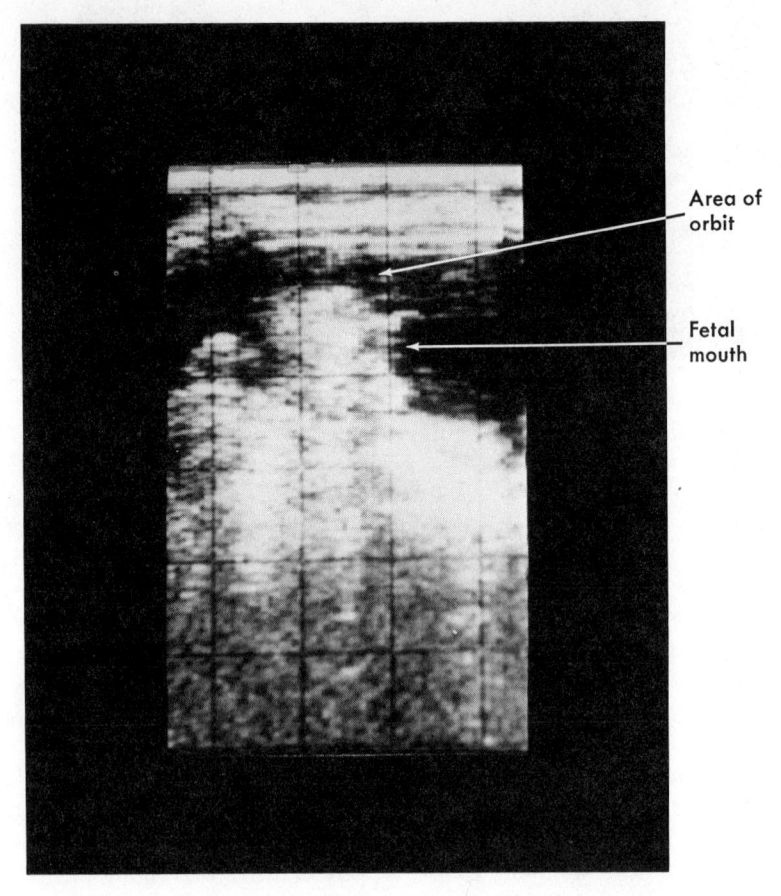

Fig. 15-12. RTBS showing anencephalic fetus — note facial features with lack of bone formation.

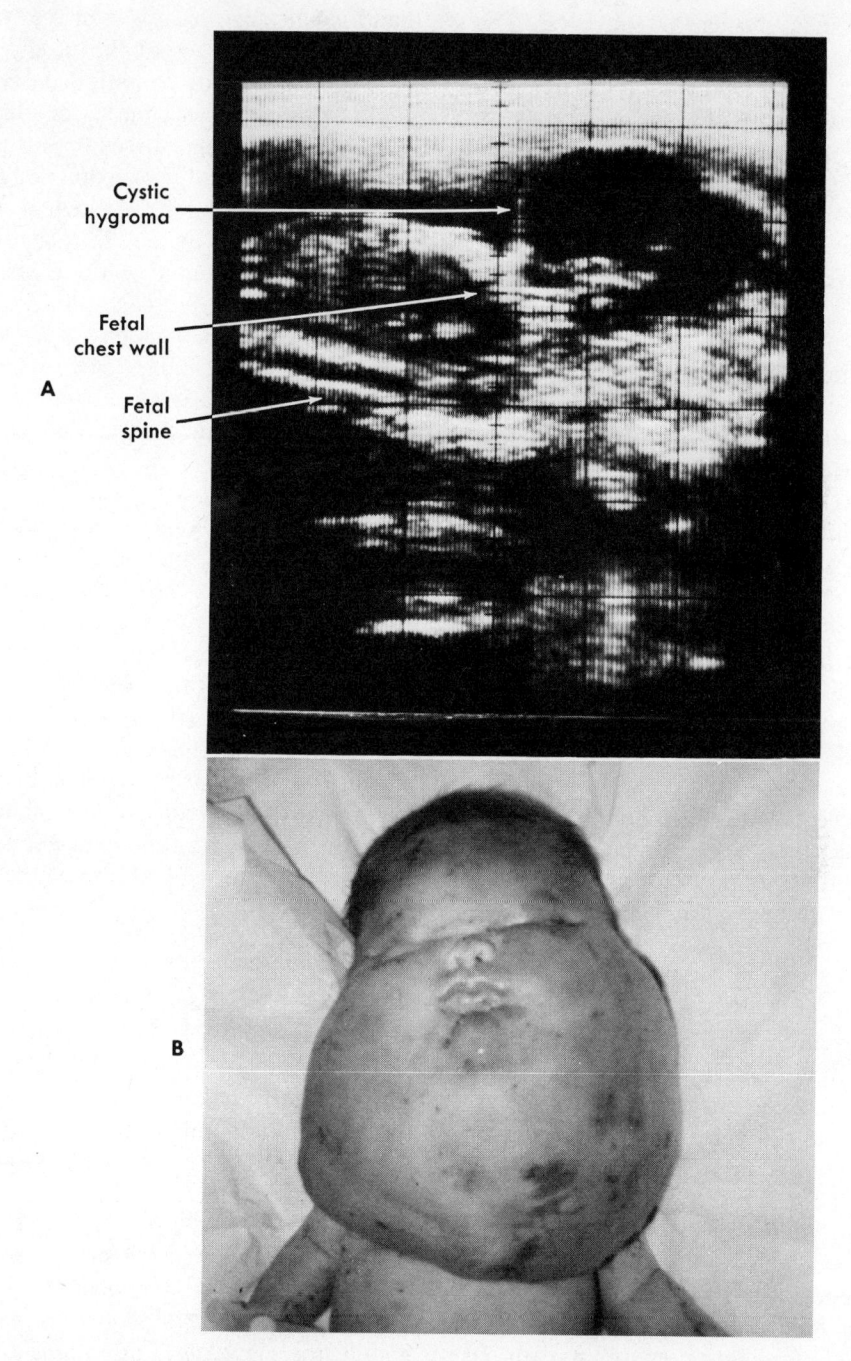

Real-time ultrasound in obstetrics and gynecology 243

Fig. 15-13. A, RTBS demonstrating fetal cystic hygroma—note large clear area anterior to fetal chest. **B,** Photograph of same infant at delivery.

in utero is measurement of the BPD. The diagnosis of hydrocephalus is generally made when the BPD at term is greater than 11.0 cm. In these cases, the BPD may be 1.5 to 2.0 cm larger than the thoracic diameter. With ultrasound scanning, one can see enlargement of the fetal ventricular system. Other anomalies such as fetal cystic hygroma can be demonstrated (Fig. 15-13).

THE FETUS AS A PATIENT

Evaluation of multiple biophysical variables is a standard method of evaluation of condition in the newborn (for example, Apgar scores) and the adult (for example, vital signs). The relative inaccessibility of the fetus in utero has made application of these principles to the fetus difficult. Until recently, the fetal heart rate and its response to stimuli (for example, fetal movement, uterine contraction) were the only dynamic fetal biophysical variables that could be readily measured. The development of RTBS ultrasound now enables the clinician to assess many additional fetal biophysical variables such as gross body movement, breathing movements, tone, and qualitative amniotic fluid volume. The correlation of these variables together with fetal heart rate response to fetal movement (nonstress testing) form the basis for a biophysical profile of the fetus that holds promise as an accurate and reliable method of differentiating the normal from the compromised fetus in utero. Using a scoring system based on these five variables, the false negative rate (that is, an abnormal test, but a normal outcome) has been reduced to less than 10%. These improvements represent a significant advance over any single test alone.[9]

Real-time ultrasound examination of the individual fetus allows for estimation of risk based on the characteristics of that fetus alone. Furthermore, the use of a constellation of fetal biophysical variables rather than a single test greatly improves the accuracy and reliability of the prediction of risk. Assessment of condition based on a single biophysical variable in an adult may be inaccurate. Thus, for example, lack of response to a stimuli (for example, a vocal command) in the adult may reflect a sleep state, coma, or even death. These states cannot be differentiated on the basis of this single variable but are easily differentiated by evaluation of other biophysical variables for example, (breathing, heart rate, movement). It seems likely that a similar principle may apply in the fetus.

ULTRASOUND IN GYNECOLOGY

The availability of real-time ultrasound has led to the introduction of several techniques that may improve the accuracy of gynecologic ultrasound examination. For example, when the clinician does the scanning, he or she has the combined ability to incorporate the findings of the bimanual examination and the scan. The ability to elevate the uterus or pelvic mass during the examination may improve identification of abnormalities. The following section discusses the basic indications for the use of RTBS in gynecology.

Intrauterine devices

The failure to identify the IUD strings may mean that the IUD has been expelled, has perforated the uterus, or remains in place with the strings drawn into the cervical canal. Ultrasound scanning is only helpful when the IUD is within the uterus.

Threatened abortion

Threatened abortion is considered when early pregnancy is complicated by vaginal bleeding. With the aid of real-time ultrasound, the clinician is often able to obtain rapid information regarding the viability of the pregnancy. If no fetal parts have been identified and the pregnancy is less than 6

Real-time ultrasound in obstetrics and gynecology 245

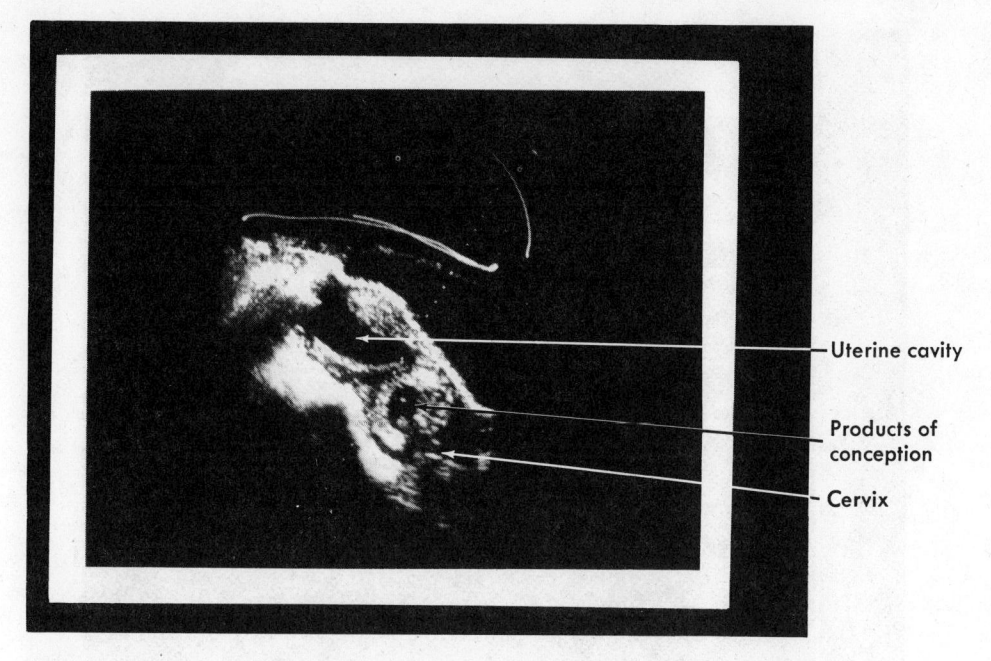

Fig. 15-14. Contact scan demonstrating threatened abortion — note fetal parts in area of lower uterine segment.

weeks from the last menstrual period, as long as the gestational sac appears intact, serial scans showing sac growth suggest that the pregnancy is still viable. Recognition of fetal movements within the sac confirms the viability of the pregnancy. In early pregnancy if the gestational sac echoes are disrupted and are implanted low in the uterine cavity, the risk of abortion is very high (Fig. 15-14).

Molar pregnancy

One out of 2000 pregnancies in the United States is associated with molar pregnancy. In cases in which early pregnancy bleeding is found, no fetal heart tones are heard, and a uterus larger than expected is present, the presence of hydatidiform mole is highly suggested. Ultrasound exam is valuable in confirming the diagnosis of molar pregnancy. The formation of multiple grapelike vesicles of the placenta are seen as a characteristic snowflake pattern on the scanner (Fig. 15-15). The diagnostic accuracy of this technique approaches 100%. Care must be taken not to mistake this finding for a degenerating myoma. Because of the serious nature of the disease, there is no excuse for an incomplete workup and history in these patients. For example, a patient with a negative pregnancy test will almost never have molar pregnancy in spite of the snowstorm appearance of the echoes. Although remote, identifying a molar pregnancy does not rule out the possibility of a mole with a coexisting normal pregnancy.[1]

Ectopic pregnancy

The patient who has a positive pregnancy test, lower abdominal pain, normal size uterus, and whose menstrual period is long overdue must be considered to have an ectopic pregnancy until proved otherwise. In these instances, a pelvic examination is of-

246 Selected Ob/Gyn problems and issues

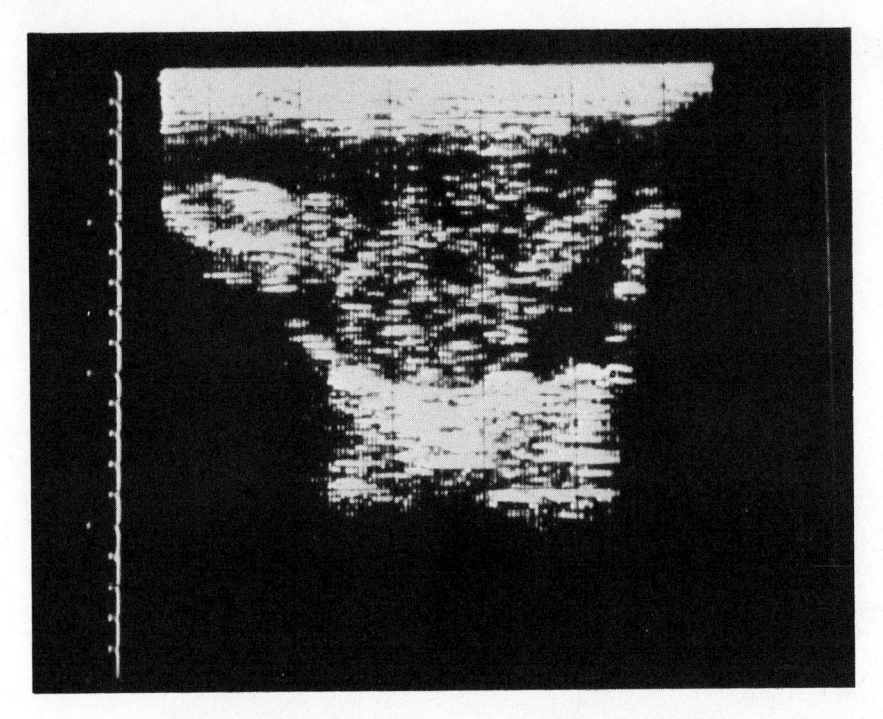

Fig. 15-15. RTBS of molar pregnancy—note snowflake-like appearance.

ten inadequate because of the patient's discomfort. RTBS may be helpful in ruling out the diagnosis if a gestational sac is seen within the uterine cavity. Sometimes the ectopic pregnancy may be seen outside the uterus if it is advanced enough. Unfortunately, while advances in ultrasound have been made, the difficulty encountered in making the precise diagnosis of ectopic pregnancy still limits the overall value of RTBS in this situation.

Ovarian masses

While visualization of the normal ovary is difficult using real-time scanners, several investigators using compound scanners have studied the normal architecture of the ovary. When a mass is felt in the adnexal area, ultrasound can often be a helpful diagnostic tool. A small ovarian cyst or a corpus luteum cyst can be followed through several menstrual cycles to determine whether or not it will regress. While large cysts may require surgical intervention regardless of the ultrasound picture, it is helpful to have some idea of the internal consistency of the cyst (Fig. 15-16). A more complex architectural structure within the cyst suggests a greater likelihood of malignancy (Fig. 15-17). In addition to the internal architecture and size of the mass, its relationship to other pelvic structures can be appreciated. With this technique, however, the scans must remain as a clinical test only. The definitive diagnosis of an ovarian mass must be left to the pathologist and a histologic evaluation.

Uterine myomas

Unlike cystic structures that allow the sound waves to pass through with very little attenuation, ultrasonic properties of sol-

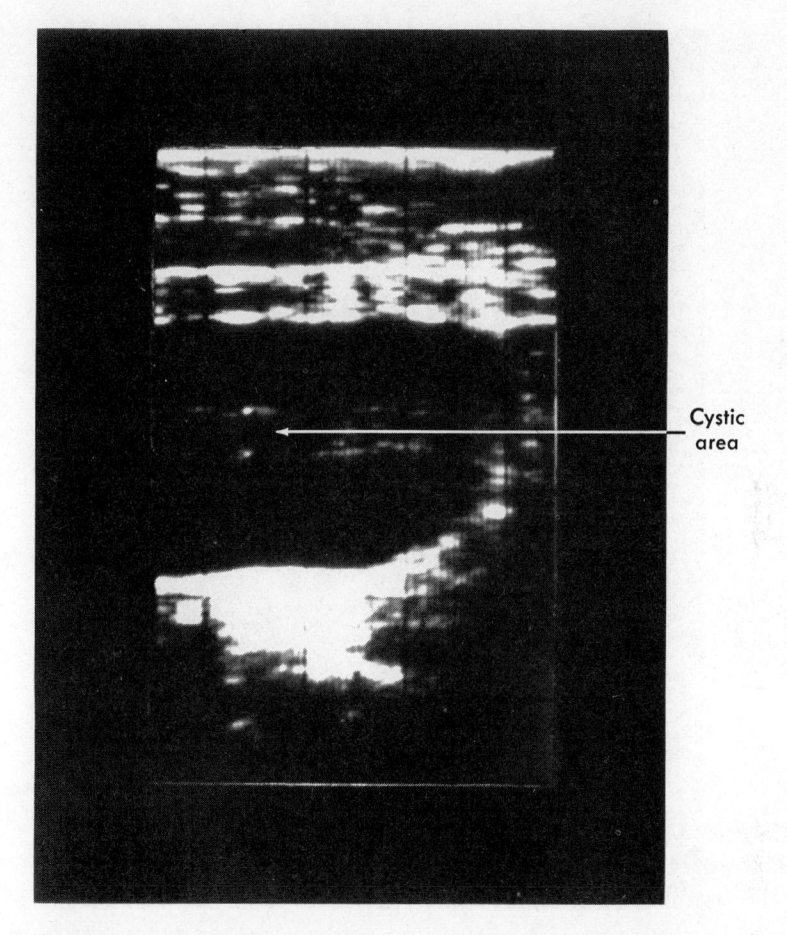

Fig. 15-16. RTBS demonstrating large ovarian cyst—note large, clear area suggesting simple cyst.

id structures are less clearly appreciated. If the structure contains both solid and cystic components, the interfaces between the two areas will serve as a reasonable reflective medium. However, because of the sound attenuation within the solid components, clear images are not always apparent and the posterior border of the mass may not be visualized.

Because these images are not always clear-cut, the use of ultrasound in myomas is, at present, of little clinical value. The difficulty encountered in identifying the exact origin of the tumor (ovaries or uterus) if seen in the adnexal area further limits its use. To state emphatically that the tumor is a benign uterine myoma when, in actuality, it is a solid ovarian neoplasm, is one of the most serious errors that can be made using ultrasound.

SUMMARY

This chapter has attempted to provide a basic understanding of the principles of ultrasound and an appreciation of the medical advances that this technology has provided. From the current applications and potential future uses discussed in this chapter, it is clear that ultrasound has become an essential tool in the field of obstetrics and gyne-

248 Selected Ob/Gyn problems and issues

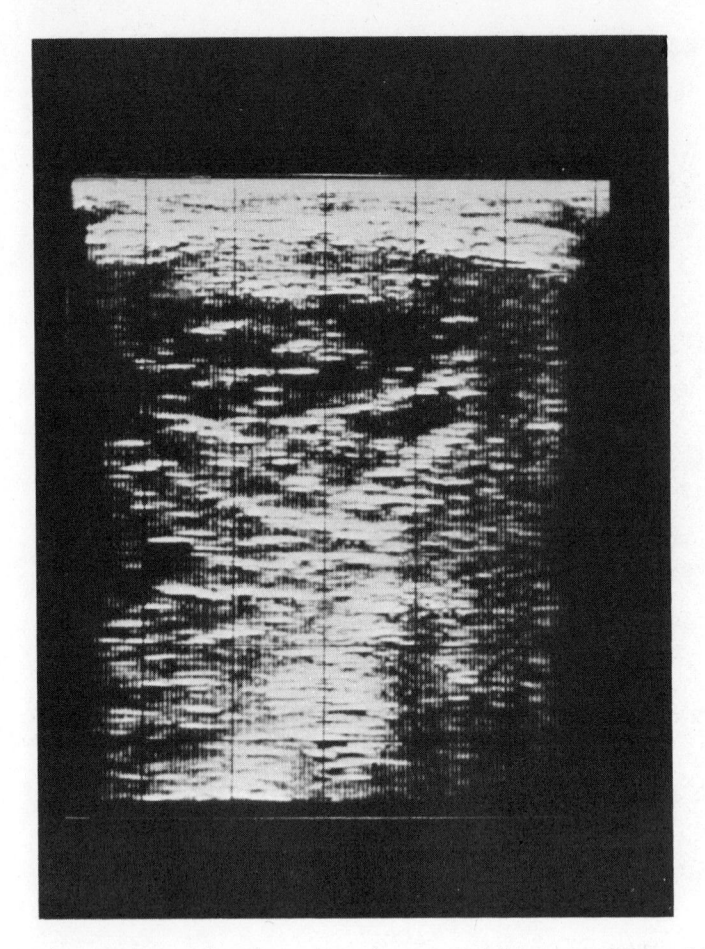

Fig. 15-17. RTBS demonstrating ovarian mass — note more complex echoes suggesting possibility of malignancy.

cology. However, discretion in the use of ultrasound is of primary importance. Clinical findings and judgments must be used in conjunction with ultrasound to determine the indication for its use and then for interpretation of the scan itself. When used by a knowledgeable and skilled operator, ultrasound scanning provides valuable information that adds to the total care of the gynecologic and obstetric patient.

REFERENCES

1. Bree, R. L., Silver, T. M., Wicks, J. D., et al.: Trophoblastic disease with coexistent fetus: a sonographic and clinical spectrum, J. Clin. Ultrasound **6:**310-315, 1978.
2. Campbell, S., and Dewhurst, C. J.: Diagnosis of the small for dates fetus by serial ultrasonic cephalometry, Lancet **2:**1002-1006, 1971.
3. Campbell, S., Pryse-Davies, J., and Coltart, T. M.: Ultrasound in the diagnosis of spina bifida, Lancet **1:**1065-1068, 1975.
4. Cooperberg, P. L., and Carpenter, C. W.: Ultrasound as an aid in intrauterine transfusion, Am. J. Obstet. Gynecol. **128**(3):239-241, 1977.
5. Donald, I.: Procedures: placental localization by sonar — a safe procedure, Br. J. Radiol. **47:**72-75, 1974.
6. Gottesfeld, K. R., Thompson, H. E., Holmes, J. H., et al.: Ultrasonic placentography — a new

method for placental localization, Am. J. Obstet. Gynecol. **96**:538-541, 1966.
7. Hobbins, J. C., Davis, C. B., and Websert, J.: A new technique utilizing ultrasound to aid in intrauterine transfusion, J. Clin. Ultrasound **4**(2): 135-139, 1976.
8. King, D. L.: Placental migration demonstrated by ultrasonography: a hypothesis of dynamic placentation, Radiology **109**:167-170, 1973.
9. Manning, F. A., and Platt, L. D.: Fetal breathing movements: antepartum monitoring of fetal condition, Clin. Obstet. Gynecol. **6**(2):335-349, 1979.
10. Martin, C. B., Jr., Murata, Y., and Rabin, L. S.: Diagnostic ultrasound in obstetrics and gynecology: experience on a large clinical service, Obstet. Gynecol. **41**:379-386, 1972.
11. Platt, L. D., Keegan, K. A., Manning, F. A., et al.: Intrauterine transfusion utilizing linear-array, real-time B-scan: a preliminary report, Am. J. Obstet. Gynecol. **135**(8):1115-1116, 1979.
12. Platt, L. D., Manning, F. A., Keegan, K. A., et al.: Unpublished data.
13. Platt, L. D., Manning, F. A., and Lemay, M.: Real-time B-scan–directed amniocentesis, Am. J. Obstet. Gynecol. **130**:700-703, 1978.
14. Robinson, H. P.: Prenatal screening for congenital abnormalities in the west of Scotland, Health Bull. (Edinb.) **34**:105-108, 1976.
15. Robinson, H. P.: Sonar measurement of the fetal crown-rump length as a means of assessing maturity in the first trimester of pregnancy, Br. Med. J. **4**:28-31, 1973.
16. Taylor, E. S., Holmes, J. T., Thompson, H. E., et al.: Ultrasound diagnostic techniques in obstetrics and gynecology, Am. J. Obstet. Gynecol. **90**:655:659, 1964.
17. Winsberg, F.: Echographic changes with placental aging, J. Clin. Ultrasound **1**:52-55, 1973.

Index

A

Abdomen, maternal, length of, 61
Abortion
 clinics, 8
 law(s), 7-8
 need for, 6-7
 procedures, 8
 relationship of, to equality for women, 6-8
 removing legal barriers to, 7-8
 Supreme Court decisions on, 7-8
 threatened, 244
Abuse, child; *see* Child abuse, statistics concerning
ACOG; *see* American College of Obstetricians and Gynecologists
Acoustic blink reflex, 77
Advertising by physicians, 12
Aggression, displaced, 123
Ahlfeld's rule, 61
American College of Obstetricians and Gynecologists
 rape bulletin published by, 20
 sterilization restriction of, 6
American Society for Prophylaxis in Obstetrics, 43
Americans
 Asian, 33-35
 Black, 31-33
 Hispanic, 28-31
 Native, 35-37
Amines, biogenic, effects of, on mood and behavior, 179, 180
Anesthesia, effects of hypnosis regarding, 49
Anger as cause of illness, 30-31
Ankle clonus reflex, 76
Anxiety, state and trait, 173
Arousal, 174
Asian Americans, 33-35
 beliefs of
  about childbearing, 35
  about health and illness, 34-35
 historical perspective of, 33-34
 traditional family life of, 34

Assault
 accessory-to-sex, 142
 sexual, 101, 136-155
Assault and battery, problems of, 101-155
Assaults between husband and wife; *see* Violence, marital
Attention focusing, 52
Attention state, 48
Automatic walk reflex, 74, 77

B

Babinski reflex, 76
Backstrom's postulate of hyperestrogenemia, 171
Battered child, 103
Battery
 infant, 101, 103-120
  early identification of, 110-111
  environmental influences on, 109-110
  families involved in, 104, 107-109
   lower-class, 108
  former attitude toward, 117
  incidence of, 104
  and parental role, 109
  perpetrators of, 107, 108
   characteristics of, 108, 109
   sensitivity of nurse to health needs of, 114
  physiologic states of women in relation to, 108
  prevention of, 113-114
  role of nurse regarding, 114-117
   in community activities, 115, 117
   in family planning, 114
   knowledge needed to perform, 114
   as observer of baby and parents, 114-115
   in professional education, 117
   as record keeper, 115
   in referral, 115
  screening high-risk families for, 113
   index of suspicion for, 115, 116
  sequelae of, 103-104, 106, 107
   influences associated with, 106

Battery—cont'd
  infant—cont'd
    intellectual, 104, 106, 107
    motor, 106, 107
    physical, 103-104, 106-107
    social-emotional, 107
  task of professional in, 108, 114-117
  treatment alternatives for, 111-112
  victims of, 104-107
    distorted perception of, 106, 109
    failure-to-thrive of, 106-107
    prematurity among, 104-105, 107
    temperament of, 105, 107
    variables associated with, 104-105, 107
    vulnerability of, 104, 107
  whiplash shaken syndrome of, 106
  wife, 121-122
    alcohol use with, 124
    assaults and injuries of, 125-127
      damage done by, 126-127
      emotional, 129
      frequency of, 125
      parts of body involved in, 126
    constraints perpetuating relationship involving, 130-132
      external, 130-131
      internal, 131-132
    continuum of, 125
    cycle of violence in, 124-125
    dynamics of, 127-130
      marriage, 128
    escalation of, 124
    evolution of, 124
    mechanisms triggering, 128-129
    nature of, 123-125
      social, 123-124
    perpetrators of, 128
    in pregnancy, 127
    reason(s) for occurrence of, 122-123
      fear of loss as, 129-130
    self-defense against, 125-126
    self-propelling aspect of, 126
    and sex-role stereotypes, 129
    verbal abuse accompanying, 124
    victims of, 127-128
      frozen fright of, 132
      internalization of blame by, 129
      isolation of, 130
    weapons used in, 126
  of women, 121-135
    helping victims of, 132-135
      Change Potential Scale for, 132-134
      by encouraging realistic appraisal, 134
      by encouraging talk about battering and injuries, 134

Battery—cont'd
  of women—cont'd
    helping victims of—cont'd
      by involving hospital social department, 134
      by keeping records, 134-135
      by knowing community resources, 134
      by remaining patient, 134
    perpetrators of, 121
B.I.A.; *see* Bureau of Indian Affairs
Bile, 30-31
Bilis, 30-31
Bing, Elizabeth, 43
Biopsies, iodine stains used with, limitation of, 205
Biparietal diameter, 62-63
  usefulness of
    in estimating gestational age, 236, 239
    in intrauterine growth retardation, 239
Birth control, motivations for, 9
Birth control clinics, 5
Birth control pill, 12-13
Birth defects, viruses associated with, 98
Biskin's postulate about hyperestrogenemia, 171
Black Americans, 31-33
  beliefs of
    about childbearing, 33
    about health and illness, 32-33
  historical perspective of, 31-32
  traditional family life of, 32
Blink reflex
  acoustic, 77
  optical, 75
Blood cells, 187
BPD; *see* Biparietal diameter
Brazelton Scales, 72, 78
Breastfeeding, 18
Breath, cleansing, 44, 45
Breathing
  abdominal, 41
  abdominal-costal, 41
  costal, 41
  exercises, 42, 44, 46-47, 50
  high-chest, 41
Bronchitis, 31
Budding, 188
Bureau of Indian Affairs, eligibility for services of, 36

C

Candida albicans; see Monilia
"The Cause," 3-4
Cervical intraepithelial neoplasia; *see* CIN
Cervical pathology, differential diagnosis of, 157, 200-215
Cervical pseudopolyp, 204
Cervicitis
  acute, 200-201

Cervicitis—cont'd
  chronic, 201-202
Cervix, 200
  abnormalities of, 157, 200-215
  adenocarcinoma of, 210
  biopsy of
    cone, 207
    random, 205
  carcinoma of
    chemotherapy in, 214
    invasive, 209-214
      adenosquamous cell, 210
      diagnosis of, 209-210
      endophytic, 210
      exophytic, 209-210
      follow-up of, 213
      infiltrating, 210
      occult, 209
      pelvic exenteration for, 214
      radiotherapy of, 212-213
      recurrence of, 213-214
      squamous cell, 210
      symptoms of, 209, 210
      treatment of, 209, 211-213
      ulcerative, 209
      workup for, 210
    microinvasive, 208-209
      diagnosing, 206, 209
    in situ, 207-208
    staging of, 210-211
  cryosurgery of, 208
  dysplasia of
    mild, 206-207
    moderate, 207
    severe, 207-208
  ectopy of, 203, 204
  erosion on, 202-203
  leiomyoma of, 203-204
  metaplasia of, 205
  polyps on, 202
  transitional zone of, 205
Child abuse, 104; *see also* Battery, infant
  current situation regarding, 117
  effect of stress on, 110
  environmental implications in, 109-110
  and failure-to-thrive, relationship of, 111
  information available about, 117
  and isolation, 110
  lay therapists treating, 112
  as low base rate phenomenon, 113
  in past, 117
  prevention of, 113-114
  signs indicating, 110-111
  statistics concerning, 103, 104
  study of, 107

Childbearing; *see also* Childbirth
  beliefs about, 31,33, 35, 37
  cultural aspects of, 27-39
    awareness of, needed by health professional, 27-28
  as developmental crisis, factors determining outcome of, 30
  reducing discomfort during, 40
Childbirth, 17-18, 19; *see also* Childbearing
  abdominal-costal breathing during, 41
  changes concerning, 19
  cultural adaptations in, 38
  educated; *see* Childbirth, psychophysical preparations for
  fear-tension-pain syndrome in, 41
  hospitalization for, 17-18
  Lamaze method for, 18, 42-45
    breathing component of, 44, 45, 46-47
      cleansing breath in, 44, 45
    childbearing team in, 44
    emphasis in, 47
    exercising component of, 44, 45, 46
    labor-support person in, 48
    relaxing component of, 43-44, 45, 46, 50
      feedback technique for, 50, 52
    setting goals in, 44
  natural, 18, 40-42, 45, 47, 50
    concept of, 41
  neo-Pavlovian method of, 42-43
  Nicolaiev method of, 42-43
  pain relief in
    methodologies of, 40-49
      effectiveness of, 54
    psychologic strategies of, 50, 52-53
  "physiologic"; *see* Childbirth, natural
  prepared; *see* Childbirth, Lamaze method for
  psychoprophylactic method of, 42-43
  psychophysical preparation(s) for, 1, 40-56
    attention focusing in, 52
    body-building exercises used in all methodologies of, 51
    cognitive rehearsal as, 52-53
    comparison between Lamaze and Read techniques of, 45, 47-48
    criticisms of, 44
    didactic element of, 49-50
    effectiveness of, 54
    hypnosuggestive method of, 48-49; *see also* Hypnosis, in childbirth
    Lamaze method of; *see* Childbirth, Lamaze method for
    Leboyer's influence on, 53-54
    nurse-practitioner's role in, 54
    physiotherapeutic element in, 50
    psychologic strategies used in, 50, 52-53

Childbirth—cont'd
  psychophysical preparation(s) for—cont'd
    Read method of, 40-42; see also Childbirth, natural
      decreasing fear and tension in, 41
      emphasis in, 45, 47
      "schools" of, 40
      elements shared by, 49-50
Children's Bureau, 17
"Chinatowns," 34
Chinese Americans; see Asian Americans
Chinese calendar, 34
Chinese New Year, 34
Chvostek's reflex, 75
CIN, 205
CIN I, 206-207
CIN II, 207
CIN III, 207-208
Client, definition of, 10
Clinics, self-help, 14
Clitoral hood, 222, 223
Cloth binder, 31
CMV; see Cytomegalovirus
Coccygeus muscle, 217
Cognitive control, 52
Cognitive rehearsal, 52-53
Cold sores among hospital personnel, 93
Colposcope, 205
Colposcopist, 205
  gaining experience as, 206
Colposcopy, 205-206
Compadres, 29
Condoms, 9
Condyloma acuminatum, 203
Consent, informed, 12-13
Contraception
  hormonal, 182
  limitations of, 6-7
  methods of
    female, development of, 9
    male, 9
  "modern," 6
  oral, risks associated with, 13, 182
  relationship of, to equality for women, 5-6, 8-10
  use of, 6, 9
"Contraceptive revolution," 6
Contraceptives, hormonal, moods produced by, 174
Corneal reflex, 75
Corynebacterium vaginalis, 193-194
  clinical course of infection with, 194
  microscopic examination of, 194
  primary complaint with, 194
  treatment for, 194
Countertransference, 167

Crabs, 196-197
  clinical course of, 196
  microscopic examination of, 196-197
  primary complaint with, 196
  treatment for, 197
Crawling reflex, 77
Cross extension reflex, 74, 76
Cultural aspects of childbearing, 27-39
  awareness of, needed by health professional, 27-28
Cultural beliefs about diseases, 30-31, 34, 37
Cultural practices, factors affecting, 38
"Cultural sensitivity" skills, need of nurses for, 27, 28
Culture, 37-38
Curandero, 30
Curranderisma, 30
Cystocele, 219
Cytomegalovirus, 91
  in fetus and newborn, 96
  history of, 87-88
  infection during pregnancy, 91-92
  isolation of, 91
  perinatal transmission of, 88, 92
Cysts, Nabothian, 202

D

Decarboxylase, 179
Deep tendon reflex, 76
Delivery
  anesthesia during, 17-18, 40
  forceps, 18
  Leboyer, 53-54
  position assumed for, 18, 38
DES, 203-204
Desensitization, systematic, 53
Development, fetal and neonatal, 57-99
Developmental profile, 71-72
  reflexes considered useful in, 75-77
Diaphragm, pelvic, 217
Dick-Read, Grantly, 18, 40, 41-42, 45, 47, 50
  childbirth method of, 40-42, 45, 50
Diethylstilbestrol; see DES
Discrimination, sexual, 3
  in education, laws prohibiting, 23
Disease(s)
  cause of, cultural ideas concerning, 30-31, 34, 37
  of dislocation of internal organs, 30
  of emotional origin, 30-31
  fetal and neonatal, 86-99
  of hot and cold imbalance, 30, 35
  of magical and folk origin, 30
  salivary gland, 88
  standard medical, 31
  vaginal and cervical, self-diagnosis and treatment of, 14

Index   255

Dislocation of internal organs, disease of, 30
Displacement, 123
Dissociation, cognitive, 52, 53
Distraction, 52
Döderlein's bacillus, 188
Doppler effect, 230
Drug risks, advising users of, 13

E

Ectopic pregnancy, 245-246
Effleurage, 44
Ejaculation
   premature, 161, 164-165
      definition of, 164
      psychologic factors contributing to, 164-165
   retarded, 161, 165
Emotional origin, diseases of, 30-31
Empacho, 30
Endocervix, 200
Endomyces albicans; see Monilia
Enterovirus infections in newborn, 98
Episiotomies, 18
   effects of, on P.C. muscle, 224
Equality for women
   biologic barriers to, 5
   health services necessary for, 5-10
Erythema, 189
Espanto, 30-31
Estrogen products, 13
Estrogens, 171, 181
Evil eye, 30
Exercises
   body-building, 41, 44, 46, 50, 51
   breathing, 42, 44, 46-47, 50
   expulsion, 47
   Lamaze psychoprophylaxis preparatory, 46-47
   neuromuscular, 43, 46
   relaxation, 42, 43-44, 46, 50
Exocervix, 200

F

Failure-to-thrive, 111
Faja, 31
Family planners, medical, feminists as "watchdogs" of, 8-10
Family planning
   motivations for, 9
   slogan, 6
   women's movement and physician involvement in, 8-9
Family planning movement, 5-6
Fang, 35
FDA informational drug-packaging requirements, 13

Fear-tension-pain syndrome, 41
   effort to control, 50
Female organs and functions, removing aura of abnormality and illness from, 16-19
Feminist goals, 5, 6
Feminists, relationship of, with medical family planners, 8-10
Fetus
   agents of infection of; *see* TORCH
   assessing size and growth of, 57, 59-68
      by abdominal palpation, 60-61
      by Ahlfeld's rule, 61
      by biparietal diameter, 60, 62-63
         accuracy of, 62
         in diabetic women, 63, 66
         distinguishing cephalic growth patterns in, 63
         during second trimester, 62
         serial measurements for, 62
         during third trimester, 66
      clinical guidelines for, 64, 66
      conditions causing errors in, 66
      by crown-rump length measurement, 60, 62
      by early bimanual exam, 60
      in first trimester, 64
      by fundal height, 60-61, 66
      importance of, 59, 66
      by MacDonald's rule, 60-61
      by menstrual history, 60
      by radiologic methods, 60, 61
      in second trimester, 66
      in third trimester, 66
      by ultrasound, 60-61
         advantages of, 61-62
         mechanism of, 62
         in third trimester, 66
      by ultrasound cephalometry; *see* Fetus, assessing size and growth of, by biparietal diameter
   calculating gestational age of, 60-61, 62-63, 66
      correlation of data in, 65
      by ultrasound, 236-239
         from biparietal diameter, 236, 238-239
         through crown-rump length measurement, 236, 237
   crown-rump measurement of, 236
   development of, 57-68, 86-99
   diseases of, 86, 87, 88, 89-99
      infectious agents suspected to cause, 98
   growth retardation of, 64, 66
      diagnosis and follow-up of, by ultrasound measurement of BPD, 239
   head to abdominal circumference ratio of, 64
   at low risk for perinatal mortality, 59
   macrosomatic, 59
      detection of, 63

Fetus—cont'd
  as patient, 244
  ultrasound image of, 235, 236
  weight of, predicting, 63-64
"Flicker fusion threshold," 174
Focal-point visualization technique of pain management, 43-44
Folk disorders, 30
Folk theories, 30, 31, 32
Fontanelle, fallen, 30
Food and Drug Administration; *see* FDA informational drug-packaging requirements
Frank's postulate about hyperestrogenemia, 171
Fright as cause of illness, 30-31
Frigidity, 161, 162
Fundus, 60
Fungus, 188, 189-190

G
Galant reflex, 76
Genital infection; *see* Vulvovaginitis
Genital relaxation; *see* Pelvic muscles, relaxation and degeneration of
Genitalia, external female, 222, 223
Gestational age inventory, 72
  delayed, 72, 74
  used immediately after birth, 72, 73
Glabellar reflex, 74, 75
Gonorrhea, 195-196, 201
  clinical course in, 196
  microscopic examination for, 196, 201
  primary complaint in, 196
  treatment of, 196, 201
Grasp reflex
  palmar, 74, 76
  plantar, 76
Greer, Germaine, 18
Guttmacher, Alan, 43
Gynecology, ultrasound in; *see* Ultrasonography, in obstetrics and gynecology

H
Habituation state, 48
Haley, Alex, 31
Hames, Margie Pitts, 7, 8, 9
Hawthorne effect, 53
Health
  assuming responsibility for one's own, 13-14
  cultural beliefs about, 28, 30, 32, 35, 37
    as relating to harmony and balance, 32-33, 34-35, 38
  Hippocratic theory of, 30
Health care, women's, 1-56
  effects of women's movement on, 1, 3-26

Health care system, sexism in, 8
Health information, alternative source of, 11-12
Health services necessary for equality for women, 5-10
Health states, perinatal, 71
Health visitors, 113, 114
Hemophilus vaginalis; *see Corynebacterium vaginalis*
Hepatitis B infection in infant, 98
Herbst, Arthur, 203
Herpes simplex virus, 92
  controlling transmission of, 93
  perinatal disease caused by, 86
    in fetus and newborn, 96-98
      diagnosis of, 97
      disseminated, 96-97
      localized, 97
      serologic assays in, 97
      treatment of, 97-98
    during pregnancy, 92-93
    transmission of, 88
  type II, 194-195
    microscopic examination with, 194-195
    primary complaint with, 194
    treatment of, 195
Hertz, 230
Hippocratic theory, 30
Hispanic Americans, 28-31
  beliefs of
    about breastfeeding, 31
    about dietary restrictions and taboos, 31
    about diseases, 30-31
    about health and illness, 30
  characteristics of, 28
  historical perspective of, 29
  subgroups of, 28
Hot and cold imbalance, diseases of, 30
HSV; *see* Herpes simplex virus
Human Sexual Inadequacy, 159
Humors, four, 30
Hymen, 186
Hyperestrogenemia, causal postulates about, 171
Hyperventilation, 44
Hypnosis
  in childbirth, 42, 48-49
    advocates of, 48
    amnesia in, 49
    contraindications for, 48
    effects of, 48-49
    history of, 42-43, 48
    instruction for, 48
    needs of patient using, 49
    somnambulism in, 49
    successful, prerequisites for, 48
    uses of, 49

Hyponosis—cont'd
  deep, 49
  second level of, 49
Hypnosuggestive method of childbirth preparation; see Hypnosis in childbirth
Hypnotic state, 48
Hysterectomy
  follow-up of, 208
  radical, 211-212
    sexual function following, 213
Hz; see Hertz

I

Iliococcygeus muscle, 217
Illness
  cultural beliefs about, 28, 30-31, 32-33, 34-35, 37
    caused by emotional experiences, 30-31
    caused by supernatural powers, 33
    as natural and unnatural, 32
Impotence, 161, 163-164, 165
  primary, 163
  secondary, 163
Infection
  CMV, 88
  genital; see Vulvovaginitis
  perinatal, TORCH syndrome of, 86-99
Informed consent, 12-13
Insulin, effect of glucose load on, 175
Interference, 52
Intrauterine device; see IUD
Intrauterine growth retardation, 239; see also Fetus, growth retardation of
Itch mite, 197
IUD, 6, 13
  use, 9
IUGR; see Intrauterine growth retardation

K

Karmel, Marjorie, 43
Kegel, Arnold H., 219-221, 222, 225, 226
  research of, 219, 220, 221, 228
Kegel exercises, 226-227; see also Kegeling
Kegeling, 221, 226-227, 228
Kinsey publications, 14-15, 159

L

Labor
  cognitive rehearsal for, 52-53
  effect of fear on, 41
  hyperventilation in, 44
  pain in, 50
    relief of; see Pain relief in labor
Lactobacillus, 185

Lamaze, Fernand, 18, 43, 47, 50
  pregnancy views of, 47
Lamaze psychoprophylaxis method for childbirth, 18, 42-45
  breathing techniques of, 43, 44
  childbearing team in, 44
  contrasted with Nicolaiev method, 43
  emphasis in, 47
  exercises for, 46-47, 50
    body-building, 44, 46, 50
    breathing, 46-47, 50
    relaxation, 43-44, 46, 50
  labor-support person in, 48
  setting goals in, 44
  support for, 43
Latido; see Palpitation
Leboyer, Charles, 53
Levator ani, 217
Lice, pubic; see Crabs
Lugol's iodine stain, 205

M

MacDonald's measurements, 60
MacDonald's rule, 60-61
Magical and folk origin, diseases of, 30
Mal ojo, 30
Massage, 44
Masseter reflex, 75
Masters, W. H., 159, 160, 161, 164, 165, 166, 167, 168
MDQ; *see* Moos' Menstrual Distress Questionnaire
Measles, 31
Medicine, male domination of, 8, 23
  overcoming, 23-24
Medicine man, 37
Menses, 173
Menstrual cramps, biologic basis for, 17
Menstrual cycle(s)
  abnormality of; see Premenstrual tension syndromes
  determining luteal phase of, 179
  food consumption during, primate studies of, 174-175
  normal, 173
    arousal variations during, 174
    body weight fluctuations during, 175
    cognitive performance in, 175
    glucose tolerance during, 175
    mood changes during, 173-174
    pain threshold during, 176
    and PMT menstrual cycles, comparison between, 173-176
      for behavioral parameters, 173-175
      for endocrine parameters, 175

Menstrual cycle(s)—cont'd
  normal—cont'd
    and PMT menstrual cycles, comparison between—cont'd
      for pain threshold, 176
      for somatic parameters, 175-176
Menstrual extraction, 14
Menstruation, 16-17; *see also* Menstrual cycle(s)
Mexican Americans, 29
  beliefs of
    about childbearing, 31
    about dietary restrictions and taboos, 31
    about health and illness, 30
  cultural traditions of, 29
  traditional family life of, 29-30
Mexicans, 29
Microorganisms, "niche" concept of growth of, 187
Molar pregnancy, 245
Mollera caida, 30
Monilia, 188-191
  associated lesions of, 189
  budding, 188, 190
  of cervix, 200
  clinical course of, 189
  dermatophytids of, 189
  in diabetic patients, 189
  diagnosis of, 190
  discharge of, 189
  history pertinent to, 189
  hyphae of, 188
  microscopic examination of, 189-190
  in pregnancy, 189
  primary complaint with, 188-189
  pruritus of, 189
  pseudohyphae of, 190
  in pseudomycelia form, 190
  reproduction of, 188
  treatment of, 190-191
Monilia albicans; see Monilia
Monilia psiloses; see Monilia
Moniliasis; *see Monilia*
Mood
  neurotransmitters and effects on, 179, 180
  nutritional influence on, 180
Mood state and behavior, 173
Moos' Menstrual Distress Questionnaire, 174, 177-179
Moro reflex, 74, 77
Mothering behaviors, adaptive and maladaptive, 80
Mott, Lucretia, 3
Muscle(s)
  coccygeus, 217
  iliococcygeus, 217
  obturatorius internus, 217
  pelvic, relaxation and degeneration of, 157, 216-217
Muscle(s)—cont'd
  piriformis, 217
  pubococcygeus, restoring or maintaining function of, 157, 216-228

N

Nabothian cysts, 202
National Center for Child Abuse and Neglect, 103
National Institute of Neurological Diseases and Stroke Collaborative Perinatal Study, 17, 18
Native Americans, 35-37
  beliefs of
    about childbearing, 37
    about health and illness, 37
  definition of, 35-36
  historical perspective on, 35-36
  racial traits of, 35
  traditional family life patterns of, 36-37
"Natural childbirth movement," 18, 40
  beginnings of, 40
Navajo, 36, 37; *see also* Native Americans
Neisseria gonorrhea, 195
Nelson, Gaylord, 13
Neonatal Behavioral Assessment Scale, 72, 78
Neonate(s)
  activity programs for, 82
  agents of infection of; *see* TORCH
  assessing behaviors of, 57, 69-85
    early, importance of, 84
    interacting with care-giver, 81-82
    process of, 70-71
    tools and implications in, 71-82
  care-giver to, characteristics of, 71
  and care-giver, interaction between, 80, 81-82
    adaptive and maladaptive, 80, 81
    feeding as source of data about, 80, 81-82
  characteristics of, 71-82
    alertness, 78
    evaluation of, 71
    hearing, 78
    motor, 78-79, 81
    rhythms, 81
    vision, 78
  development of, 57, 69-99
    importance of family in planning and facilitating, 82
    nursing interventions in
      demonstrating complete learning loops, 82-84
      principles of, 82
    profile of, 69-85
  diseases of, 86-88, 89-99
    infectious agents suspected to cause, 98
    examinations of, variables influencing, 69

Neonate(s)—cont'd
  hypotonia in, 78-79
  low–birth weight, 59, 64
  mothering of, adaptive and maladaptive, 80
  neurologically at-risk
    early identification of, 69-70
      through proneness and assessment, 70-71
    factors compounding difficulties of, 69
    home visits by nurse-practitioners to, 71
  perinatal health states of, 71
  precursor reactions of, 69-70
  premature
    alertness "transition state" in, 78
    development of muscular tone in, 72
    developmental profile for, 71-72
    fostering appropriate sensory environment for, 82
    gestational age inventory of, 72
      delayed, 72, 74
      used immediately after birth, 72, 73
    hearing in, 78
    motor development of, 79, 81
    and Neonatal Behavioral Assessment Scale, 72
    neurologic examination of, 72
    nursing assessment and intervention programs for, 71-84
    stimulation of, 82-84
      vestibular, 82
    vision testing of, 78, 79
  proneness screening of, 70, 71
  reflexes of, 75-77
  stimulation programs for, 82
Neonatology: Physiology and Management of the Newborn, 71
Neuromuscular exercises, 43, 46
Neurotransmitters, effects of, on mood, 179-180
  dietary precursors of, 180
Newborn; *see* Neonate
"Niche" concept of growth of microorganisms, 187
Normal, definitions of, 173
Nurse-midwifery, 22
  medical and legal support for, 23
Nurse practice acts, expansion of, 22
  opposition to, 23
Nurse-practitioner and nurse-midwife movement, 22-23
Nurses
  "cultural sensitivity" of, 27, 28, 38
  roles of, 1
Nursing
  cross-cultural, implications of, 37-38
  development of, 20-21
  effect of women's movement on, 21
  status basis of, 21
  struggle to upgrade, 21-23

Nutrition
  influence of, on mood and behavior, 180
  research in, 179

O

Ob/gyn problems and issues, 157-249
Obstetric care, prenatal, history of, 17
Obstetrics
  anesthesia for, 17-18, 40
  ultrasound in; *see* Ultrasonography in obstetrics and gynecology
Obturatorius internus muscle, 217
Oidium albicans; see Monilia
Optical blink reflex, 75
Orgasms, women's, 15
Our Bodies, Ourselves, 11-12, 13-14, 221
Ovarian mass, diagnosis of, 246
Ovulation, 173
Oxytocin, action of, 18

P

Pacing reflex, 77
Pain, primal, theory of, 53
Pain relief in labor
  cognitive control for, 52
  cognitive rehearsal for, 52-53
  and Hawthorne effect, 53
  methodology(ies) of, 40-49
    body-building exercises used in all, 51
    elements shared by, 49-50
    Lamaze, 42-45
      through breathing techniques, 44
      by focal-point visualization, 43-44
      physiologic mechanism of, 50
    major, 50
    neo-Pavlovian, 42-43
    psychologic strategies used in, 50, 52-53
      most successful of, 52
    Read, 40-42
  systematic desensitization for, 53
  systematic relaxation for, 50, 52
  theoretical framework of, 49-53
Pain threshold, effect of anxiety on, 176
Palmar grasp reflex, 74, 76
Palpitation, 30
Pap smear, 204
  abnormal, 204-205
    workup of, 204-206
      by colposcopy, 205-206
      by cone biopsy, 206
      by random biopsy, 205
  results of, 204-205
Parental role, 109
Parents Anonymous, 112

Partera, 31
Pathogens, opportunistic, 187
Patient, definition of, 10
"Patient package inserts," 13
Pavlov's theory of conditioned reflexes, 42-43
P.C. muscle; *see* Pubococcygeus muscle
Pediculus pubis; see Crabs
Pelvic diaphragm, 217
Pelvic examination, 222-226
   exterior, 222
   internal, 222-226
     digital, 222, 223-225
     speculum, 222-223
Pelvic exenteration, 214
Pelvic muscles
   "lack of awareness of function" of, 219
   relaxation and degeneration of, 157, 216-217
     cause of, 216-217
     classification of cases involving, 221
     diagnosis of, by pelvic examination, 222-226
     passive and stimulative exercises for, 219
     remedies for, 217, 219, 220, 221, 226
     results of, 218-219, 226, 228
Perez reflex, 76
Perinatal health states, 71
Perinatal infection
   with herpes simplex virus, 86, 92, 93
   TORCH syndrome of, 86-99
   with toxoplasma, 86, 89-90
Perinatal study, 17, 18
Perineal floor, 217
Perineometer, 220, 225
   reliability of, 226
   use of, 225-226, 227
Physician(s)
   advertising by, 12
   female, influence of, on medicine, 24
   role, 10
     changing, 12
Physician-patient relationship
   changing, by changing patients, 10-14
     means of, 11
     reasons for, 11
     through acknowledgment of rights, 12-13
     through assumption of responsibilities, 13-14
     through providing information, 11-12
   stereotypic, 10
Pica, 33
Piezoelectric crystals, 230
Pill, birth control, 12-13
Piriformis muscle, 217
Placenta previa, change in position of, 240-241
Plantar grasp reflex, 76
PMT; *see* Premenstrual tension; Premenstrual tension syndrome

Pneumonia, 31
Polyp, 202
Pope Pius XII, 43
Pregnancy, 17
   causes of apparent excessive uterine enlargement in, 60
   ectopic, 245-246
   exercises during, 46-47, 51
     purposes of, 41, 43, 44, 46, 47, 51
   low back pain in, 51
   molar, 245
   study of, 17, 18
   traditional and cultural beliefs about, 28-38
Premenstrual discomfort, 177, 179
Premenstrual molimina, 177, 179
Premenstrual syndromes, 170
Premenstrual tension, 170
Premenstrual tension syndromes, 157, 170-184
   and birth control, 182
   classification of, 172-177
   evaluation of, 177-179
     by basal body temperature, 179
     form for, 177-179
   glucose tolerance in, 175
   hormonal imbalance theory of, 170-171
   hormone changes found in, 175
   hyperestrogenemia, causal postulates of, 171, 181
   magnesium nitrate effect on, 171-172
   moods in, 173-174
   nutritional deficiencies theory of, 171-172
   and pain threshold, 176
   postulated pathophysiologies of, 170-172, 176-177, 181
   pyridoxine effect on, 172
   and stress, 172
   stress susceptibility in, 181-182
   subgroups of, 176-177
   symptoms of, 176, 177
   treatment of, 179-182
     by controlling environmental stress, 180-181
     with hormones, 182
     with nutrition, 179-180, 181-182
       by pyridoxine (B_6) therapy, 181-182
     symptomatic, 182
     testing of, 179
   weight gain in, 175
Prepuce, 222, 223
Primal pain, theory of, 53
Progestogens, products containing, 13
The Prosecutors, 138
Psychoprophylactic method of childbirth, 42-43
Psychoprophylaxis, 42, 43
Pubic lice; *see* Crabs
Pubococcygeus muscle, 217-219, 227-228
   effects of episiotomy on, 224

Pubococcygeus muscle—cont'd
  evaluation of, 222-226, 228
  location of, 217-218
  in normal tone, 218
  restoring or maintaining function of, 216-228
    with exercises, 226, 227
    historical research on, 219-222
    phases of, 221
  shape of, in intravaginal palpation, 224
Pulmonia, 31
"Pulse-echo" system; *see* Ultrasonography, pulsed
Punishment, physical, of babies, 110
Pupil reflex, 74, 75
Pyrimethamine, antifolic effects of, 95

Q

Quakers, influence of, on women's rights movement, 3

R

Radiation shelf, 213
Rape, 19-20, 137; *see also* Sexual assault
Rape crisis counseling services, 20
Rape trauma syndrome, 142-144
  acute phase of, 143
  in children and adolescents, 144
  definition of, 143
  factors determining distress level experienced in, 142-143
  long-term phase of, 143-144
Rapist
  as opportunist, 142
  profile of, 140
RDS; *see* Respiratory distress syndrome
Read method of childbirth preparation, 40-42, 45, 47, 50
Rectocele, 219
Reflexes
  neonatal, 75-77
  primitive, 69
Relaxation
  kinds of, 50
  systematic, as pain control method, 50, 52, 53
Reproduction, control of, 5-10
Resolution, theoretical limit of, 230
Respiratory distress syndrome, elective intervention as cause of, 59-60
Rooting reflex, 74, 75
RTBS; *see* Ultrasonography, real-time B-scan
Rubella
  abortion counseling of pregnant women affected by, 91
  in fetus and newborn, 95-96
  prevention of, 88-89, 91
  risk to fetus from, 90
Rubella syndrome, expanded, 87

Rubella virus, 87, 90-91
  testing for, 88, 90-91
  transmission of, to fetus and newborn, 87, 88
Rule
  Ahlfeld's, 61
  MacDonald's, 60-61

S

Salivary gland disease, 88
Sanger, Margaret, 5-6, 8, 9
Sarampion, 31
Sarcoptes scabiei, 197; *see also* Scabies
Scabies, 197
  clinical course of, 197
  microscopic examination of, 197
  primary complaint with, 197
  treatment of, 197
Schiller's solution, 205
Self-diagnosis and treatment of vaginal and cervical disease, 14
Self-help clinics, 14
"Sensate focusing," 166
Sex as natural function, 166-167
Sex counselors and therapists, feminist-oriented, development of, 15-16
Sex roles, 139
Sexism
  gaining understanding of, 11
  in health care system, 8
Sexist socialization, reasons for, 5
Sex-stress assault, 142
Sexual assault, 101
  aspects of, 136-155
  attitudes toward, 136, 144-147
    of counseling resources, 147
    of family and friends, 146
    law enforcement, 144-145
    legal system, 146-147
    medical system, 145-146
  choice of term, 137
  counseling and advocacy groups, 136, 147, 154
  as crime of opportunity, 142
  as crisis, 136
  definitions of, 137
  experiences, range of, 137
  female-on-female, 136-137
  female-on-male, 136-137
  forcible
    and assailant, 140-141
    victim's part in, 141
  general profiles of, 139-140
  incidence of, 137-139
    general statistics on, 137
  male-on-female, 136-155
  male-on-male, 136

Sexual assault—cont'd
  management of, 147-150
    by counseling personnel, 150
    by family and friends, 149, 154
    law enforcement, 147-148, 154
    legal system, 149-150, 154
    medical system, 148-149, 154
  nonforcible, 142
  physical force used in, 139
  prevention of, 152-154
    by education, 152
    precautions for, 152-153
    when attack is unavoidable, 153-154
  problems in reporting, 138
  spurious complaints of, 142
  state laws regarding, 137, 147, 148, 152
  statistics on, 138-139
  victim
    "conscientious harassment" of, 145
    dictum for dealing with, 145
    dreams of, 144
    feelings of, 142-144, 154
    as "good witness," 147
    phobias of, 144
    unique role of nurse regarding, 150-152
      guidelines for, 151-152
      in prevention of further victimization, 151, 154
      in providing support and communication, 150-151, 154
  "whys" of, 139-142
Sexual behavior, double standard for, 14
Sexual dysfunction, 157, 159-169
  as conditioned response, 166
  etiology of, 161
  historical perspectives on, 159
  male, 161, 163-165
    erectile, 163-164; see also Impotence
    involving ejaculatory overcontrol (incompetence), 161, 165
    involving inadequate ejaculatory control, 164-165; see also Ejaculation, premature
  nurses' role regarding, 159, 160
  treatment of
    basic goal of, 167
    categories of, 165
    couple-oriented, 165, 166
    dual-therapy team in, 167
    patient considerations in, 165-166
    principles of, 165-168
    procedural considerations in
      of couples, 167-168
      of individuals, 168
    referral for, 169
    results of, 168-169

Sexual dysfunction—cont'd
  treatment of—cont'd
    therapist considerations in, 166-167
    transference in, 167
    work of Masters and Johnson in, 159, 165, 166, 167
  of women, 161-163
    categories of, 161
    causes of, 15
    general, 161
    orgastic, 161, 162
    physiologic and psychologic etiology of, 162
Sexual functions of women, normalizing, 14-19
Sexual people, women as, 14-16
Sexual response, physiology of, 160-161
Sexual satisfaction in women
  enhancing, 15
  judging, 15
  lack of, 14-15
  misinformation about, 15
Sexuality, female, goals of women's movement regarding, 15
Shaman, 37
Sheppard-Towner Act, 17
Sick role, 10
Smallpox, 98
Socialization, sexist, reasons for, 5
Somnambulism, 49
Soul loss, 37
Sound, 229
Sound velocity, 229
Sound waves, 229
  frequency of, 230
  wavelength of, 229-230
Spanish Americans, 29
Spanish-speaking Americans; see Hispanic Americans
Sperm, 188
Spirit intrusion, 37
Spirochetes, 195
Squamocolumnar junction; see Cervix
Stanton, Elizabeth Cady, 3
Sterilization, 6
  informed consent for, 10, 13
  involuntary, 9-10
  legislation preventing, 10
  male, 9
Stevens, R., 50, 52, 53
  research findings of, 50, 52-53
Steptococci chains, 188
Stress, effect of, on synthesis of catecholamines, 180
Subcultures, impact of, on nurse and client, 1
Suck reflex, 74, 75
Suffrage, women's, fight for, 3-4

Suggestibility, 49
Surfeit, 30
Susto, 30-31
Syndrome(s)
  expanded rubella, 87
  male dysfunctional, 161
  premenstrual tension, 157, 170-184
  rape trauma, 142-144
  respiratory distress, 59-60
  TORCH, of perinatal infection, 57, 86-99
  whiplash shaken, 106
Syphilis, 195
Syringospora albicans; see Monilia

T

Theory of primal pain, 53
Threadworm vaginitis, 197
TIUV; *see* Total intrauterine volume
TORCH, 86
  birth of, 88
  "O" of, 98-99
TORCH agents, 86, 98-99
  transmission of, 88
TORCH infections
  in fetus and newborn, 93-98
    evaluation of, 94
    follow-up for, 94
    rehabilitation after, 94
  outcome and clinical findings associated with, 87, 93-94
  before pregnancy, 88-89
  during pregnancy, 89-93
TORCH syndrome, 57, 86-99
Tos ferina, 31
Total intrauterine volume, determination of, 64
Toxoplasma antibodies in pregnant women, 90
Toxoplasmosis, 89
  in fetus and newborn, 94-95
    findings in, 87, 94
  perinatal, 86
  during pregnancy, 89-90
    testing for, 90
  transmission of, 89, 90
Transducer, ultrasound, 230
Transference, 167
Tribe, definition of, 36
Trichomonas, 191
Trichomonas vaginalis, 191-193
  extravaginal sites of, 192
Trichomoniasis, 191, 200-201; *see also Trichomonas vaginalis*
  clinical course of, 192
  examination for, 192
  microscopic examination of, 192-193

Trichomoniasis—cont'd
  and other venereal disease, 192
  phases of, 191-192
  in pregnancy, sequelae of, 192
  primary complaint in, 192
  "strawberry marks" of, 192
  treatment of, 192, 193, 201
Tryptophan, effect of, on brain neurotransmitters, 179
Tumor, cancerous, radical surgery for, basis behind, 211

U

Ultrasonography
  B-scan, 230
  continuous wave Doppler, 230
  for diagnostic purposes, types of, 230
  frequency used in medical application of, 230
  in obstetrics and gynecology, 61-62, 235-248
    prior to amniocentesis, 241, 242
    detection of congenital malformations by, 242-244
      demonstrating fetal cystic hygroma in, 243, 244
      diagnosing anencephaly in, 242
      diagnosing hydrocephaly in, 242, 244
    displays used in, 230
    fetal position determination through, 235-236
    fetal viability or demise and missed abortion confirmation by, 235
    frequency used in, 230
    gestational age determination by, 236-239
      from biparietal diameter, 236, 238-239
      through crown-rump length measurement, 236, 237
    for intrauterine transfusion, 241
    locating intrauterine devices with, 244
    nursing responsibilities in, 231, 235
    placenta localization by, 239-241
      anterior, 239, 240
      with decreased amniotic fluid, 240
      placenta previa diagnosis in, 240-241
      posterior, 240
    precautions to use in, 248
    real-time, 157, 229-249
      clinical test of ovarian masses by, 246, 247, 248
      confirming diagnosis of molar pregnancy by, 245, 246
      confirming viability of pregnancy with, 244-245
      ectopic pregnancy diagnosis with, 246
      fetal biophysical variables assessed by, 244
      and maternal-infant bond, 235
      prediction of fetal risk by, 244
      for suspected multiple gestation, 236, 237
      techniques to improve accuracy of ultrasound examination through, 244

264 Index

Ultrasonography—cont'd
  in obstetrics and gynecology—cont'd
    real-time—cont'd
      in threatened abortion, 244-245
      record keeping for, 231, 233-234
        form used for, 234
      technique of, 231
      use of, to identify myomas, 246-247
  principles of, 229-230
  production of, 230
  pulsed, 230
  real-time B-scan, 230, 233
  visualization with
    cystic structure, 246
    solid structure, 246-247
Ultrasound scanner, real-time, 231
  ADR, 232
Ultrasound scanning; see Ultrasonography
Ultrasound shadowing, 240
Umbilicus, position of, 61
Urinary stress incontinence, 219
  relief of, 219, 220, 221, 226-227, 228
    historical research into, 219-221
Uterus
  fundus of, MacDonald's measurements of, 60
  prolapsed, 219, 224

V

Vaccinia, 98
Vagina, 186
  adenosis of, 203-204
  bacterial proliferation in, 187
  "contracting" of, 226
  flora of, 186, 187
  "gaping introitus" of, 222
Vaginal and cervical disease, self-diagnosis and treatment of, 14
Vaginal discharge, historical diagnosis and treatment of, 185; see also Vulvovaginitis
  normal and abnormal, 186
Vaginal epithelial cells, 188
Vaginal mucosa, 186
Vaginal Politics, 8, 18-19
Vaginal secretions, 186
Vaginal sphincter, exercise of, 51
Vaginismus, 161, 162-163
Vaginitis
  caused by
    antibiotics, 198
    Shigella flexneri, 197
    threadworm, 197
Varicella-zoster virus, effects of, on fetus or newborn, 98
Vestibular reflex, 77

Violence, 101-155
  marital, 121-122
    patterns of, 123-125
  on media, 110
  private, discovery of, 103
  responses to, 141
  tendency toward, 140
Vulvar area, anatomy of, 185-188
Vulvitis, allergic salivary, 198
Vulvovaginitis, 157
  allergic seminal, 197-198
  in children, 187
  diagnosis of, 185-199
    differential, 187-188
    guidelines for, 198
  intrauterine contraceptive devices as cause of, 198
  potential sources of, 198
  psychosomatic, 198
  and sexual intercourse, 191
  treatment guidelines for, 198
  types of, 188-198
  unusual conditions accounting for, 197-198

W

Weddington, Sarah, 7, 8, 9
The Well Body Book, 221
"Wetback," 29
Whooping cough, 31
Wife battering; see Battery, wife
Witchcraft, 30
  relating to animal intrusion, 33, 36
Women
  battered, 101, 121-135
  equality for
    biologic barriers to, 5
    health services necessary to, 5-10
  evaluation of, 139
  health care role of, 12
  orgasms of, 15
  premenopausal, health services required by, 10-11
  sexual functions of, normalizing, 14-19
  as sexual people, 14-16
  sexual satisfaction of, 14-15
  sexuality of, 14-16
Women's groups, 11
Women's health care, 1-56
  effects of having more women physicians on, 24
  effects of women's movement on, 1, 3-26
    in future, 24-25
  role of women in, 12
  trend to change in, 1
    by changing care providers, 20-24
      effect of, on nursing profession, 20-23
      effect of, on medical profession, 23-24

Women's movement
  contributions of, to fertility control, 5-6, 7, 8
  as cure for sexual problems, 15
  early, 3-4
  effects of, on women's health care, 1, 3-26
  goals of, regarding female sexuality, 15, 16
  health-related goals of, 5-20
  main participants of, 4, 18
  modern, 4, 23
  organization of, 3
  and physician involvement in family planning, 8-9
  pregnancy and childbirth attitudes of, 17, 18, 19

Women's movement — cont'd
  purpose of, 3
  re-emergence of, 4
  and reproduction, 5
  societal factors related to, 4-5
  and women's magazines, 16
Women's suffrage, fight for, 3-4

Y

Yang, 34
Yeast; *see Monilia*
Yin, 34-35